Davidso

167329

615.535
Mur

100
Super Supplements
for a Longer Life

167329

DISCARD

100
Super Supplements
for a Longer Life

Frank Murray

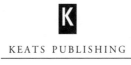

KEATS PUBLISHING

LOS ANGELES

NTC/Contemporary Publishing Group

The purpose of this book is to educate. It is sold with the understanding that the publisher and author shall have neither liability nor responsibility for any injury caused or alleged to be caused directly or indirectly by the information contained in this book. While every effort has been made to ensure its accuracy, the book's contents should not be construed as medical advice. Each person's health needs are unique. To obtain recommendations appropriate to your particular situation, please consult a qualified health care provider.

Library of Congress Cataloging-in-Publication Data

Murray, Frank, 1924–
    100 super supplements for a longer life / by Frank Murray.
      p. cm.
    Includes bibliographical references and index.
    ISBN 0-658-00973-7 (pbk.)
     1. Dietary supplements. I. Title: One hundred super supplements for a longer life.
  II. Title.

  RM258.5 .M87 2000
  613.2—dc21

                                    00-058650

Published by Keats Publishing
A division of NTC/Contemporary Publishing Group, Inc.
4255 West Touhy Avenue, Lincolnwood, Illinois 60712, U.S.A.

Copyright © 2000 by Frank Murray.

All rights reserved. No part of this work may be reproduced, stored in a retrieval system, or transmitted in any form or by any means electronic, mechanical, photocopying, recording, or otherwise, without prior permission of NTC/Contemporary Publishing Group, Inc.

Managing Director and Publisher: Jack Artenstein
Executive Editor: Peter Hoffman
Director of Publishing Services: Rena Copperman
Managing Editor: Jama Carter
Editor: Claudia McCowan

Design by Andrea Reider

Printed in the United States of America
International Standard Book Number: 0-658-00973-7
00 01 02 03 04 DHD 18 17 16 15 14 13 12 11 10 9 8 7 6 5 4 3 2 1

Contents

CONTENTS

CONTENTS

Foreword

Many people believe that in order for medicine to be effective, it must include expensive procedures and complicated technological equipment operated by highly trained specialists who perform in extravagant, templelike hospitals. In many instances, doctors using highly technical conventional modalities *can* accomplish miracles: the specialties of plastic or facial maxillary surgery, for example. Modern doctors, however, are often helpless in their efforts to treat complicated cancers or other life-threatening conditions. Frequently, no amount of chemotherapy, surgery, or radiation will increase a patient's chances of long-term survival if the disease is widespread throughout the patient's body. I often wonder why many patients opt for expensive, painful treatments even though their doctors tell them that there is no hope for recovery, and especially when

more effective therapies might be found in the realm of natural products.

Twenty-three years ago, when I was a medical resident at a large university-affiliated hospital, Dr. Fred Bartter of the National Institutes of Health introduced me to a natural and highly effective therapy for serious liver disease. At the time, four patients had been assigned to me with "irreparable" liver damage and I was told by my instructors that there was no hope for their recovery. I called Dr. Bartter for his advice. He informed me that Czechoslovakian doctors had been successfully using a natural product called alpha-lipoic acid (thioctic acid) to regenerate livers. I quickly arranged to have the lipoic acid shipped to me by air. After I administered it to my patients, I was astounded by their rapid and complete recovery from their "terminal" disease. Dr. Bartter and I published our findings on 79 people with almost complete liver destruction; 75 of them recovered quickly. These extraordinary results were almost completely ignored by the American medical community. When I shared my experience with my colleagues and patients, I was repeatedly asked, "How could a simple, inexpensive, and natural substance be more effective than an expensive and extensively researched drug?"

Although many continue to ask the same question today, knowledgeable academics, clinical medical doctors, and patients alike now understand the role of natural products in treating illness. They take natural medicine seriously, and most realize its potential for treating severe disease.

In this volume, Frank Murray, a pioneer in his field and a highly experienced health and nutrition writer, does a superb job of explaining how and why natural treatments work by furnishing the reader with comprehensive amounts of information on natural supplements for preventing and treating disease conditions. This book also contains abundant and easy-to-use references to scientific studies that support the text. It provides both layperson and professional practically all they need to know about using simple and inexpensive natural substances for preventing serious illness and promoting good health.

Burt Berkson, M.D., Ph.D.
President, Integrative Medical Center
   of New Mexico
Las Cruces, New Mexico

1

Alpha-Lipoic Acid

An essential cofactor in energy metabolism in organisms from microbes to human beings, alpha-lipoic acid (ALA)—also referred to as lipoic acid and thioctic acid—provides sufficient protection against arthritis, cataracts, diabetes, heart disease, aging, heavy-metal poisoning, liver cirrhosis, kidney damage, AIDS, and other health conditions. ALA is found in spinach and other foods, but it is unlikely that a food source will contain enough of the product to be effective.

Unlike other antioxidants, such as vitamin C, which is water soluble, and vitamin E, which is fat soluble, ALA is both water and fat soluble, making it bioavailable in a variety of locations in the body. ALA and dihydrolipoic acid (DHLA), its reduced form, are effective against a variety of free radicals, those wayward molecules that accelerate aging and contribute to many health problems.

Interviewed by John McKenzie on *World News Tonight* in September 1997, Lester Packer, Ph.D., of the University of California, Berkeley, said ALA could be a missing link in the treatment and prevention of disease. He added that it is probably the most potent naturally occurring antioxidant known to man.[1]

Packer, who with his associates has published more than 60 studies on ALA, explained that the product has its own antioxidant properties and is more potent than other antioxidants, including vitamin C and vitamin E. In addition, it increases the effectiveness of both vitamins.

Type 2 (non-insulin-dependent) diabetics may improve their insulin function and glucose metabolism with ALA supplements. Researchers gave 10 thin and 10 obese patients with Type 2 diabetes 600 mg of oral alpha-lipoic acid twice daily for four weeks. During that time, insulin function, glucose, and lactate and pyruvate levels were measured to determine glucose metabolism. The ALA supplements were found to be beneficial to both groups. The thin diabetics registered better insulin function and decreases in fasting glucose—suggesting a shift toward normalization—while the obese patients had improvements in insulin function. In both groups, levels of lactate and pyruvate decreased, indicating more normal glucose metabolism. ALA seems to work by stepping up the burning of glucose.[2]

Diabetics often have an increased risk of neuropathy, which is characterized by reduced heart-rate variability. In a study called Alpha-Lipoic Acid in Diabetic Neuropathy (ALADIN), 328 patients with diabetic neuropathy were given either 100, 600, or 1,200 mg of ALA or a placebo or look-alike pill daily for three weeks. Researchers in the Deutsche Kardiale Autonome Neuropathie (DEKAN) Studie gave 73 patients with cardiac autonomic neuropathy either 800 mg of ALA or a placebo daily for four months. In the ALADIN study, pain and other symptoms decreased significantly with dosages of 600 or 1,200 mg daily for 19 days. ALA also improved heart-rate variability in the diabetics with cardiac autonomic neuropathy. With this and other confirmation, researchers believe that ALA exerts a protective antioxidant effect on nerve cells.[3]

ALA is being used successfully to treat alcohol-induced liver damage, amanita mushroom poisoning, and metal toxicity. It has also been found useful in treating diabetic polyneuropathy, a type of nerve damage.

ALA acts as a natural supplement, somewhat like vitamin E, in preventing many diseases, especially those influenced by free radicals.[4]

To test the value of ALA in treating diabetics, researchers in Germany and elsewhere gave ALA and gamma-linolenic acid (GLA) to diabetic laboratory animals in an attempt to improve nerve function and blood flow. Each substance was found to cause modest improvements in the animals, and when combined, showed a marked synergistic effect.[5]

ALA assumes some of the biochemical functions of glutathione—a primary antioxidant containing three amino acids—including maintaining high blood levels of vitamin C and recycling vitamin E. According to animal experiments, ALA may prevent cataracts, which are caused by oxidative stress in the lens of the eye.[6]

ALA and DHLA have substantial antioxidant properties, including the ability to quench a variety of reactive oxygen species, inhibit reactive oxygen-generators, and spare other antioxidants. A number of clinical studies, including some reported here, address the use of ALA as a therapeutic agent for such diverse conditions as myocardial and cerebral ischemia-reperfusion injury, heavy-metal poisoning, radiation damage, diabetes, neurodegenerative diseases, and AIDS.[7]

Burton Berkson, M.D., Ph.D., of the Integrative Medical Center in Las Cruces, New Mexico, has seen firsthand how ALA can save lives. A 35-year-old woman with severe hepatitis C was informed by her physicians that she probably would die without a liver transplant. After Berkson treated her with ALA, she was able to avoid the transplant.[8]

"A number of recent studies have also shown alpha-lipoic acid to be effective in treating diabetic neuropathy," explained Berkson, who is principal FDA investigator for intravenous ALA treatments in acute liver diseases and a consultant to the National Centers for Disease Control and Prevention. "A 55-year-old man with adult-onset diabetes was informed by his doctors that there was practically nothing they could do about his incapacitating burning feet and pins and needles in his hands. After months of treatment, including ALA, this man no longer suffers these symptoms. Alpha-lipoic acid should be considered in the same class as vitamin E, based on its remarkable benefits and impressive research."

Berkson became interested in ALA after treating a patient with hepatic necrosis caused by eating toxic mushrooms. An intravenous infusion of ALA 30 hours after the patient had ingested the mushrooms brought an improvement within one hour, and the patient was soon discharged. Berkson prescribed ALA for two additional patients with mushroom poisoning, and within a short time they were feeling better and had almost normal liver function.[9] Since then he has prescribed ALA, both orally and intravenously, to more than 100 patients.

ALA acts as a coenzyme for the production of acetyl coenzyme alpha-dihydrolipoic acid, which in turn recycles other antioxidants such as vitamin C. Like other researchers, Berkson has found ALA to inhibit HIV replication in cultured T cells, prevent cataracts, protect the kidney from amino-glycoside damage, protect islet cells in the pancreas from inflammatory attack, and increase helper T cells in the blood, among other benefits. In addition, ALA reduces the toxic side effects of some forms of chemotherapy. ALA crosses the blood-brain barrier easily and plays a significant role in a variety of neural metabolic processes.

Berkson has successfully treated three patients with chronic hepatitis C who are now thriving and did not require a liver transplant. Most researchers report that there are no effective treatments for chronic hepatitis C, and that interferon and antiviral drugs have less than a 30 percent response rate. For those who do undergo a transplant, the new liver often becomes infected, Berkson said. One year of antioxidant therapy as prescribed by Berkson costs less than $2,000, compared to $300,000 for a liver transplant.[10]

The three patients were selected at random from a group of about 50 chronic hepatitis C subjects at Berkson's Integrative Medical Center. Each day they were given 600 mg of ALA in two divided doses; 900 mg of silymarin (from milk thistle) in three divided doses; and 400 mcg of selenomethionine (selenium) in two divided doses. Patient No. 1 was also treated with B complex vitamins, vitamin C, vitamin E, and coenzyme Q10. Patient No. 2 was also given medication for insomnia. Patient No. 3 was also treated for other health problems. All three show no signs of hepatitis.

By helping recycle vitamin E in the body, ALA and DHLA keep the concentration of the vitamin high so that it can perform its antioxidant functions adequately, according to M. Podda and colleagues at the University of California, Berkeley. ALA and DHLA have also been shown in vitro to possess potent antioxidant activity and may even substitute for vitamin E. Research supports the idea that the major effect of ALA in vitamin E–deficient animals is to replace the vitamin rather than recycle it. In any case, it cannot be ruled out that ALA antioxidant activity may be acting through other antioxidants—such as coenzyme Q10 or vitamin C—where in vitro recycling has been described.[11]

For athletes, ALA helps prevent muscle and tissue damage during intense workouts and speeds muscle recovery, according to Dallas Clouatre, Ph.D., and Will Brink. ALA regenerates not only vitamins C and E but also glutathione in the cytoplasm of the cell, and coenzyme Q10 within the mitochondria. ALA quenches an unmatched variety of free radicals and also regenerates other antioxidant and free radical quenching systems.[12]

"If you are an endurance athlete," Clouatre and Brink wrote, "you are pumping many times the amount of oxygen through your system when you are exercising than when you are at rest. Burning glucose and fats for fuel (as we do during exercise) generates free radicals, and pushing so much oxygen through your system allows this source of oxidation and free radicals greater access to your tissues."

Similarly, an athlete performing resistance exercise such as weight training may be causing countless small tears in the muscle (microtrauma) and other forms of tissue damage. Microtrauma leads to localized inflammation, pain, and swelling as the immune system attempts to clear out damaged tissue by generating free radicals to destroy both bacteria and cells that are to be replaced.

Spinach is the richest source of lipoyllysine, which is protein-bound ALA. Large amounts of the substance are also found in broccoli, kidney, heart, and liver. There is little or no lipoyllysine in garden peas, Brussels sprouts, rice bran, or bananas. Researchers do not yet know if the protein-bound form of ALA has as much activity as "free" ALA found in supplements.[13]

According to a number of studies, patients with HIV have a compromised antioxidant defense system. Therefore, blood antioxidants are decreased and peroxidation products of fats and proteins are increased in these patients, reported Michael Murray, N.D. This blood profile may contribute to the progression of AIDS, since antioxidants such as glutathione prevent viral replication while reactive oxidants tend to stimulate the virus.[14]

"A small pilot study was designed to determine the short-term effect of ALA supplementation (150 mg three times daily) in HIV positive patients," Murray said. "The supplementation increased plasma ascorbate (vitamin C) in 9 of 10 patients, total glutathione in 7 of 7 patients, total plasma sulfur groups in 8 of 9 patients, T-helper lymphocytes and T-helper/suppressor cell ratio in 6 of 10 patients; while the level of free radical damage decreased in 8 of 9 patients. This pilot study indicated that lipoic acid supplementation led to significant beneficial changes in the blood of HIV infected patients."

For general antioxidant support, the recommended dosage is 20 to 50 mg/day, Murray wrote. In the treatment of diabetic neuropathy, the recommended dose is now 400 to 800 mg/day. For the treatment of AIDS, the recommended amount is 150 mg three times a day.

"Lipoic acid supplementation appears to be very safe as there have not been any reports of adverse effects in over three decades of use in the treatment of diabetic neuropathy," Murray said. "In addition, animal studies have shown it to be of very low toxicity."

In addition to sparing vitamins C and E and other antioxidants, ALA works synergistically with two B vitamins—B_1 and B_3—in cellular energy production. ALA also may improve blood sugar control in diabetes, resulting in a reduction in the dosage of insulin or oral blood sugar–lowering drugs.

ALA is available in tablets and capsules. According to Dr. Packer, it is probably the most potent naturally occurring antioxidant known to humankind.

References

1. McKenzie, John, "Health Report," *World News Tonight with Peter Jennings,* Sept. 29, 1997.
2. Konrad, T., et al., "Alpha-Lipoic Acid Treatment Decreases Serum Lactate and Pyruvate Concentrations and Improves Glucose Effectiveness in Lean and Obese Patients with Type 2 Diabetes," *Diabetes Care* 22: 280–87, 1999.
3. Ziegler, D., and F. A. Gries, "Alpha-Lipoic Acid in the Treatment of Peripheral and Cardiac Autonomic Neuropathy," *Diabetes* 46 (Suppl. 2): S62–S66, 1997.
4. Bustamante, J., et al., "Alpha-Lipoic Acid in Liver Metabolism and Disease," *Free Radical Biology and Medicine* 24: 1023–39, 1998.
5. Cameron, N. E., et al., "Effects of Alpha-Lipoic Acid in Neurovascular Function in Diabetic Rats; Interaction with Essential Fatty Acids," *Diabetologia* 41: 390–99, 1998.
6. Maitra, I., et al., "Alpha-Lipoic Acid Prevents Buthionine Sulfoxamine-Induced Cataract Formation in Newborn Rats," *Free Radical Biology and Medicine* 18: 823–29, 1995.
7. Packer, Lester, et al., "Alpha-Lipoic Acid as a Biological Antioxidant," *Free Radical Biology and Medicine* 19(2): 227–50, 1995.

8. Berkson, Burton M., "The Remarkable Benefits of Alpha-Lipoic Acid," Paper presented at 1998 World Congress, Oxygen Club of California, Santa Barbara, 1998.

9. Berkson, Burton M., "Alpha-Lipoic Acid (Thioctic Acid): My Experience with This Outstanding Therapeutic Agent," *Journal of Orthomolecular Medicine* 13(1): 44–48, 1998.

10. Berkson, Burton M., "A Conservative Triple Antioxidant Approach to the Treatment of Hepatitis C," *Medizinische Klinik* 94 (Suppl. III): 84–89, Oct. 15, 1999.

11. Podda, M., et al., "Alpha-Lipoic Acid Supplementation Prevents Symptoms of Vitamin E Deficiency," *Biochemical and Biophysical Research Communications* 204(1): 98–104, Oct. 14, 1994.

12. Clouatre, Dallas, and Will Brink, "Alpha-Lipoic Acid for Total Performance," *Let's Live,* Oct. 1997, 65–67.

13. Lodge, J. K., et al., "Natural Sources of Lipoic Acid: Determination of Lipoyllysine Released from Protease-Digested Tissues by High Performance Liquid Chromatography Incorporating Electrochemical Detection," *Journal of Applied Nutrition* 49: 3–11, 1997.

14. Murray, Michael, "Lipoic Acid—A 'New Breed' of Antioxidant," *Natural Medicine Journal* 1(3): 20–21, April 1998.

2

Beta-Carotene

Carotenoids are naturally occurring compounds found in the pigments in plants. Although more than 600 carotenoids have been isolated, only a small number are found in appreciable amounts in human blood and tissue. The most notable carotenoids are alpha-carotene, beta-carotene, lutein, zeaxanthin, cryptoxanthin, and lycopene. Carotenoids work in tandem to prevent and control free radicals and to limit free radical/oxidative damage. Companion antioxidants for fighting free radicals include vitamins C and E, alpha-lipoic acid, polyphenols, and the enzymes superoxide dismutase, catalase, and glutathione peroxidase.[1]

A great deal has been written about the dangerous free radicals, by-products of metabolic processes that originate from environmental pollutants (nitrogen dioxide and ozone in polluted air), heavy metals (cadmium, mercury, etc.), halogenated hydrocarbons, ionizing radiation, and cigarette smoke. Unless destroyed by antioxidants, these wayward free radicals attack cell walls and cell constituents such as DNA. Another likely target is polyunsaturated fatty acids (PUFAs). Reacting with PUFAs, free radicals can generate chain reactions in profusion, damaging the structure and function of cells, nucleic acids, and electron-dense regions of proteins. Oxidative damage due to free radical attacks is linked to many degenerative diseases and conditions, including cancer.

Carotenoids have various diverse biological functions. For example, certain carotenoids such as beta-carotene are precursors of vitamin A and can be metabolically converted into fat-soluble vitamin A in the body. Alpha-carotene and cryptoxanthin are also provitamin A carotenoids.

Carotenoid absorption is generally between 10 and 30 percent and decreases with increased intake. Dietary fat influences absorption, since carotenoids are absorbed only when bile salts are present. Dietary fiber can inhibit absorption. Carotenoids are transported along with lipoproteins, and adipose tissue (body fat) is the primary storage depot for them. But carotenoids are also found in the liver, lung, and other tissues, such as the corpus luteum (in the ovary), adrenal glands, prostate, and macula of the eye.

Apricots, cantaloupe, carrots, leafy green vegetables, pumpkin, sweet potatoes, and winter squash are rich sources of beta-carotene. Alpha-carotene is found in carrots and pumpkin. Lutein and zeaxanthin are available in leafy green vegetables, pumpkin, and red peppers. Guava, pink grapefruit, tomatoes and tomato products, and watermelon are good sources of lycopene. Mangoes, nectarines, oranges, papayas, peaches, and tangerines provide cryptoxanthin. Natural mixed carotenoid supplements contain various carotenoids naturally found in fruits and cruciferous, yellow, and dark green vegetables. Synthetic carotenoid supplements contain only beta-carotene.

Based on dietary guidelines from government agencies, a daily intake of 6 mg of beta-carotene is recommended. The Alliance for Aging Research, a citizens advocacy organization, recommends a dosage of 10 to 30 mg/day.

A research team analyzed the dietary habits of more than 83,000 women in the Nurses' Health Study to find out how long-term intake of certain carotenoids might affect risk of breast cancer. Women who consumed foods with the highest amounts of beta-carotene, lutein, zeaxanthin, vitamin C, and vitamin A had a relatively low risk of breast cancer. Premenopausal women who had an established family risk of developing the disease benefited the most. Vitamin E supplements and foods rich in this vitamin provided a somewhat reduced risk for breast cancer.[2]

In a related trial, researchers analyzed the relationship between dietary consumption of carotenoids and the risk of developing colorectal adenomatous polyps. Although these polyps are usually benign intestinal growths, they can become precancerous. Women with the highest blood levels of beta-carotene were 38 percent less likely to develop polyps, compared to those with low beta-carotene levels. Women with high levels of alpha-carotene had a 41 percent lower risk. Women with the highest levels of total carotenoids, such as beta-carotene, alpha-carotene, beta-cryptoxanthin, lutein, zeaxanthin, and lycopene, had a 34 percent reduced risk.[3]

Researchers evaluated data from the 12-year Physician's Health Study, in which more than 22,000 male doctors were given either 50 mg of beta-carotene or a placebo every other day. Beta-carotene–deficient doctors who took the supplement were 36 percent less likely to develop prostate cancer than those deficient in the vitamin who did not take the supplement.[4]

In a case-control study involving 273 women with breast cancer and 371 controls, it was found that increased intake of beta-carotene was associated with a decreased risk of breast cancer among postmenopausal women. Postmenopausal women who had been consuming diets rich in beta-carotene for 20 to 45 years had a decreased risk of breast cancer when compared to women with low intakes of the vitamin.[5]

Studies have shown that foods rich in beta-carotene enhance immune function and therefore reduce the risk of cancer. Using 50 volunteers, researchers gave 30 mg/day of beta-carotene for three months either to patients being treated for colon cancer or colonic polyps or to healthy controls. The cancer patients had lower percentages of CD4, interleukin-2 (IL-2), and interleukin-2 positive (IL-2R) immune cells, which help prevent and fight cancer. Beta-carotene was found to increase the number of IL-2R and CD4 cells in the patients with colon cancer. IL-2R and CD4 cells increased slightly in the patients with polyps.[6]

In another study, researchers analyzed levels of 10 antioxidants in the blood and cervical tissue of three groups of women: those diagnosed with cervical cancer, those diagnosed with precancerous tissue changes, and healthy women with no signs of cancer. Of the 10 antioxidants measured, only low levels of beta-carotene in the blood and tissue were associated with an increased risk of cervical cancer. As might be expected, the women with cancer had the lowest levels of antioxidants in their blood.[7]

Like its cousin beta-carotene, alpha-carotene is a common plant pigment and accounts for almost one-third of the carotenoids found in carrots and over half of the carotenoids in pumpkins. Researchers in Finland evaluated 4,545 men ranging in ages from 20 to 69, and found that diets high in alpha-carotene were associated with a 67 percent lower risk of lung cancer among nonsmokers and a 30 percent lower risk among smokers. Diets high in beta-carotene were related to a 62 percent reduced risk of cancer in nonsmokers and a slight reduction in risk among smokers. Also, a high fruit and vegetable intake was associated with a 40 percent lower risk for lung cancer, while root vegetables such as carrots were associated with a 44 percent lower risk.[8]

When cancer patients are given high doses of beta-carotene and vitamins C and E, this combination seems to protect normal cells from the effects of chemotherapy and radiation, according to Kedar N. Prasad, Ph.D., of the University of Colorado Health Sciences Center at Denver. High doses of multiple antioxidants not only protect normal cells during cancer treatment, but also improve the efficacy of the treatment. The antioxidants protect normal cells as well as cancer cells from free radical damage caused by chemotherapy and radiation.[9]

Using human lung cells, researchers determined that beta-carotene provided significant protection against ultraviolet (UV) light rays (which can generate free radicals), whereas vitamins C and E did not. A combination of all three antioxidants, however, was significantly more protective than beta-carotene alone.[10]

Although certain amounts of UV radiation from sunlight are beneficial—for example, it helps the body to produce vitamin D—too much exposure can suppress the immune system and lower the body's resistance to infection and cancer. In one study, researchers placed 31 men ranging in age from 55 to 79 on a low-carotenoid diet and gave them either 30 mg/day of beta-carotene or a placebo for 47 days. Twenty-eight days into the study, half of the men in each group were exposed to large amounts of UV radiation. Although the exposure compromised immune function in all of the men, those with the highest blood levels of beta-carotene were most resistant to the radiation.[11]

Radiation exposure disrupts the body's cells, generating harmful free radicals that go on to damage even more cells. Israeli researchers measured "conjugated dienes," which are markers of free radical damage, in 262 children who were exposed to radiation during the 1986 Chernobyl nuclear accident, but who later moved to Israel and thus avoided additional exposure. The researchers gave 99 of the children a daily dose of 40 mg of natural beta-carotene (from algae) for three months. Initially the children had higher than normal levels of conjugated dienes, suggesting that their exposure to radiation had increased free radical damage in their bodies. After three months of beta-carotene therapy, however,

levels of conjugated dienes had declined significantly.[12]

It has been suggested for some time that diet, particularly a high intake of refined carbohydrates and sugars, is a principal risk factor for adult-onset (Type 2) diabetes. Researchers analyzed blood levels of various carotenoids in 1,665 people ranging in age from 40 to 74 to determine correlations between carotenoid levels and the risk of diabetes and prediabetic symptoms. Those with the highest beta-carotene levels were among the volunteers with normal glucose levels, but levels declined substantially among those with impaired glucose tolerance and diabetes. As an example, those with impaired glucose tolerance had beta-carotene levels 13 percent below normal, and those who had recently been diagnosed with diabetes had beta-carotene levels 20 percent below normal. Antioxidants such as beta-carotene may protect against insulin-damaging free radicals.[13]

Beta-carotene and vitamin E can reduce the oxidation (free radical damage) of LDL-cholesterol, thereby lowering the risk of developing coronary heart disease. Obesity is a known risk for heart disease, and low levels of beta-carotene and vitamin E may also be risk factors. In studying 6,000 children, researchers found that obese children had significantly lower blood levels of beta-carotene and vitamin E, compared to their peers with normal weight. Thus, low blood levels of the two vitamins may well contribute to the long-term risk of heart disease in overweight children.[14]

Researchers at Erasmus University Medical School in Rotterdam, the Netherlands, and at other facilities in the Netherlands and Germany, after reviewing epidemiological evidence that antioxidants provide protection against ischemic heart disease, decided to test this theory on a group of elderly volunteers ranging in age from 55 to 95. They found that a high dietary intake of beta-carotene provided protection against cardiovascular disease. When the volunteers took beta-carotene supplements, the risk of myocardial infarction (heart attack) was slightly more pronounced.[15] "Whether the association may be ascribed to beta-carotene–containing products, or to dietary patterns and lifestyle behavior closely linked to a diet rich in vegetables and fruit remains to be determined," the researchers said.

At the University of Michigan at Ann Arbor, 45 patients with cardiovascular disease were evaluated during a 12-week study. The volunteers were randomly assigned to either a placebo group; a group getting 400 IU of vitamin E, 500 mg of vitamin C, and 12 mg of beta-carotene; or a group receiving 800 IU of vitamin E, 1,000 mg of vitamin C, and 24 mg of beta-carotene. The higher doses of antioxidants reduced the susceptibility of LDL cholesterol in patients with cardiovascular disease, compared to controls. It was suggested that this therapy might be an ideal preventive measure.[16]

In the Atherosclerosis Risk in Communities Study, dietary and disease patterns were analyzed among 12,773 men and women. For both genders, carotenoid-rich foods brought a substantially lower prevalence of cholesterol deposits in the carotid, a major blood vessel. Women seemed to benefit more than men. Overall, women with diets high in beta-carotene had a 16 percent lower risk of developing cholesterol deposits on their carotids. Women smokers had the greatest benefits, with a 33 percent reduction risk when compared with smokers on low-carotenoid diets.[17]

At Wageningen Agricultural University in the Netherlands, researchers studied the relationship between beta-carotene and vitamins C and E and lung function and respiratory symptoms. High intakes of beta-carotene and vitamin C were found to increase lung capacity. While vitamin E was not associated with lung function, it was linked to a greater likelihood of "productive cough," which helps to expel phlegm.[18]

A research project involving Baltimore's Johns Hopkins University and other facilities analyzed blood levels of beta-carotene, vitamin C, and vitamin A from patients who developed rheumatoid arthritis and systemic lupus erythematosus—both autoimmune disorders—2 to 15 years after the initial blood samples were taken. Low antioxidant levels of these nutrients were a risk factor for both diseases. On average, those who developed rheumatoid arthritis had blood levels of beta-carotene that were 29 percent lower than those in healthy people.[19]

Strenuous exercise can generate DNA damage. To test this theory, researchers gave 30 mg/day of beta-carotene to 14 sedentary men ranging in age from 19 to 22, for one month. Six other volunteers were given a placebo. Beta-carotene levels increased 17-fold in the supplement group, but decreased in both groups after strenuous exercise. While neither group showed an increase in DNA damage, exercise did increase some markers of oxidative stress. The postexercise decline in levels may suggest that beta-carotene is used up in preventing free radical damage during exercise.[20]

Another study found that beta-carotene is essential in preventing lipid peroxidation, and that 1 mg of beta-carotene per kg of body weight is necessary for correcting the oxidant-antioxidant imbalance in cystic fibrosis patients. In theory, lipid peroxidation suggests that while oxygen is necessary for life, the oxidation of cell membranes causes the destruction of the outer coating of a cell, filling it with waste matter.[21] Pancreatic insufficiency, found in 85 to 90 percent of cystic fibrosis patients, causes fat malabsorption and severe deficiencies in fat-soluble vitamins, such as vitamin A, beta-carotene, and vitamin E. The study determined the efficacy of giving these patients 1 mg per kg of beta-carotene up to 50 kg, or 50 mg for those with body weight over 50 kg, for 12 weeks, followed by 10 mg for another 12 weeks, or a placebo. The volunteers were also given pancreatic enzymes and supplements of vitamins A, C, and E.

In analyzing the cognitive function of almost 1,800 middle-aged and elderly men and women in Austria, researchers found that those with the poorest cognitive scores had the lowest levels of beta-carotene and vitamin E. Subsequent analysis showed that high levels of vitamin E were strongly associated with normal cognitive function. It was suggested that adequate lifelong intake of vitamin E may help maintain normal brain function in middle and old age and possibly ward off Alzheimer's disease.[22]

Numerous beta-carotene supplements are available over the counter, in individual dosages, or combined with other nutrients. A relatively new carotenoid supplement is Betatene. Extracted from *Dunaliella salina* algae, it is a mixture of alpha-carotene, cryptoxanthin, zeaxanthin, and lutein. A companion product also contains lycopene.

References

1. Lanvik, Sharon, manager, VERIS Research Summary, La Grange, Illinois, Aug. 1997.
2. Zhang, S., et al., "Dietary Carotenoids and Vitamins A, C, and E and Risk of Breast Cancer," *Journal of the National Cancer Institute* 91: 547–56, 1999.
3. Smith-Warner, S. A., et al., "A Prospective Study of Plasma Carotenoids and Colorectal Adenomatous Polyps," *American Journal of Epidemiology,* 1998, 147–49.
4. "Prostate Cancer and Beta-Carotene," *Nutrition Week* 27(23): 7, June 13, 1997.

5. Jumaan, A. O., et al., "Beta Carotene Intake and Risk of Postmenopausal Breast Cancer," *Epidemiology* 10: 49–53, 1999.

6. Kazi, N., et al., "Immunomodulatory Effect of Beta-Carotene on T Lymphocyte Subsets in Patients with Resected Colonic Polyps and Cancer," *Nutrition and Cancer* 28: 140–45, 1997.

7. Peng, Y. M., et al., "Concentrations of Carotenoids, Tocopherols, and Retinol in Paired Plasma and Cervical Tissue of Patients with Cervical Cancer, Precancer, and Noncancerous Diseases," *Cancer Epidemiology, Biomarkers, and Prevention* 7: 347–50, 1998.

8. Knekt, P., et al., "Role of Various Carotenoids in Lung Cancer Prevention," *Journal of the National Cancer Institute* 91: 182–84, 1999.

9. Norton, Amy, "Antioxidants' Role in Cancer Prevention Explored," *Medical Tribune,* March 18, 1999, 20.

10. Bohm, F., et al., "Enhanced Protection of Human Cells Against Ultraviolet Light by Antioxidant Combinations Involving Dietary Carotenoids," *Journal of Photochemistry and Photobiology* 44: 211–15, 1998.

11. Herraiz, L. A., et al., "Effect of UV Exposure and Beta-Carotene Supplementation on Delayed-Type Hypersensitivity Response in Healthy Older Men," *Journal of the American College of Nutrition* 17: 617–24, 1998.

12. Ben-Amotz, A., et al., "Effect of Natural Beta-Carotene Supplementation in Children Exposed to Radiation from the Chernobyl Accident," *Radiation and Environmental Biophysics* 37: 187–93, 1998.

13. Ford, E. S., et al., "Diabetes Mellitus and Serum Carotenoids: Findings from the Third National Health and Nutrition Examination Survey," *American Journal of Epidemiology* 149: 168–76, 1999.

14. Strauss, R. S. L., "Comparison of Serum Concentrations of Alpha-Tocopherol and Beta-Carotene in a Cross-Sectional Sample of Obese and Nonobese Children (NHANES III)," *Journal of Pediatrics* 134: 160–65, 1999.

15. Klipstein-Grobusch, Kerstin, et al., "Dietary Antioxidants and Risk of Myocardial Infarction in the Elderly: The Rotterdam Study," *American Journal of Clinical Nutrition* 69(2): 261–66, Feb. 1999.

16. Mosca, Lori, et al., "Antioxidant Nutrient Supplementation Reduces the Susceptibility of Low Density Lipoprotein to Oxidation in Patients with Coronary Artery Disease," *Journal of the American College of Cardiology* 30(2): 392–99, Aug. 1997.

17. Kritchevsky, S. B., et al., "Provitamin A Carotenoid Intake and Carotid Artery Plaques: The Atherosclerosis Risk in Communities Study," *American Journal of Clinical Nutrition* 68: 726–33, 1998.

18. Grievink, Linda, et al., "Dietary Intake of Antioxidant (Pro) Vitamins, Respiratory Symptoms, and Pulmonary Function: the MORGEN Study," *Thorax* 53: 166–71, 1998.

19. Comstock, G. W., et al., "Serum Concentrations of Alpha-Tocopherol, Beta-Carotene, and Retinol Preceding the Diagnosis of Rheumatoid Arthritis and Systemic Lupus Erythematosus," *Annals of the Rheumatic Diseases* 56: 323–25, 1997.

20. Sumida, S., et al., "Effect of a Single Bout of Exercise and Beta-Carotene Supplementation on the Urinary Excretion of 8-Hydroxy-Deoxyguanosine in Humans," *Free Radical Research* 27: 607–618, 1997.

21. Rust, P., et al., "Effects of Long-Term Oral Beta-Carotene Supplementation on Lipid Peroxidation in Patients with Cystic Fibrosis," *International Journal of Vitamin and Nutrition Research* 68: 83–87, 1998.

22. Schmidt, R., et al., "Plasma Antioxidants and Cognitive Performance in Middle-Aged and Older Adults: Results of the Austrian Stroke Prevention Study," *Journal of the American Geriatrics Society* 46: 1407–10, 1998.

3

Bilberry

During World War II, British Royal Air Force pilots often munched bilberries to sharpen their night vision during bombing raids. Later studies showed that bilberry extract given to healthy volunteers resulted in improved nighttime visual acuity, quicker adjustment to darkness, and faster restoration of visual acuity after exposure to glare, according to Michael T. Murray, N.D.[1] In Europe, he added, bilberry extracts are part of the conventional medical treatment for many eye problems, including cataracts, macular degeneration, retinitis pigmentosa, diabetic retinopathy, and night blindness.

Bilberry, or European blueberry *(Vaccinium myrtillus)*, belongs to the *Vaccinium* family, which includes almost 200 species of berries, such as American blueberry, cranberry, and cowberry. Researchers have long known that the pharmacologically active constituents in bilberries are flavonoids

known as anthocyanosides. These important constituents help prevent free radical damage with their potent antioxidant and free radical scavenging action.

"The origin of many eye diseases, including cataract formation and macular degeneration, is ultimately related to damage caused by free radicals," Murray said. "Free radical or 'oxidative' damage is what makes us age. In addition to their role in causing cataracts and macular degeneration, free radicals have also been shown to be responsible for the initiation of many diseases, including the two biggest killers of Americans—heart disease and cancer."

Bilberry extract may also play a significant role in the prevention and treatment of glaucoma via its effect on collagen structures in the eye. Bilberry anthocyanosides may protect against degeneration of the macula, the portion of the eye that distinguishes fine details in a person's vision. In one study, 31 patients with various types of retinopathy (20 with diabetic retinopathy, 5 with retinitis pigmentosa, 4 with macular degeneration, 2 with hemorrhagic retinopathy due to anticoagulant therapy) were treated with bilberry extract. A tendency toward reduced permeability and reduced tendency to hemorrhage was observed in all of the patients, especially those with diabetic retinopathy.

Murray also reported that bilberry has been used to treat varicose veins. In one study, 47 patients with varicose veins were given 480 mg/day, and significant improvements were found in abnormal capillary permeability, swelling, feelings of heaviness, tingling sensations, pain, skin dystrophy, and changes in skin color. The bilberry anthocyanosides improved vein function by reducing capillary flow.

Recommended dosages, which should be taken three times daily, are 20 to 40 mg of anthocyanosides (calculated as anthocyanidin) and 80 to 160 mg of bilberry extract (25 percent anthocyanidin content). In a study published by James A. Duke, Ph.D., 400 mg/day of bilberry and 20 mg/day of beta-carotene improved night vision and enlarged visual fields in the volunteers who were tested. Duke quoted Daniel Mowry, Ph.D., as saying that the anthocyanosides in bilberry strengthen the capillaries in the retina of the eye. Mowry suggests a tea including bilberry, butcher's broom, centella, and ginger for the prevention and treatment of several types of mac-

ular degeneration. Steep the herbs in boiling water for 15 minutes and drink one cup up to four times daily.[2]

Duke added that a group of Italian researchers used a mixture of bilberry anthocyanosides and vitamin E to halt the progression of lens clouding in 97 percent of patients with early-stage cataracts. Naturopaths recommend a standardized bilberry extract at a dose of 80 to 160 mg three times a day. German herbalists recommend a tea containing 2 to 4 tablespoons of crushed bilberries.

Writing in *Clinical Pearls 1998 with The Experts Speak,* Kirk Hamilton interviewed Merrill J. Allen, O.D., Ph.D., professor emeritus of the Indiana University School of Optometry at Bloomington, who has been studying retinitis pigmentosa since 1941. Allen is convinced that bilberry, zinc, and taurine (an amino acid) play an important role in preventing that eye condition.[3] About 20 years ago, Allen prescribed zinc for a young man with retinitis pigmentosa. The prescription brought a sensational improvement in the young man's vision. After reading a report from Australia concerning a national epidemic of cat blindness similar to retinitis pigmentosa, Allen was convinced that this disorder is not genetic, as had previously been thought. The cause of the cat blindness epidemic was dog food mistakenly labeled as cat food. Dog food does not contain taurine, which cats need to prevent the disease. When Allen was in the military, he read that bilberries were known to improve night vision, which is the first area that retinitis pigmentosa attacks.

Years later, at the Mayo Clinic, a 15-year-old girl was diagnosed with retinitis pigmentosa and was advised to learn Braille. Allen and a colleague, Ray Lowry, M.D., decided to give the girl nutritional supplements and electrical stimulation. Beginning in December 1992, the supplements included 300 mg of bilberry and 750 mg of taurine daily. At her last eye exam in December 1997, her right eye registered 20/20 and the left 20/40. The girl's peripheral vision is reasonably normal beyond 55 degrees, she has reasonably good night vision, and she now has a driver's license.

Another of Allen's patients, a 37-year-old female, was diagnosed with retinitis pigmentosa. After four years of electrical stimulation and nutritional supplements, she is able to drive comfortably once more and maintains that she has no vision problems. The daily supplements, given to all patients with retinitis pigmentosa, include bilberry, taurine, 50 mg of zinc, and a multiple vitamin/mineral formula.

According to Ralph Golan, M.D., bilberry flavonoids are often used in the treatment or prevention of hardening of the arteries, rheumatoid and osteoarthritis, gout, periodontal disease, varicose veins, venous insufficiency, and microscopic hematuria caused by capillary fragility in the kidneys.[4]

References

1. Murray, Michael T., "Bilberry (*Vaccinium myrtillus*)," *American Journal of Natural Medicine* 4(1): 18–22, Jan./Feb. 1997.
2. Duke, James A., *The Green Pharmacy* (Emmaus, Pa.: Rodale Press, 1997), 128, 318ff.
3. Hamilton, Kirk, *Clinical Pearls 1998 with The Experts Speak* (Sacramento, Calif.: ITServices, 1998), 58. Merrill J. Allen, "Successful Reversal of Retinitis Pigmentosa," *Journal of Orthomolecular Medicine* 13(1): 41–43, 1998.
4. Golan, Ralph, *Optimal Wellness* (New York: Ballantine, 1995), 447.

4

Biotin

Those who consume egg whites to avoid the cholesterol in the yolks may be at risk for a biotin deficiency. Biotin, a B vitamin, appears to be an essential component of a coenzyme in carbon dioxide fixation, an important reaction in intermediary metabolism and a requirement for purine synthesis. Raw egg white contains the protein avidin, which combines with biotin to prevent its absorption. However, cooking seems to inactivate avidin.[1]

At the University of Georgia, Virgil Sydenstricker and colleagues produced experimental deficiency in biotin by feeding volunteers large amounts of raw egg whites. Such a deficiency causes dry, scaly skin, as well as changes in skin color. Other abnormalities included nervous symptoms, tongue lesions, and changes in the electrocardiogram, findings consistent with a deficiency in other members of the B complex.

Researchers at the University of Iowa at Iowa City determined that a biotin deficiency is associated with altered metabolism of fatty acids and cholesterol. For example, patients given parenteral alimentation developed fatty acid compositions in their blood, including changes in phospholipids, cholesterol, triglycerides, and free fatty acids that responded to biotin supplements. This effect on fatty acid metabolism may help to explain the development of hair loss, dermatitis and other skin rashes, central nervous system abnormalities, and other conditions affecting those with a biotin deficiency. The research team was unable to determine whether or not a biotin deficiency might affect cholesterol metabolism in such a way as to increase the risk of developing hardening of the arteries or heart disease.[2]

Oral biotin is absorbed almost completely even in large doses. Given in a large dose, however, most of the biotin may be eliminated from the body through the kidneys. Utilization might be improved if supplements are given in two or three smaller doses during the day.[3]

A Japanese infant who was fed a standard cow's-milk formula developed diaper rash and vomiting at 39 days of age. He lost 12 percent of his body weight over the next two days and was admitted to the hospital, where it was determined that his blood levels of biotin were low. After the infant was given 1 g/day of biotin orally, the diaper rash subsided within two weeks.[4]

An 11-month-old Japanese infant developed a biotin deficiency after being diagnosed with cow's-milk and soybean allergies. Researchers administered an amino acid formula and a hypoallergenic rice concoction. Although the infant's zinc and essential fatty acids were in the normal range, biotin levels were below normal. Symptoms of mouth lesions, lethargy, muscle spasms, and hair loss eventually cleared after the infant was given 1 g/day of biotin. The researchers recommended that biotin should be added to Japanese amino acid formulas to avoid a biotin deficiency.[5]

Acquired biotin deficiency and the two congenital disorders of biotin metabolism—biotinidase and holocarboxylase synthetase—can lead to the excretion of an acid urine and severe life-threatening illness. Symptoms include feeding difficulties, neurologic abnormalities, and changes in the skin.

Newborn screening for biotinidase deficiency has uncovered those with partial deficiency as well as those with a profound deficiency. Ten milligrams per day or less are sufficient to treat a profound deficiency, and the prognosis is good if these disorders are discovered early on. If treatment does not come until later, there can be irreversible neurological damage. However, some patients with holocarboxylase synthetase deficiency have responded only partially to vitamin therapy, even when given 100 mg/day of biotin.[6]

Those with brittle nails may want to have their biotin reserves monitored. In a study conducted by Columbia University College of Physicians and Surgeons in New York and Thomas Jefferson University Hospital in Philadelphia, 2,000 mcg/day of biotin were found to be helpful in most patients with brittle nails.[7]

When Japanese researchers studied the biotin and blood sugar levels of patients with Type 2 (non-insulin-dependent) diabetes, they reported that those with high blood sugar levels had low blood levels of biotin. After giving 9 mg/day (9,000 mcg) of biotin to 18 of these patients for a month, blood sugar levels fell to nearly half of their original levels.

Biotin, which is manufactured in the intestines by gut bacteria, is necessary for the manufacture and utilization of carbohydrates, fats, and amino acids, according to Michael Murray, N.D., and Joseph Pizzorno, N.D. A vegetarian diet, however, may inhibit the intestinal bacterial flora, compromising the absorption of biotin. In addition, biotin supplements are thought to enhance insulin sensitivity and increase the action of glucokinase, the enzyme responsible for the utilization of glucose by the liver.[8]

Seborrheic dermatitis often begins in infancy as cradle cap. While this is not primarily an allergic disease, it has been associated with food allergy, since 67 percent of children with cradle cap develop some form of allergy by age 10, Murray and Pizzorno added. "The underlying factor in infants appears to be a biotin deficiency," the authors said. "A syndrome clinically similar to seborrheic dermatitis has been produced by feeding rats a diet high in raw egg white. A large portion of the human biotin supply is provided by intestinal bacteria, and it has been postulated that, since newborns are born with a sterile gastrointestinal tract, the absence of normal intestinal flora may be responsible for biotin deficiency in infants. A number of studies have demonstrated successful treatment of seborrheic dermatitis with biotin in both the nursing mother and the infant."

Biotin is distributed rather widely in foods of both plant and animal origin. It occurs in a free state in fruits, vegetables, milk, and rice bran, and it is found partly in a form bound to protein in meats, egg yolk, plant seeds, and yeast. Leading biotin sources include brewer's yeast, chicken liver, torula yeast, beef liver, pasteurized American cheese, soybean flour, rice bran, wheat bran, rice polish, calf liver, and eggs.[9]

No toxic effects of oral biotin have been reported in humans or animals, and no adverse reactions have been reported when infants were given injections of up to 10 mg for six months or from adult oral intakes of up to 10 mg/day. The lack of reported toxicity at an intake of 2,500 mcg (2.5 mg) per day suggests that this is a safe intake.[10]

References

1. Goldsmith, Grace A., "Vitamins of the B Complex," *The Yearbook of Agriculture 1959* (Washington, D.C.: U.S. Department of Agriculture, 1959), 149.
2. Mock, D., et al., "Effects of Biotin Deficiency on Serum Fatty Acid Composition: Evidence for Abnormalities in Humans," *Journal of Nutrition* 118: 342–48, 1988.
3. Zempleni, Janos, and Donald M. Mock, "Bioavailability of Biotin Given Orally in Humans in Pharmacologic Doses," *American Journal of Clinical Nutrition* 69: 504–8, 1999.
4. Higuchi, R., et al., "Intractable Diaper Dermatitis as an Early Sign of Biotin Deficiency," *Acta Paediatrica* 87: 228–29, 1998.
5. Higuchi, R., et al., "Biotin Deficiency in an Infant Fed with Amino Acid Formula and Hypoallergenic Rice," *Acta Paediatrica* 85: 872–74, 1996.
6. Baumgartner, E. Regula, and Terttu Suormala, "Multiple Carboxylase

Deficiency: Inherited and Acquired Disorders of Biotin Metabolism," *International Journal for Vitamin and Nutrition Research* 67: 377–84, 1997.

7. Feinstein, Alice, *Healing with Vitamins* (Emmaus, Pa.: Rodale Press, 1996), 4.

8. Murray, Michael, and Joseph Pizzorno, *Encyclopedia of Natural Medicine,* 2nd ed. (Rocklin, Calif.: Prima Publishing, 1998), 419, 794–95.

9. Ensminger, A., et al., *Foods & Nutrition Encyclopedia* (Clovis, Calif.: Pegus Press, 1983), 210ff.

10. Hathcock, John N., *Vitamin and Mineral Safety: A Summary Review* (Washington, D.C.: Council for Responsible Nutrition, 1997), 17.

5

Black Cohosh

Also called black root, rattle root, and squawroot, black cohosh *(Cimicifuga racemosa)* is a native North American plant whose chief constituent is cimicifugin. Its bitter taste is caused by a crystalline principle called racemosin.[1]

Black cohosh has an ancient reputation as a remedy for what were known as "female complaints," and as such was one of the ingredients in the famous proprietary medicine called Lydia E. Pinkham's Vegetable Compound. Studies have shown that the herb suppresses hot flashes in menopausal women by reducing the secretion of luteinizing hormone (LH), which is involved in the egg-releasing stage of reproduction. Black cohosh contains the isoflavone formononetin, thought to be the basis of its estrogenic activity, since it is converted in the body by the gastrointestinal microbial flora to compounds that bind to the estrogen receptor, initially as diadzein and then as the more active isoflavan equol. The herb occasionally causes stomach upset in susceptible people.[2]

In one study reported by James A. Duke, Ph.D., involving 110 menopausal women, half were given black cohosh root extract, while the other half took a placebo. After eight weeks of therapy, blood tests showed significant estrogenic activity in those receiving the herb. In another study, women experiencing vaginal dryness due to menopause experienced similar relief whether taking black cohosh or a pharmaceutical estrogen. Duke quotes herbalist Deb Soule, who told an anecdotal story of how a neighbor gained relief after taking black cohosh for tinnitus (ringing in the ears).[3]

Black cohosh is recommended by *The Complete German Commission E Monographs* for premenstrual discomfort, dysmenorrhea (painful menstruation), and other menopausal complaints. The commission recommends extracts corresponding to 40 mg of the root. It suggests that the extract should not be used longer than six months without consulting a professional.[4]

At a meeting of the American College of Obstetricians and Gynecologists, Maida Taylor, M.D., explained that many botanicals have both positive and adverse effects. Black and blue cohosh are used for menopausal hot flashes and irregular menstrual bleeding, since they contain phytosterols with estrogenic-like activity.[5]

Today herbalists still recommend black cohosh for menstrual problems. It is also sometimes used as a sedative and for treating rheumatoid arthritis, edema, and sore throat. Its main claim to fame, however, has been its ability to relieve menstrual cramps and the pain of childbirth. Using it for the latter application, Native Americans called the herb squawroot.[6]

Dried roots and rhizomes are good estrogenic constituents of black cohosh because they act specifically on the uterus to reduce cramps and congestion as well as hot flashes. Since the herb contains two antirheumatic compounds, it is said to be an excellent herb for relieving muscular pain and cramping. It is also believed to reduce cholesterol levels and blood pressure. Some researchers recommend 250 mg in tablet or capsule form, two to four times daily, or one-half teaspoon of tincture twice a day.[7]

Black cohosh was used by G. Vorberg, a Munich physician, to treat 50 women ranging in age from 45 to 60 who had menopausal complaints. The women were given 40 drops per day (equivalent to two tablets). After four weeks of therapy, Vorberg noticed a significant decrease in hot flashes, sweating, nervousness, irritability, and headache. After 12 weeks of treatment, most of the symptoms, except lack of concentration and arthritis pain, had eased.[8]

Another physician, Ernst Wolrad Schotten, M.D., gave menopausal patients 20 drops (equivalent to one tablet) of black cohosh extract three times daily, but noted that the effects were not immediately apparent. However, giving the treatment for three to four weeks was so successful that he was able to reduce the dose to 10 drops three times daily. He discontinued the sedatives he had previously prescribed and reported a normalization of blood pressure in some of the women.[9]

After prescribing black cohosh extract for four years for 517 female patients, one physician concluded that the extract has a hormonelike and slightly euphoric effect. He reviewed a number of case histories and found that black cohosh extract is usually prescribed at 20 to 30 drops or one tablet three times a day. Since the effectiveness does not kick in immediately, short-term use is pointless.[10]

Eva-Maria Dueker and colleagues at the University of Goettingen in Germany found that cessation of ovarian function during menopause is characterized by reduced estrogen production and increased LH and FSH (follicle-stimulating hormone) secretion. These endocrine changes bring on hot flashes, depression, and so forth, which are often treated with estrogen. However, Dueker said, although estrogen replacement therapy can be effective, alternative treatments such as black cohosh are necessary, because some women refuse to take steroid hormone replacement or because these therapies are contraindicated.[11]

"We have evidence that a preparation made from *Cimicifuga racemosa* is able to suppress LH secretion in menopausal women," the researchers said. "Since LH secretion and the occurrence of hot flashes are closely related, measurement of LH levels is a suitable parameter to study the potency of plant extracts in regard to the reduction of hot flashes. To the best of our knowledge, this is the first report about a plant extract affecting LH secretion in both humans and [rats]."

In addition to menopausal complaints, black cohosh is used by herbalists for a variety of gynecological complaints, such as premenstrual syndrome.

References

1. Grieve, Maude, *A Modern Herbal* (New York: Dover Publications, 1982), 211.

2. Robbers, James E., and Varro E. Tyler, *Tyler's Herbs of Choice* (New York: Haworth Herbal Press, 1999), 191.

3. Duke, James A., *The Green Pharmacy* (Emmaus, Pa.: Rodale Press, 1997), 323–24, 422.

4. Blumenthal, Mark, senior ed., *The Complete German Commission E Monographs* (Boston: Integrative Medicine Communications; Austin, Texas: American Botanical Council, 1998), 90.

5. Scarbeck, Kathy, "Botanicals Used in Menopause," *Family Practice News,* Jan. 15, 1996, 46.

6. Guinness, Alma E., *Family Guide to Natural Medicine* (Pleasantville, N.Y.: Reader's Digest Association, 1993), 298.

7. Cabot, Sandra, *Smart Medicine for Menopause* (Garden City, N.Y.: Avery Publishing Group, 1995), 110.

8. Murray, Frank, *Remifemin: Herbal Relief for Menopausal Symptoms.* (New Canaan, Conn.: Keats Publishing, 1996), 40.

9. Ibid., 41.

10. Ibid., 42–43.

11. Ibid., 36–37. Also, E. M. Dueker, et al., "Effects of Extracts from *Cimicifuga racemosa* on Gonadotropin Release in Menopausal Women and Ovariectomized Rats," *Planta Medica* 57(5): 420–24, 1991.

6

Black Elderberry

The flu, which is caused by a family of three viruses—A, B, and C—known as the myxoviruses influenzae, no longer ravages the world as it did during the 1918 epidemic, which killed hundreds of thousands in the United States and an estimated 20 million worldwide. Today, however, it is still responsible for an estimated 20,000 fatalities each year in this country. Those especially susceptible are people over 65 years of age and those with weakened immune systems.

A new weapon in nature's armamentarium—black elderberry extract—is now available commercially in a syrup and lozenges, although it has been used for more than 2,500 years to treat flu, coughs, and colds. Black elder *(Sambucus nigra L.)* was highly praised by the physicians Hippocrates and Dioscorides and the scholar Pliny for its effectiveness on upper respiratory infections.

The berries are rich in thiamine, riboflavin, pyridoxine, calcium, and phosphorus.

To be effective, viruses cannot replicate on their own, but instead must invade living cells and alter their function. Therefore, if you can stop the virus from entering the cell, you have defeated the disease.

"The flu virus invades cells by puncturing their walls with tiny spikes called hemagglutinin that cover its surface," explains Madeleine Mumcuoglu, Ph.D., an Algerian-born, French-educated virologist now practicing in Israel. "The active ingredients in elderberry actually disarm the spikes, binding to them, and thus preventing them from piercing the cell membrane. The viral spikes are covered with an enzyme called neuraminidase, and this enzyme acts to break down the cell wall. Bioflavonoids, which are present in high concentrations in elderberries, may inhibit the action of this enzyme."[1]

In 1992, a team of Israeli researchers developed a syrup and a lozenge containing the active elderberry ingredients combined with other natural components, and gave them to a group of flu patients during an epidemic in southern Israel. Half of the patients received 4 tablespoons of the syrup daily, while the other half were given a placebo. Within 24 hours, fever, cough, and muscle pain had significantly subsided in 20 percent of the patients receiving the syrup. After the second day, another 75 percent of the patients were much improved, and within three days a complete cure was registered in over 90 percent of the patients. For the control group, only 8 percent showed an improvement after 24 hours, and for the remaining 92 percent, improvement did not take place for six or more days. The level of antibodies was higher in those receiving the elderberry extract in contrast to those getting a look-alike syrup.

In 1993, researchers at Hebrew University–Hadassah Medical School in Jerusalem and other facilities in Israel conducted a placebo-controlled, double-blind trial in which volunteers at an agricultural community (kibbutz) were administered either a placebo or a standardized plant extract from the fruit of the black elder to fight an outbreak of influenza B/Panama flu.[2] A significant improvement in symptoms, including fever, was noted in 93.3 percent of those getting the black elderberry within two days, compared to 91.7 percent in the control group in six days. A complete recovery was achieved within two to three days in almost 90 percent of the elderberry-treated volunteers, compared to about six days in the placebo group.

"No satisfactory medication to cure influenza A and B is available," the researchers said. "However, considering the efficiency of elderberry extract in laboratory tests on all strains of the influenza virus tested, the clinical results, its low cost, and absence of side effects, the extract could offer a possibility for treatment for influenza A and B."

Because black elderberry stimulates the immune system, it has shown some activity in preliminary trials against other viruses, such as Epstein-Barr, herpes, and HIV, according to James A. Duke, Ph.D. "If I had HIV, I'd eat lots of elderberries," he wrote.[3]

Researchers at Hebrew University–Hadassah tested whether black elderberry would inactivate an HIV infection. Using test tubes, the researchers placed black elderberry extract in cultures containing HIV isolates from patients infected with HIV and controls who were not infected. HIV-antigen was not detected five and nine days after treatment with black elderberry. This approach may have a practical application in designing a simple or combined viral intervention therapy for those already exposed to the virus.[4] The researchers also tested black elderberry extract against four strains of herpes simplex virus, type 1, which causes cold sores. The success of this trial may be of significance and deserves further in vitro and in vivo testing.[5]

As a preventive measure, the recommended dosage for black elderberry is either 1 tablespoon syrup or one lozenge four times daily, according to Bob Arnot, M.D.[6]

References

1. Mumcuoglu, Madeleine, *Sambucus: Black Elderberry Extract. A Breakthrough in the Treatment of Influenza* (Skokie, Ill.: RSS Publishing, 1995).

2. Zakay-Rones, Zichria, et al., "Inhibition of Several Strains of Influenza Virus in Vitro and Reduction of Symptoms by an Elderberry Extract *(Sambucus Nigra L.)* During an Outbreak of Influenza B Panama," *Journal of Alternative and Complementary Medicine* 1(4): 361–69, 1995.

3. Duke, James A., *The Green Pharmacy* (Emmaus, Pa.: Rodale Press, 1997), 136–37, 146, 270–71.

4. Shapira-Nahor, O., et al., "The Effect of Sambucol on HIV Infection In Vitro," paper presented at Congress of Microbiology, Jerusalem, Feb. 6–7, 1995.

5. Morag, A., et al., "Inhibition of Sensitive and Acyclovir-Resistant HSV-1 Strains by an Elderberry Extract In Vitro," paper presented at 10th International Congress of Virology, Jerusalem, Aug. 11–16, 1996.

6. Arnot, Bob, "Health Check," *Good Housekeeping,* Feb. 1996, 58.

7

Boron

Boron is not considered a true antioxidant, but it does possess some antioxidant properties, according to Jason Theodosakis, M.D. The mineral is important in maintaining joint health and keeps some cells from releasing harmful free radicals. In geographic areas where boron intakes are low, osteoarthritis incidence is high, and vice versa. Also, studies have shown that boron supplements have a beneficial effect on osteoarthritis.[1]

"The mineral boron has proved helpful for my patients," said Robert M. Giller, M.D. "Boron naturally elevates estrogen levels, and I originally recommended it to help fight osteoporosis. Many women told me that it had an immediate beneficial effect on their hot flashes."[2]

Researchers at Winthrop University at Rock Hill, South Carolina, conducted a study involving 28 female students, 18 to 25 years of age. Seventeen of the women were recruited from the university's athletic program and some were sedentary. In addition to their typical diets, the women were given 3 mg/day of boron or a placebo to test the mineral's relationship to other minerals and bone health.[3]

Calcium excretion increased in all the groups tested, and boron excretion increased in those getting the boron supplement. Boron supplementation modestly affected mineral status, and exercise modified the effects of boron supplementation on serum minerals. Magnesium levels tended to be on the low end to normal, and researchers suggested that young female athletes in the study who showed low serum magnesium concentrations and who were consuming a low-magnesium diet might be at risk for developing bone metabolism disorders. The boron supplements reduced the amount of phosphorous in the blood.

The researchers added that increasing dietary calcium and boron may be beneficial in balancing blood minerals to optimize bone mineralization during the final developmental period and in building a bone mineral bank for later years. Although much research has centered on calcium and bone health, this interest should be extended to optimal intakes of all minerals known or suspected of affecting bone density, such as boron, calcium, phosphorus, and magnesium.

In a double-blind study in Britain comparing 6 mg/day of boron with a placebo in treating arthritis, researchers found that of the 10 patients given the mineral, five improved while only one in the placebo group had any relief. The trial lasted for eight weeks, and no side effects were reported. The boron was administered in two tablets and was observed to have a significant effect on severe osteoarthritis.[4]

Parris M. Kidd, Ph.D., in a general review article on the role of nutrition, lifestyle, and bone loss, stated that boron is an ultra trace element that may play a role, via the kidneys, in preventing urinary loss of calcium. Boron supplements given to postmenopausal women not on estrogen therapy raised their serum calcium to levels comparable with a control group of women receiving estrogen replacement therapy.[5]

Only 3 mg/day of boron has been shown to reduce calcium excretion by almost half. Boron, like magnesium, may be necessary for the conversion of vitamin D in the kidneys to its most active form. In one study, the mineral dramatically increased levels of 17 beta-estradiol, the most biologically active form of estrogen. Boron supplements have been shown to mimic the effects of estrogen therapy in some postmenopausal women.[6]

Melvyn Werbach, M.D., of the UCLA School of Medicine, reported that studies in various countries have found that the lower the level of boron in the soil, the more people in that area develop osteoarthritis. He quoted one physician who said that in his experience, 90 percent of his osteoarthritis patients improved after they were given boron supplements, and that most experienced complete remission of their symptoms.[7] Although Werbach does not prescribe boron supplements, he does urge everyone to eat ample amounts of the mineral. Food sources include alfalfa, cabbage, lettuce, peas, snap beans, soy, apples, dates, prunes, raisins, almonds, hazelnuts, and peanuts.

French researchers have reported that although an absolute dietary requirement for boron has not been officially established in humans and animals, experiments with boron supplements and low-boron diets show that the mineral is involved in calcium and bone metabolism. Its effects are more pronounced when other nutrients (cholecalciferol, magnesium, etc.) are deficient. Cholecalciferol is one form of vitamin D.[8] The researchers went on to say that boron supplements increase the serum concentrations of 17 beta-estradiol and testosterone, but that an excess of the mineral has toxic effects on reproduction. Boron may be involved in cerebral function through its effects on the transport of the mineral across membranes. It is believed to affect the synthesis of the extracellular matrix, as well as aid in wound healing. The average diet is thought to contain from 1 to 2 mg/day of boron. Boronated compounds have been shown to be potent antiosteoporotic, anti-inflammatory, anticoagulant, and antitumor substances in both humans and animals.

References

1. Theodosakis, Jason, Brenda Adderly, and Barry Fox, *The Arthritis Cure* (New York: St. Martin's Press, 1997), 109.

2. Giller, Robert M., and Kathy Matthews, *Natural Prescriptions* (New York: Carol Southern Books, 1994), 245.

3. Meacham, Susan L., et al., "Effects of Boron Supplementation on Blood and Urinary Calcium, Magnesium, and Phosphorous, and Urinary Boron in Athletic and Sedentary Women," *American Journal of Clinical Nutrition* 61: 341–45, 1995.

4. Travers, Richard L., "Boron and Arthritis: The Results of a Double-Blind Pilot Study," *Journal of Nutritional Medicine* 1: 127–32, 1990.

5. Kidd, Parris M., "An Integrative Lifestyle: Nutritional Strategy for Lowering Osteoporosis Risk," *Townsend Letter for Doctors,* May 1992, 400–05.

6. Whitaker, Julian, *Dr. Whitaker's Guide to Natural Healing* (Rocklin, Calif: Prima Publishing, 1995), 320.

7. Werbach, Melvyn, *Healing with Food* (New York: HarperPerennial, 1993), 283, 367.

8. Benderdour, M., et al., "In Vivo and In Vitro Effects of Boron and Boronated Compounds," *Journal of Trace Elements and Medical Biology* 12: 2–7, March 1998.

8

Bovine Colostrum

Colostrum is a thick, milklike secretion produced by mammary glands in women and female animals, particularly during the first few days after giving birth. A high-calorie fluid, it contains protein and fat to nurture the newborn. Its yellow color signifies its high content of beta-carotene, or provitamin A. In contrast to mature breast milk, it has more protein and less milk sugar and fat.[1]

Colostrum is an excellent nutritional supplement since it is high in nutrient density, rich in the basic building blocks of protein and nucleic acids, and a good source of vitamins and of sufficient calorie content to satisfy basic nutritional needs, according to David J. Hurley, Ph.D., of South Dakota State University at Brookings. Colostrum can be used to either stimulate or satisfy the appetite, and the combination of fats, amino acids, and sugars starts the gastric activity in the neonate or restarts that activity after illness or antibiotic therapy.[2]

Many studies of the activity of colostrum in protection against infections that occur in or enter through the digestive tract have been completed. In the 1950s, Albert Sabin, M.D., developer of the polio vaccine, suggested feeding bovine colostrum to children with polio.

Hurley noted that several studies have shown antiviral effects of colostrum. Kuhl et al. examined the ability of colostral cells to kill herpes viruses, and reported that a combination of colostral antibodies and leukocytes effectively killed herpes-infected cells. Similar results were obtained with bovine colostrum by Rouse et al. in 1976.

Neil V. MacKay, D.C., wrote that several factors in colostrum prevent the success and survival of pathogens in the gut. These factors work synergistically to slow or halt pathogen survival. They are the

Immune Component, which contains immuglobulin proteins that bind to and assist in killing pathogens; the Growth Factor Component, which stimulates repair and recovery of damaged intestinal lining; the Specialized Protein Component, which contains immunologically active cytokines and such antimicrobial proteins as lactoferrin; and the Glycoconjugate Component, composed of sugar molecules that confuse pathogens as to where they might attach themselves.[3] Cytokines are immunoregulatory substances secreted by cells of the immune system.

Researchers in Guatemala City evaluated 12 patients with either rheumatoid arthritis or osteoarthritis. Their average age was 52.5 years. The volunteers were taking between one and five medications and were started on Infopeptides (bovine colostrum) as adjuvant therapy. The treatment lasted for three months, and each person received a dose of 5 ml/day orally. After two to six weeks of treatment, 10 of the 12 patients reported a reduction or disappearance of pain, swelling, and inflammation.[4]

At that point, 10 osteoarthritis patients, average age of 58.4 years, entered the study. All were taking nonsteroidal anti-inflammatory drugs. Between 15 and 21 days into the therapy, 9 of the 10 volunteers reported a significant reduction in pain and inflammation. Colostrum-derived products contain one or more immunomodulating agents that promote anti-inflammatory, cytokine-type activity similar to anti-inflammatory activity of cytokines 4, 10, 13, 15, and 16. The Infopeptides seem to act non-specifically, allowing the organism to regain normal functioning patterns. Bovine colostrum products are low in cost compared to other agents, and their most profound effect is on pain relief.

Bovine colostrum may be useful in the treatment of patients with immunodeficiency disorders, as reported in the *British Medical Journal*. Researchers studied a small boy who had trouble gaining weight. He was found to have diarrhea and was infected with *Pneumocystis carinii,* the microorganism that causes pneumocystis pneumonia in debilitated patients. The research team suggested that bovine colostrum is safer than most drugs, which is a consideration when treating debilitated patients.[5]

A research team from Frankfurt, Germany, reported that an immunoglobulin supplement prepared from bovine colostrum has a high antibacterial antibody strength, as well as a high capacity for the neutralization of bacterial toxins. Bovine colostrum is well tolerated and is effective in the treatment of severe diarrhea such as that found in AIDS patients.[6]

Immunoglobulins (IgG, IgM, and IgA) are found in high concentrations in colostrum and exhibit antibacterial and antiviral effects against a range of microorganisms, according to a research team from Germany and France.[7] The study involved seven volunteers, six female and one male, ranging in age from 20 to 42. The researchers said that, like other scientists, they found that immunoglobulin concentrate from bovine colostrum improved virus-associated diarrhea in imunodeficient patients.

An eight-week study of 40 Australian athletes found that those who took daily doses of colostrum had more stamina than those who took a placebo. Jon Buckley, project leader from the University of South Australia, said that the athletes taking colostrum ran longer and covered greater distances.[8]

Daniel Gastelu and Fred Hatfield, Ph.D., emphasize that colostrum's many benefits are to the digestive system, since it helps keep the lining of the digestive system healthy. Its constituents also assist with the maintenance of the intestine's "good bacteria," which inhibits the production of "bad bacteria." In athletes, colostrum normalizes the gastrointestinal system and reduces diarrhea, resulting in better digestion and absorption of nutrients. The immunoglobulins in colostrum also boost the athlete's immune system, which is constantly challenged during exercise.[9] "The muscle-building and connective-tissue-repair of IGF-I and IGF-II are biochemically unsurpassed," the authors said. "They are essential ingredients in muscle growth, primarily through their roles in the repair and conversion of broken-down muscle fibers."

Bovine colostrum is available over the counter in capsules, chewable tablets, liquids, and powders, as well as in energy bars. It is now gaining wider acceptance in the alternative medicine community.

References

1. Ronzio, Robert A., *The Encyclopedia of Nutrition and Good Health* (New York: Facts on File, 1997), 107.

2. Hurley, David J., "A Summary of Research Studies on the Biological Properties of Colostrum," June 1994, unpublished.

3. MacKay, Neil V., "Bovine Colostrum: The Natural Cure for Diarrhea," *Let's Live,* March 1996.

4. Nitsch, A., and F. P. Nitsch, "The Clinical Use of Bovine Colostrum," *Journal of Orthomolecular Medicine* 13(2): 110–18, 1998.

5. Tzipori, S., et al., "Remission of Diarrhoea Due to Cryptosporidosis in an Immunodeficient Child Treated with Hyperimmune Bovine Colostrum," *British Medical Journal* 293: 1276–77, Nov. 15, 1986.

6. Stephan, W., et al., "Antibodies from Colostrum in Oral Immunotherapy," *Journal of Clinical Chemistry and Clinical Biochemistry* 28: 19–23, 1990.

7. Roos, N., et al., "15-N-Labeled Immunoglobulins from Bovine Colostrum Are Partially Resistant to Digestion in Human Intestine," *Journal of Nutrition* 125: 1238–44, 1995.

8. *Nando Times,* Oct. 1998.

9. Gastelu, Daniel, and Fred Hatfield, *Dynamic Nutrition for Maximum Performance* (Garden City, N.Y.: Avery Publishing Group, 1997), 103–4.

9

C-MED-100

With the growing encroachment of civilization on the world's rain forests, scientists are in a race against time to catalog as many healing plants as possible before they disappear forever. In underdeveloped countries, farmers are clearing more and more land to raise feed for their cattle. This deforestation leaves fewer acres for food production, which can contribute to global warming, depletion of the world's water supply, and consequently an adverse effect on public health.[1]

One of the plants that has drawn considerable interest from scientists is cat's claw *(Uncaria tomentosa),* which the Campa Indians and other natives indigenous to the Amazon basin in South America have utilized for centuries for its health-promoting constituents. Also referred to as *una de gato,* the English name is derived from the branches of the plant, which resemble the claws of a cat.

While the natives have consistently used cat's claw to treat cancer, arthritis, and infectious diseases, there has been limited research on the plant's antitumor properties. Researchers have long theorized that apoptosis (programmed cell death) is a likely approach to treating cancer. Apoptosis is best described as a naturally occurring form of cell death or suicide that provides a defense against cancer, viral infections, AIDS, and autoimmune and neurodegenerative disorders.[2]

At the University of Lund in Sweden, Ronald W. Pero, Ph.D., Yezhou Sheng, and Carl Bryngelsson have observed that a significant repair of DNA has been recorded after supplementation with a combination of carotenoids, nicotinamide (vitamin B_3), and zinc. Using a similar methodology with laboratory animals, the researchers found that supplementation with a newly discovered water-soluble extract of cat's claw (C-MED-100) enhanced DNA repair and immune response in the animals, and no toxicity was found with the dose range tested.

DNA repair is necessary for maintaining both cell vitality and stability of genetic material of an organism. Cells respond to DNA damage in three ways: (1) by absorbing the damage; (2) by repairing the damage; and (3) by undergoing apoptosis. The researchers confirmed that C-MED-100 is effective in killing leukemic cells, and that the extract may have antitumor, anti-inflammatory, and immune-stimulating properties. In another experiment involving two human leukemic cells, the research team confirmed the first direct evidence for the antitumor properties of the cat's claw extract.[3]

Writing in *Whole Foods*, Richard A. Passwater, Ph.D., asked Pero about any human trials. At that time Pero's team had completed one study involving four volunteers whose white blood cell counts were monitored for four weeks.[4] White blood cells, or leukocytes, defend the body against disease-causing bacteria, viruses, and fungi. Following treatment with the cat's-claw extract, three of the four volunteers showed increases in white blood cell counts, while the fourth remained unchanged. But as a group, the white blood cell levels were increased significantly, Pero noted.

While cat's-claw extract continues to be investigated, biological analysis shows that C-MED-100 contains a previously unrecognized class of neutraceuticals called carboxyl alkyl esters. These constituents are said to influence membrane integrity, which programs a cell to attack invaders.[5]

C-MED-100 products are now available. Recommended dosage is two 350-mg servings daily for a month. As a maintenance dose, the suggested amount is 5 mg/kg of body weight. That translates to about 350 mg daily for a 150-pound person.

See the cat's claw entry in this book for more information.

References

1. Lewis, Stephen, "An Opinion on the Global Impact of Meat Consumption," *American Journal of Clinical Nutrition* 59 (Suppl.): 1099S, 1994.

2. Sheng, Yezhou, et al., "Enhanced DNA Repair and Reduced Toxicity of C-MED-100, a Novel Aqueous Extract from *Uncaria tomentosa*," *Journal of Ethanopharmacology* (In press, 2000).

3. Sheng, Yezhou, et al., "Induction of Apoptosis and Inhibition of Proliferation in Human Tumor Cells Treated with Extracts of *Uncaria Tomentosa*," *Anticancer Research* 18: 3363–68, 1998.

4. Passwater, Richard A., "Vitamin Connection: An Interview with Dr. Ronald Pero," *Whole Foods*, Feb. 1999.

5. "Ingredients in the Spotlight," *Nutritional Outlook*, Jan./Feb. 1999.

10

Calcium

A simple calcium supplement could prevent hip fractures caused by osteoporosis in more than 100,000 people and save billions of dollars in medical costs annually, according to the Council for Responsible Nutrition in Washington, D.C. The complete study was published in the June 1999 issue of *Clinical Therapeutics.* Approximately 300,000 American men and women over the age of 45 are hospitalized each year with osteoporotic hip fractures. An estimated 10 million Americans have osteoporosis, and 18 million more are at risk for developing the disease. Further, the National Institute for Child Health and Human Development in Washington, D.C., speculates that 41 million Americans could develop osteoporosis or low bone mass by 2015 unless measures are taken to detect, prevent, and treat the disease. Many of these fractures could be prevented with the consumption of the recommended levels of calcium and vitamin D, weight-bearing exercise, a nonsmoking lifestyle, and medication where appropriate.[1]

The average daily intake of dietary calcium is woefully less than the minimum recommended amount of 1,200 mg for older adults. A sampling of U.S. households found that only half of adults aged 60 to 94 drank one glass of milk daily, which would provide 300 mg of calcium. Another survey found that only 2 percent of adults aged 50 and older consumed a calcium supplement.

The effectiveness of calcium supplements at a particular dosage is ultimately dependent on a woman's diet and lifestyle. Bone is dependent on a constant supply of various nutrients, and a deficiency in any one of them affects bone health. The effective calcium dosage for most women is 800 to 1,200 mg/day. However, if there is significant bone loss, the dosage may need to be increased to 1,200 to 1,700 mg/day.[2]

Calcium also has been associated with a reduced risk of colon cancer and high blood pressure in some individuals. Despite the benefits, many Americans, especially women, are not getting the recommended dietary allowance. As for bone health, individuals must build up a substantial "bone bank" in the early years to carry them throughout their lives. For example, approximately 90 percent of the total bone mass in females is achieved by 16.9 years of age; 95 percent by age 19.8; and 99 percent by age 26.2.[3]

A research team at Purdue University reported that dietary intakes of calcium and milk at early ages may influence bone mineral measures at specific sites during development of peak bone mass. Dietary calcium intakes decline from childhood to adolescence, which leads to suboptimal intakes of calcium during this critical period.[4]

In a three-year study at Tufts University in Boston, men and women aged 65 and older supplementing with calcium and vitamin D moderately reduced their bone loss in the femoral neck, spine, and total body and reduced the incidence of nonvertebral fractures. The 176 men and 213 women were given either 500 mg/day of calcium and 700 IU/day of vitamin D or a placebo.[5]

Calcium supplements produce beneficial effects on bone mass throughout postmenopausal life and may reduce fracture rates by as much as 50 percent. Some of the most substantial reductions in fractures have been due to calcium and vitamin D supplements. Vitamin D is necessary for the absorption of calcium. Vitamin D status can be normalized in the frail elderly by encouraging them to walk outdoors for 15 to 30 minutes in sunlight, which is one source of the vitamin. Of course, they can't be bundled up in clothing.[6]

A study in Paris and Amiens, France, determined that calcium supplementation can decrease the concentrations of biochemical markers of bone turnover in postmenopausal women with low dietary calcium intake. This agrees with previous studies showing that added calcium impedes bone loss and vertebral fractures in postmenopausal women who consume a low-calcium diet.[7]

Researchers at St. Luke's–Roosevelt Hospital Center and other facilities in New York reported that calcium supplementation is a simple and effective treatment for premenstrual syndrome (PMS). This condition results in a major reduction in overall luteal (egg-releasing) phase symptoms, according to a study of women aged 18 to 45, who were recruited from 12 outpatient centers. The women were given either 1,200 mg/day of calcium or a placebo for three menstrual cycles. By the third treatment cycle, water retention symptoms were reduced by 36 percent in the calcium-treated group, compared to 24 percent in the controls; food cravings were reduced 54 percent in the calcium group, compared to 34 percent for the placebo group; pain symptoms were reduced by 54 percent, compared with 15 percent for the controls. Calcium supplementation resulted in an approximately 50 percent reduction in total mean symptom scores, with a significant benefit for such symptoms as depression, mood swings, headache, and irritability. The researchers suggest that calcium should be considered an alternative therapeutic approach in the management of PMS.[8]

In evaluating 1,309 women between the ages of 20 and 92, researchers at the University of Michigan at Ann Arbor found that the incidence of kidney stones was 3.4 percent. But renal stone formation was not associated with calcium intake, high blood pressure, bone mineral density, fractures, high-oxalate food consumption (spinach, etc.), or vitamin C from food supplements. In fact, women with kidney stones consumed almost 250 mg/day less of calcium than women without stones. The data suggest that increased dietary calcium is not associated with a greater prevalence of kidney stones, and the stones are not a risk factor for low bone mineral density.[9]

Calcium supplementation during pregnancy leads to an important reduction in systolic (beating) and diastolic (resting) blood pressure and preeclampsia, according to a research team from McMaster University, Hamilton, Ontario, Canada, and other facilities. Preeclampsia is high blood pressure that usually develops in pregnant women during the 20th week of gestation.[10]

Women who take calcium supplements during pregnancy may reduce the risk of high blood pressure in their newborns. Researchers found that three-month-old infants whose mothers had taken 2,000 mg/day of calcium from 20 weeks of gestation to term had slightly lower blood pressure than the infants whose mothers took a placebo.[11]

A research team at the University of Southern California School of Medicine at Los Angeles and Louisiana State University School of Medicine at New Orleans has found that calcium supplements can lower diastolic blood pressure in African-American adolescents with low dietary intakes of the mineral. The study involved 65 girls and 51 boys, mean age of 15.8 years, who were given 1,500 mg/day of calcium or a look-alike pill for eight weeks. The supplement brought a drop of 2 mmHg in the treatment group, compared to a decrease of 5 mmHg in those eating a low-calcium diet, according to lead researcher James H. Dwyer, M.D.[12]

At Dartmouth-Hitchcock Medical Center in Lebanon, New Hampshire, and various facilities in the United States, calcium supplements were found to provide a significant reduction in large-bowel adenomas, which are likely precursors of most colorectal cancers. In the double-blind study, 930 volunteers were given either 3 g/day of calcium or a placebo, with follow-up colonoscopies one and four years after the initial examination. Seventy-two percent of the men had a recent history of colorectal adenomas. After four years, the overall incidence of polyps was 52 percent in the control group and 45 percent in the calcium-treated group.[13]

Researchers at the Arizona Cancer Center at Tucson evaluated the use of 2 or 13.5 g/day of wheat bran fiber and 250 or 1,500 mg/day of calcium. The higher amounts reduced the risk of colorectal cancer. Calcium is thought to "soak up" bile acids associated with the growth of tumors.[14]

In January 1997, the National Resources Defense Council, a California-based consumer action group, reported that some over-the-counter calcium supplements and antacids contain too much lead. Annette Dickinson, Ph.D., of the Council for Responsible Nutrition responded that the council had analyzed five brands of calcium supplements and found that the lead content ranged from 3.1 to 6.9 mcg per 1,000 mcg. Since calcium kicks out some of the lead, only about 0.25 mcg of that amount is probably absorbed.[15] Dickinson added that the FDA had analyzed lead content in some foods. In whole milk, the lead content ranged from 1.7 to 6.7 mcg. There were 2.4 mcg of lead in a serving of fresh spinach; 8.5 mcg in canned spinach; and 7.7 mcg in a glass of wine.

The new calcium dosages recommended by the Food and Nutrition Board in Washington, D.C., as well as the 1994 optimal calcium intakes recommended by an advisory group for the National Institutes of Health, are now higher for many age groups and exceed the intakes of most Americans:

500 mg/day for children aged 1 to 3.
800 mg/day for children aged 4 to 8.
1,300 mg/day for adolescents aged 9 to 18, including pregnant and breast-feeding females.
1,000 mg/day for adults aged 19 to 50, including pregnant and lactating females.
1,200 mg/day for adults over 50.[16]

The elderly's generally low intake of calcium and vitamin D places them especially at risk for osteoporosis. In one study involving 1,765 women in their 80s, those who consumed a low-calcium diet (514 mg/day) lost hip-bone density at a rate of 3 percent a year. When they increased their calcium intake by 1,200 mg/day and consumed an additional 800 IU/day of vitamin D for 18 months, hip-bone density increased, and hip fractures and nonvertebral fractures were reduced.

At the Institute of Food Research in Norwick, United Kingdom, the short-term effect of 1,200 mg/day of calcium supplements on daily nonheme iron absorption was measured in 14 healthy adults. Supplementation with calcium did not reduce plasma ferritin concentrations in iron-replete adults consuming a Western-style diet that contained moderate to high amounts of calcium. Ferritin is the major form of iron stored in the body.[17]

Leif Hallberg of the University of Goteborg, Sweden, in commenting on the study, said that those with high iron requirements (adolescents and pregnant and menstruating women) should try to restrict calcium intake with main meals, which contain most of the dietary iron, and that calcium supplements, when needed, should be taken when going to bed.

A study has found that organically grown tomatoes have a higher concentration of calcium and vitamin C than tomatoes not grown organically. Organically grown tomatoes had lower concentrations of iron, but potassium and phosphorus amounts were the same in both types of production.[18] In addition to milk and dairy products, calcium is found in nuts, carob flour, dried whey, kelp, soybean flour, kale, collards, dandelion greens, mustard greens, and sesame seeds, among other foods.

A number of years ago it was reported that *all* present-day teenage girls would eventually develop osteoporosis. This was based on the fact that many girls do not drink milk because they are afraid that the milk sugar will cause them to gain weight. Girls also consume a lot of soft drinks that contain phosphorus, which washes out calcium from the body.

Most Americans are apparently deficient in calcium and should eat more calcium-rich foods, perhaps adding a calcium and vitamin D supplement. Many products are available to choose from.

References

1. "Calcium Supplement Has Potential to Save Billions," *CRN News,* Aug. 1999, 3.

2. Murray, Michael T., "Calcium vs. Osteoporosis in Postmenopausal Women," *Natural Medicine Journal* 1(1): 16–17, Feb. 1998.

3. Weaver, Connie M., "Meeting Optimal Calcium Requirements," paper presented at the Workshop on the Role of Dietary Supplements for Physically Active People, Bethesda, Maryland, June 3–4, 1996.

4. Teegarden, Dorothy, et al., "Previous Milk Consumption is Associated with Greater Bone Density in Young Women," *American Journal of Clinical Nutrition* 69: 1014–17, 1999.

5. Dawson-Hughes, Bess, et al., "Effect of Calcium and Vitamin D Supplementation on Bone Density in Men and Women 65 Years of Age and Older," *New England Journal of Medicine* 337: 670–76, 1997.

6. Reid, I. R., "The Roles of Calcium and Vitamin D in the Prevention of Osteoporosis," *Endocrinology and Metabolism Clinics of North America* 27(2): 389–98, June 1998.

7. Fardellone, Patrice, et al., "Biochemical Effects of Calcium Supplementation in Postmenopausal Women: Influence of Dietary Calcium Intake," *American Journal of Clinical Nutrition* 67: 1273–78, June 1998.

8. Thys-Jacobs, Susan, et al., "Calcium Carbonate and the Premenstrual Syndrome: Effects of Premenstrual and Menstrual Symptoms," *American Journal of Obstetrics and Gynecology* 179(2): 444–52, August 1998.

9. Sowers, M. R., et al., "Prevalence of Renal Stones in a Population-Based

Study with Dietary Calcium, Ocalate, and Medication Exposures," *American Journal of Epidemiology* 147(10): 914–20, 1998.

10. Bucher, Heiner C., et al., "Effect of Calcium Supplementation on Pregnancy-Induced Hypertension and Preeclampsia," *Journal of the American Medical Association* 275: 1113–17, April 10, 1996.

11. Modica, Peter, "Prenatal Calcium Has Anti-hypertensive Effect on Infant," *Medical Tribune,* June 4, 1998, 8.

12. Dwyer, James H., et al., "Dietary Calcium, Calcium Supplementation, and Blood Pressure in African-American Adolescents," *American Journal of Clinical Nutrition* 68: 648–55, 1998.

13. Baron, J. A., et al., "Calcium Supplements for the Prevention of Colorectal Adenomas," *New England Journal of Medicine* 340(2): 101–07, Jan. 14, 1999.

14. Alberts, David S., et al., "Randomized, Double-Blinded, Placebo-Controlled Study of Effect of Wheat Bran Fiber and Calcium on Fecal Bile Acids in Patients with Resected Adenomatous Colon Polyps," *Journal of the National Cancer Institute* 88(2): 81–91, Jan. 17, 1996.

15. Burnett, Mary, "Calcium Supplements Are Beneficial and Safe, Tighter Standards Would Produce No Medical or Scientific Advantage," *CRN News,* Jan. 27, 1997, 1.

16. McBean, Lois D., "Emerging Dietary Benefits of Dairy Foods," *Nutrition Today* 34(1): 47–53, Jan./Feb. 1999.

17. Minnihane, Anne Marie, et al., "Effect of Calcium Supplementation on Daily Noheme-Iron Absorption and Long-Term Iron Status," *American Journal of Clinical Nutrition* 68(1): 96–102, July 1998. Also, Leif Hallberg, "Does Calcium Interfere with Iron Absorption?" ibid., 3–4.

18. "Organic Tomatoes, Vitamin C, and Calcium," *Nutrition Week* 28(24): 7, June 19, 1998.

11

Canola Oil

A monounsaturated vegetable oil derived from rapeseed *(Brassia rapus),* canola oil contains 34 percent polyunsaturated fatty acids, 62 percent monounsaturated fatty acids, and only 6 percent saturated fatty acids. Monounsaturates are believed to be more healthful than saturated fats (animal fat, coconut oil, and palm oil), since they tend to lower LDL cholesterol, the harmful kind, and raise HDL cholesterol, the beneficial kind.[1] The name *canola oil* is derived from Canada, the country in which a new species of rapeseed was developed to produce canola oil. Naturally occurring rapeseed is said to contain 45 percent erusic acid, which is thought to be harmful, but this specially bred variety has very little of this substance.

In 1991 the average American ate 15 pounds of seafood, a 26 percent increase since 1970, and also consumed an average of 112 pounds of meat and 58 pounds of poultry. Health professionals continue to urge people to eat two servings of fish, particularly deep-water fish, each week as a means of decreasing heart disease. Fish is a rich source of omega-3 fatty acids, especially eicosapentaenoic acid (EPA) and docosahexaenoic acid (DHA), which may also reduce the likelihood of blood clots. Omega-3 fatty acids are converted into EPA from canola oil, flaxseed oil, and walnuts, all rich sources of alpha-linolenic acid, an omega-3 fatty acid that is almost as health protective as the omega-3 fish oils.[2]

As mentioned earlier, canola (at 6 percent) is lower in saturated fat than any other vegetable oil, compared to 10 percent for safflower oil. Canola also contains about 56 percent oleic acid, roughly the same as olive oil and genetically modified sunflower oil. While canola contains 32 percent polyunsaturated fatty acid, olive oil has only between 7 and 8 percent. Of the 32 percent polyunsaturated fatty acids, almost 10 percent of canola is alpha-linolenic acid. Canola oil has a bland flavor and a light color and flows easily. It is stable at high temperatures, making it an excellent oil for sautéing and other cooking purposes.[3]

Ninety-six men who had suffered strokes and 96 controls were studied for their intake of alpha-linolenic acid. Researchers found that for every 0.13 percent increase of alpha-linolenic acid in the blood, there was a 37 percent decrease in the risk of stroke. They concluded that increased amounts of omega-3 fatty acids are important in the prevention of stroke.[4]

At the University of Uppsala in Sweden 22 patients with high cholesterol levels in their blood were evaluated in two consecutive 3.5-week treatment periods. The volunteers consumed either canola oil or olive oil, both of which showed similar lipid-lowering effects. The two oils may be interchangeable in a lipid-lowering diet.[5]

A research team at Tufts University in Boston studied three diets given to 15 volunteers whose mean age was 61. The study mirrored the Step 2 National Cholesterol Educational Program Guidelines but substituted canola, corn, and olive oils. Two-thirds of the fat calories were from the three oils, which were used in a randomized, double-blind test that lasted 32 days. Plasma cholesterol concentrations declined by 12 percent with the canola oil diet; 13 percent with the corn oil diet; and 7 percent with the olive oil diet. LDL cholesterol went down by 16, 17, and 13 percent, respectively, with the canola, corn, and olive oil diets.[6] HDL cholesterol dropped by 7 percent with the canola oil diet and 9 percent with the corn oil diet. The findings demonstrated that significant reductions in LDL cholesterol and apoprotein-B levels can be obtained in middle-aged men and women with LDL-cholesterol levels greater than 130 mg/dl by reducing dietary saturated fat and cholesterol intake and by incorporating vegetable oils rich in monounsaturated fatty acids, such as canola and olive oils.

During a 13-week evaluation by Australian researchers, a group of 23 explorers in the Antarctic had canola margarine (containing 28 percent saturated fat) and canola cooking oil (polyunsaturated margarine and vegetable oil) substituted for butter. Total cholesterol and low-density lipoprotein cholesterol concentrations fell by 7 and 10 percent, respectively, with the canola products.[7]

Long-chain omega-3 fatty acid is necessary for optimal brain development, visual function, motor development, and other parameters, especially in newborns. Ingesting alpha-linolenic acid over an extended period may offer adequate conversion to the respective long-chain fatty acid products. Dietary alpha-linolenic acid can reduce triglyceride and cholesterol levels. Alpha-linolenic acid from canola or flaxseed oils can alter EPA platelet content without affecting DHA levels. Omega-3 fatty acids can also have major physiological effects on immune function, platelet aggregation, and amelioration of inflammation, and possibly enhance antitumor activity.[8]

In human infants, primates, and other animals, omega-3 fatty acids (especially DHA) are heavily concentrated in the brain and retinal tissues. The acid accumulates during the late fetal and early neonatal life. If the mother's diet is deficient in omega-3 fatty acids, this can result in reduced levels of DHA in erythrocytes and brain and retinal tissues, resulting in abnormal eye function that might be irreversible. Premature infants lose DHA from body stores unless they are given breast milk or formula supplemented with DHA. Expectant mothers are urged to consume more fish and canola and olive oils, which may help to avoid extreme ratios of omega-6 and omega-3 fatty acids and will utilize alpha-linolenic acid more favorably.[9]

References

1. Ronzio, Robert A., *The Encyclopedia of Nutrition and Good Health* (New York: Facts on File, 1997), 74.

2. Liebman, Bonnie. "Seafood: Fishing for Omega-3s," *Nutrition Action Health Letter,* Nov. 1992, 10–11.

3. Kronhausen, Eberhard, et al., *Formula for Life: The Anti-Oxidant, Free-Radical Detoxification Program* (New York: William Morrow and Co., 1989), 449–50.

4. "Fatty Acid Reportedly Lowers Stroke Risk," *Medical Tribune,* June 8, 1995, 20.

5. Nydahl, M., et al., "Similar Effects of Rapeseed Oil (Canola Oil) and Olive Oil in a Lipid-Lowering Diet for Patients with Hyperlipoproteinemia," *Journal of the American College of Nutrition* 14(6): 643–51, 1995.

6. Lichtenstein, Alice H., et al., "Effects of Canola, Corn, and Olive Oils on Fasting and Postprandial Plasma Lipoproteins in Humans as Part of a National Cholesterol Education Program Step 2 Diet," *Arteriosclerosis and Thrombosis* 13: 1533–42, 1993.

7. Matheson, Bronwyn, "Effect of Serum Lipids on Monounsaturated Oil and Margarine in the Diet of an Antarctic Expedition," *American Journal of Clinical Nutrition* 63: 933–38, 1996.

8. Kinsella, John E., "Alpha-Linolenic Acid: Recent Overview," *Nutrition* 8(3): 195–96, May–June 1992.

9. Nettleton, Joyce A., "Are Omega-3 Fatty Acids Essential Nutrients for Fetal and Infant Development?" *Journal of the American Dietetic Association* 93(1): 58–64, January 1993.

12

Capsaicin

Pain is a message carried to the brain by nerves near the surface of the skin or in the body's interior. Whether acute or chronic, the message is often a warning of injury, organic disorder, or stress on body functions. Understanding the neurochemistry of the brain's own painkillers—the endorphins—has brought a plethora of medications that often bring relief.[1]

One of the most successful topical medications for pain is capsaicin, the active pungent ingredient in chili peppers. In a study of approximately 100 patients with moderate to severe postsurgical pain following cancer treatments, those who rubbed an 0.075 percent capsaicin cream around the incision during eight weeks following surgery had a 53 percent reduction in pain, compared with a 17 percent reduction in those who used a placebo or look-alike cream.[2] Neil Ellison, M.D., of the Geisinger Clinical Oncology Program in Danville, Pennsylvania, one of the investigators in this study, believes a peptide called substance P causes neuropathic pain. Capsaicin apparently relieves the pain by releasing substance P, which initially causes a burning sensation but eventually depletes the peptide in the body. Commenting on the study, James S. Gordon, M.D., director of the Center for Mind-Body Medicine and a professor of psychiatry and family medicine at Georgetown University, Washington, D.C., said "This is the kind of study that pleases me very much, since it shows that natural products can be easily integrated into the health-care system."

Ten patients with pain associated with diabetes mellitus, neuralgia near the liver, HIV infection, or complex regional pain syndrome were instructed to coat their lower legs and feet with a cream containing 7.5 percent to 10 percent capsaicin. Over several weeks of treatment, there was a greater than 50 percent pain relief in six of the patients. The patients were given a counteracting therapy for the cream's acute burning sensation.[3]

Women with vulvar vestibulitis experience a burning and stabbing pain at the entrance of the vulva and are often unable to have intercourse. Ten patients with such a history were enrolled in a double-blind study for an average of 55 months to test the effectiveness of capsaicin. The volunteers were first treated with 2 percent topical lidocaine, a local anesthetic, for three minutes. The lidocaine was then washed off, followed by the application of either 0.025 percent topical capsaicin or a placebo. Four of the women in the treatment group reported having a 77 percent reduction in pain after six weeks of therapy. The five placebo patients experienced no difference in pain after six weeks. For an additional six weeks, all patients were treated with capsaicin, and all achieved relief from their pain.[4]

In another study, eight of nine patients with hemodialysis-related itching experienced relief by applying a capsaicin cream. Twenty patients with upper-back pain reported that capsaicin was more effective in reducing their pain than the placebo.[5]

At the Miami Hospital for Veterans Affairs in Florida, researchers said that a topically applied 0.025 percent capsaicin cream may be a first-line therapy for osteoarthritic pain. During a 12-week, double-blind, randomized study, 113 patients were given either the cream or a placebo four times daily. The cream was superior to the placebo in providing relief from osteoarthritic pain: 81 percent of the patients using the cream had less pain, compared to 54 percent using a placebo. The capsaicin-treated volunteers reported a greater reduction in pain during motion, as well as while touching the joints. One-half of the treated patients experienced mild to moderate burning and stinging after applying the cream.[6]

Capsaicin cream maybe a useful therapy for treating pain associated with primary fibromyalgia, a common cause of chronic musculoskeletal pain and fatigue. In a study, 45 patients with the disorder were evaluated for four weeks in a double-blind trial using a 0.025 percent capsaicin cream. The treated patients were given the cream four times daily, while the controls used a placebo. After four weeks, the patients using the cream felt less tenderness, and a significant increase in grip strength was noted after two weeks.[7]

Capsaicin cream is readily available over the counter in health food stores and other outlets. Patients experiencing chronic pain should consult their physicians before using this therapy.

References

1. Subak-Sharpe, Genell J., ed., *The Physicians' Manual for Patients* (New York: Times Books, 1984), 224ff.

2. McKinney, Merritt, "Capsaicin Cream Said to Ease Post-Op Pain in Cancer Patients," *Medical Tribune*, Sept. 4, 1997, 32.

3. Nidecker, Anna, "High-Dose Capsaicin Eases Neuropathic Pain," *Family Practice News*, Jan. 15, 1998, 11.

4. Baker, Barbara, "Topical Capsaicin Relieves Pain of Severe Vulvar Vestibulitis," *Family Practice News*, May 15, 1997, 62.

5. Mauer, Katherine, "Topical Anti-Itch Agents Offer Alternative Therapies," *Family Practice News*, April 15, 1996, 43.

6. Altman, Roy D., et al., "Capsaicin Cream 0.025 Percent as Monotherapy for Osteoarthritis: A Double-Blind Study," *Seminars in Arthritis and Rheumatism* 23(6/Suppl. 3): 25–33, June 1994.

7. McCarty, Daniel J., et al., "Treatment of Pain Due to Fibromyalgia with Topical Capsaicin: A Pilot Study," *Seminars in Arthritis and Rheumatism* 23(6/Suppl. 3): 41–47, June 1994.

13

Carnitine

Synthesized from two essential amino acids—lysine and methionine—L-carnitine is an amino acid necessary for the oxidation of fats and for energy production. However, carnitine may not be synthesized in the body at an adequate rate for the following: kidney patients on dialysis; patients with liver disorders; strict vegetarians, since meat and dairy products are the best dietary sources of carnitine; premature and low-birth-weight infants; pregnant and breast-feeding women; and those with a genetic predisposition to carnitine deficiency.[1]

Carnitine deficiency is related to muscle weakness, chest pain, high blood levels of cholesterol, congestive heart failure, cardiac enlargement, and chronic fatigue syndrome. Although the heart normally stores carnitine, its level may drop if there is not sufficient oxygen. Carnitine supplements raise the amount of the amino acid in the heart, permitting the heart to use a limited oxygen supply, and are often used to treat hardening of the arteries, angina, and coronary heart disease. Acetyl-L-carnitine, a derivative of carnitine, also provides protection.

In a double-blind study at the University of Pittsburgh, researchers evaluated 7 probable Alzheimer's disease patients who were given 3 g/day of L-carnitine for one year; 5 probable Alzheimer's patients who were given a placebo; and 21 controls. The Alzheimer's patients showed significantly less deterioration in various test scores than did the placebo group. It was said to be the first human study at that time to show a beneficial effect of a supplement on both the clinical and central nervous system neurochemical parameters in Alzheimer's disease.[2]

A research team at the University of Modena in Italy studied 481 people from 44 geriatric and neurologic clinics who were treated with L-acetylcarnitine supplements at 1,500 mg/day for three months. L-acetyl-carnitine has a structure similar to acetylcholine and may provide protection against oxidative damage caused by free radicals. The supplement brought improvement in mental, memory, emotional behavior, and depression.[3]

In a study evaluating 24 geriatric patients hospitalized with depression at Catholic University in Rome, clear evidence was found that L-carnitine was especially effective in patients with more serious clinical symptoms.[4] At the Instituto Mario Negri in Milan, 13 of 14 patients with Alzheimer's disease who were given L-carnitine supplements exhibited a slower rate of deterioration than did the controls. The adverse side effects were mild.[5] Researchers at the Ospedale Generale di Imola in Bologna, Italy, reported that 40 patients judged to be senile were given 500 mg tablets of L-carnitine three times daily. The study revealed that short-term, intensive carnitine treatment can significantly improve mental parameters of the senile brain without any side effects.[6]

Carnitine and its derivatives have been used to treat angina pectoris, acute myocardial infarction, congestive heart failure, peripheral vascular disease, diabetes, and other conditions. Although the trials have generally been small, the results have been favorable. Most studies involving cardio-vascular disease and other health problems often use 1 to 4 g/day of carnitine. No major toxicity has been reported.[7]

At the University of Federico in Naples, Italy, researchers evaluated 245 patients from 13 centers, 40 years of age and older, who had a history of intermittent claudication. This condition is caused by restricted blood flow to the legs, causing extreme pain, especially while walking. Seventy-six patients completed the therapy, which consisted of 1 g/day of L-carnitine. A small but significant improvement was seen in the treatment group compared to the controls. Patients walking less than 250 meters at the beginning of the study showed the most improvement. There was no significant improvement in those walking a farther distance.[8]

While some researchers remain skeptical, another study at Catholic University found that L-carnitine improves insulin sensitivity in Type 2 diabetics. Using 15 volunteers with Type 2 diabetes and 20 healthy controls, researchers gave the treatment group intravenous infusions of L-carnitine, which brought an 8 percent increase in glucose uptake, compared with the controls, who got a saline solution.[9]

In evaluating 235 men at the University Clinical Center in Belgrade, Yugoslavia, researchers found that levels of carnitine and glucosidase, an enzyme, were lower in seminal fluid from men with low sperm counts.[10]

Carnitine has been shown to lower both triglyceride and cholesterol levels, according to Seattle physician Ralph Golan, M.D. The amino acid can also decrease angina (chest pain) and blood pressure, as well as increase the metabolic efficiency of the liver and heart, making it ideal for treating congestive heart failure. Golan usually recommends 750 mg taken twice daily.[11]

Researchers at the University of Pretoria in South Africa found that 2 g/day of carnitine positively influenced aerobic capacity and normal lipid levels in seven marathon athletes. The volunteers completed two treadmill tests to exhaustion, separated by a six-week supplement period with carnitine. Peak treadmill running speed increased by 5.8 percent, and average oxygen consumption and heart rate decreased.[12]

Carnitine enhances exercise performance in a number of ways:

- It enhances oxidation of fatty acids, which is important during exercise.
- It preserves muscle glycogen during exercise, a factor involved in preventing fatigue.
- By shifting fuel substrate use to glucose, it decreases the amount of oxygen required for adenosine triphosphate (ATP) in the body. ATP supplies energy for many biochemical processes.
- It replaces the carnitine depleted by acetylcarnitine formation.
- It improves muscle fatigue resistance.
- It replaces carnitine losses that occur during aerobic training.
- It increases oxidative capacity in skeletal muscle.

Carnitine is well tolerated in humans. The only side effects of note have been diarrhea and cramping in susceptible people.[13]

A 32-year-old with sickle cell anemia developed ulcerations on both ankles and feet. His doctor, Henry L. Harrell Jr., M.D., prescribed 2 g of L-carnitine orally twice daily. Within two weeks the patient's condition had improved significantly. After getting the same dosage in a transfusion, all ulcers healed and his ankle pain subsided within an additional two weeks.[14]

Researchers at Children's Memorial Hospital in Chicago studied 23 infants with cystic fibrosis who were treated with carnitine and a predigested formula for 6 to 12 months. At the time of diagnosis, carnitine concentrations in the treated children were much less than in the 48 controls. The nutritional supplements normalized carnitine concentrations but, at three years of age, the carnitine metabolites in the children with cystic fibrosis were significantly less than in the controls, despite a carnitine-containing diet. Carnitine may be an alternation in fatty acid metabolism in the womb.[15]

L-carnitine at 50 mg/kg per day was effective in treating a 17-year-old female with Rett syndrome, a progressive and incurable neurological disorder. Within two months, she became more alert, developed good eye contact, began reaching for objects with both hands, and answered a few simple questions. When L-carnitine was discontinued, she relapsed within one week. She began improving after L-carnitine supplementation was resumed. Carnitine has two significant functions: transporting long-chain fatty acids in the mitochondria and helping to regulate the intramitochondrial ratio of acetyl-coenzyme A to free coenzyme A.[16]

Hirohiko Kuratsune, M.D., of Osaka University Medical School in Japan, and his colleagues administered acetyl-L-carnitine to 10 patients with chronic fatigue syndrome (CFS) in Japan and China. Improvement was observed in half of the patients. A 21-year-old patient with CFS was admitted to the hospital. She had been given drugs, tranquilizers, and Chinese herbal medicines but was unable to perform light tasks. Because her blood acyl-carnitine stores were low, she was given 4 g/day of acetylcarnitine for five days. Her symptoms began to subside after two weeks, and she was able to walk from her home to the store. Two months after the treatment was halted, however, her fatigue became worse and she had to stay in bed for half the day. Kuratsune said that acetylcarnitine supplements are not a treatment for acylcarnitine deficiency, but there is a possibility that the supplementation of acetyl-L-carnitine might become a useful new treatment for CFS patients with acylcarnitine deficiency.[17]

In addition to meat and dairy products, tempeh and avocados contain some carnitine. Most fruits, vegetables, and grains are poor sources of the amino acid.

References

1. Ronzio, Robert A., *The Encyclopedia of Nutrition and Good Health* (New York: Facts on File, 1997), 80.

2. Pettegrew, Jay W., et al., "Clinical and Neurochemical Effects of Acetyl-L-Carnitine in Alzheimer's Disease," *Neurobiology of Ageing* 16(1): 1–4, 1995.

3. Salvioli, G., and M. Neri, "L-Acetylcarnitine Treatment of Mental Decline in Elderly," *Drugs, Experimental, and Clinical Research* 20(4): 169–76, 1994.

4. Tempesta, E., et al., "L-Acetylcarnitine in Depressed Elderly Subjects: A Cross-Over Study versus Placebo," *Drugs, Experimental and Clinical Research* 13(7): 417–23, 1987.

5. Spagnoli, A., et al., "Long-Term Acetyl-L-Carnitine Treatment in Alzheimer's Disease," *Neurology* 41: 1726–32, Nov. 1991.

6. Bonavita, E., et al., "Study of the Efficacy and Tolerability of L-Acetylcarnitine Therapy in the Senile Brain," *International Journal of Clinical Pharmacology, Therapy, and Toxicology* 24(9): 511–16, 1986.

7. Arsenian, Michael A., "Carnitine and Its Derivatives in Cardiovascular Disease," *Progress in Cardiovascular Disease* 40(3): 265–86, Nov.–Dec. 1997.

8. Brevetti, G., et al., "Propionyl-L-Carnitine for Intermittent Claudication," *American Journal of Cardiology* 79: 777–80, 1997.

9. Leigh, Suzanne, "Amino Acid Improves Insulin Sensitivity in Patients with Type 2 Diabetes," *Medical Tribune* 40(6): 25, March 18, 1999.

10. Micic, Sava R., et al., "Seminal Carnitine and Glucosidase in Oligospermic and

Azoospermic Men," *Journal of Andrology* 15: 77(Suppl.), 1984.

11. Golan, Ralph, *Optimal Wellness* (New York: Ballantine Books, 1995), 334.

12. Swart, I., et al., "The Effect of L-Carnitine Supplementation on Plasma Carnitine Levels and Various Performance Parameters of Male Marathon Athletes," *Nutrition Research* 17(3): 405–14, 1997.

13. Brass, Eric P., "Supplemental Carnitine and Exercise," paper presented at Workshop on the Role of Dietary Supplements for Physically Active People, National Institutes of Health, Bethesda, Maryland, June 3–4, 1996.

14. Harrell, Henry L., Jr., "L-Carnitine for Leg Ulcers," *Annals of Internal Medicine* 113(5): 412, Sept. 1, 1990.

15. Lloyd-Still, John D., et al., "Carnitine Metabolites in Infants with Cystic Fibrosis: A Prospective Study," *Acta Pediatrica* 82: 145–49, 1993.

16. Plioplys, Audrius V., and Irene Kasnicka, "L-Carnitine as a Treatment for Rett Syndrome," *Southern Medical Journal* 86(12): 1411–12, Dec. 1993.

17. Hamilton, Kirk, "Chronic Fatigue Syndrome and Acylcarnitine," *Clinical Pearls with The Experts Speak* (Sacramento, Calif.: Health Associates Medical Group, 1998), 28–29. Also, Kuratsune, Hirohiko, "Acylcarnitine and Chronic Fatigue Syndrome," *Carnitine Today,* chapter 10, 195–213, 1997.

14

Cat's Claw

In its 1999 annual report, the environmental group Greenpeace predicted that the Amazon rain forest will be wiped out in 80 years if multinational logging companies continue to deforest at the current rate. The group added that illegal commercial loggers cut down 80 percent of the trees that disappear from the rain forest annually.[1] Thousands of beneficial plants may disappear before they are even discovered.

One of the products of Peru's forest is *Uncaria tomentosa,* known locally as *una de gato* and referred to in English as cat's claw. Decoctions of the bark are used in folk medicine for the treatment of arthritis, intestinal disorders, cancer, and certain epidemic diseases. Phytochemical studies of the root bark resulted in isolating the main alkaloids, including isopteropodine, pteropodine, isomitraphylline, uncarine F, mitraphylline, and speciophylline. In studies using cell cultures, researchers found that uncarine F may be considered as a possible drug for the treatment of patients with acute leukemia.[2]

Using laboratory animals, researchers at the LSU Medical Center in New Orleans conducted a study on cat's claw to determine its purported anti-inflammatory properties. They were aware that among the many factors associated with chronic gut inflammation are the production of oxidants and free radicals, integral components of cell and tissue injury. Antioxidants in the body may be depleted during chronic inflammation, which partly explains the therapeutic efficacy of mesalamine and glucocorticoids.[3] Mesalamine is a salicylate used to treat ulcerative colitis and other disorders. Glucocorticoids are anti-inflammatory drugs.

It is not clear if the present findings on antioxidant properties and transcriptional inhibition with cat's claw are due to the active ingredients or to novel chemical entities. In any event, the study offers definitive evidence that the anecdotal reports of anti-inflammatory properties of the herb are based in fact and are sufficiently diverse to be considered an important therapeutic agent. For developing countries in which health care funds are stretched, herbal medicines such as cat's claw deserve serious consideration.

In 1991, researchers analyzing the glycosides in the root of cat's claw discovered a new quinovin acid glycoside not seen in nature before, reported Alexander G. Schauss, Ph.D. This glycoside had pronounced anti-inflammatory properties. Using an animal model, researchers found that the new glycoside was a compound responsible for the anti-inflammatory activity of cat's claw. This finding may help to explain the pain-relieving benefits patients have experienced, especially those with arthritis, Schauss said.[4]

In a study of the potential antiviral activity of cat's claw, researchers demonstrated that these same nonalkaloid glycosides show anti-inflammatory properties and moderate antiviral activity in laboratory glassware against the rhinovirus type 1B (flu virus) and the vesicular stomatitis virus.

Schauss added that cat's claw is not recommended for women planning a pregnancy, women who are pregnant or breastfeeding, or patients scheduled for an organ transplant or skin graft, since the herb can cause the immune system to reject transplanted cells. Schauss recommends 250 to 750 mg/day. The dosage should provide a minimum intake of 10 to 30 mg total alkaloids and should be taken on an empty stomach. If gastrointestinal disturbances occur, empty the capsule into a cup of cold water, heat for about 10 minutes, and let cool before drinking.

In his newsletter, *Health and Healing,* Julian Whitaker, M.D., wrote that unique alkaloids in cat's claw seem to enhance the immune system. These alkaloids apparently help the white blood cells engulf and digest harmful microorganisms. One of these alkaloids reduces platelet aggregation, which reduces clot formation and would help prevent stroke and heart attacks.[5]

In the last decade, a great deal of interest has developed in substances that directly or indirectly reduce or eliminate the mutagenic activity of other chemicals. These substances, called antimutagens, occur naturally in food and are predominantly of plant origin. Antioxidants are one of the most important classes of antimutagens, since the involvement of active oxygen species and free radicals has been demonstrated in a number of pathological events such as cancer and the aging process. Cat's-claw extracts and fractions exhibited a significant antimutagenic activity, probably due to their antioxidant effect.[6]

The antimutagenic power of cat's claw in lab glassware may be due to the antioxidant property of bark components acting to quench singlet oxygen and to scavenge the other oxyradicals generated by various components under ultraviolet-A irradiation. Singlet oxygen is the most devastating free radical and is associated with cancer, hardening of the arteries, and various degenerative diseases.

Cancer patients who have experienced relief after using cat's claw have given numerous public testimonies, and high rates of tumor remission have been claimed by Peruvian phytotherapists, reported Federico R. Leon, Ph.D., and Fernando Cabieses, M.D. Cat's claw raises the cancer patient's immunoglobulin count, and its extracts exhibit cytostatic activity in some human tumors. Cytostatis is the slowing of movement and accumulation of blood cells.[7] Leon and Cabieses wrote that Peluso et al. (1993) showed an inhibitory effect on normal cellular proliferation due to direct action on DNA.

The authors also reported that conventional anti-inflammatory drugs rely on diverse action mechanisms, yet share severe gastrointestinal side effects. However, cat's claw is a more efficient anti-inflammatory and does not appear to bring undesirable side effects. Rigorous, long-term follow-up studies are needed.[8]

One of the complications of Alzheimer's disease is the deposition of beta-amyloid protein in the brain, which is thought to contribute to neuronal death and memory dysfunction. In laboratory animals, a constituent of cat's claw (PTI-00703) has inhibited the formation of plaques in the brain and prevents some of the damage caused by Alzheimer's disease. Research is continuing in this interesting application.[9]

Cat's claw is available over the counter in capsules, extracts, teas, and a variety of combinations. As scientists continue to unravel all of the mysteries of this herb, you may find it useful in dealing with your specific health problem. Ask your health care provider for guidelines.

References

1. "Fears for Amazon Forest," *The New York Times,* August 18, 1999, A4.
2. Stuppner, H., et al., "A Differential Sensitivity of Oxindole Alkaloids to Noral and Leukemic Cell Lines," *Planta Medica* 59/Suppl. A: 583, 1993.
3. Sandoval-Chacon, M. et al., "Anti-inflammatory Actions of Cat's Claw: The Role of NF-kB," *Alimentary Pharmacology Therapeutics* 12: 1279–89, 1998.
4. Schauss, Alexander G., "Cat's Claw (Uncaria tomentosa)," *Natural Medicine Journal* 1(2): 16–19, March 1998.
5. Whitaker, Julian, *Health and Healing* 5(5), May 1995, 4.
6. Rizzin, Renato, et al., "Mutagenic and Antimutagenic Activities of *Uncaria tomentosa* and Its Extracts," *Journal of Ethnopharmacology* 38: 63–77, 1993.
7. Leon, Federico R., and Fernando Cabieses, "Relevance of *Uncaria*

tomentosa (Cat's Claw) for Cancer Prevention and Treatment," *Bulletin of the National Institute of Traditional Medicine,* April 15, 1995, 1–4.

8. Leon, Federico R., and Fernando Cabieses, "Anti-inflammatory Effects of *Uncaria tomentosa* (Cat's Claw)," *Bulletin of the National Institute of Traditional Medicine,* May 15, 1995, 1–4.

9. Snow, A. D., et al., "Further Efficacy of PTI-00703: A Dietary Supplement Which Causes a Dose-Dependent Inhibition of Alzheimer's Disease Amyloid Deposition in a Rodent Model," paper presented at meeting of Federation of American Societies for Experimental Biology, April 17–21, 1999, Washington, D.C. Also, the *FASEB Journal* 13(4): March 12, 1999.

15

Chondroitin Sulfate

Osteoarthritis, or rheumatism, is an age-related degenerative disease that affects cartilage and bone in the joints of the hips, knees, and lower spine. The problem is exacerbated by those who are obese and can result from injuries, infections, and diseases affecting the joints. Stress is another aggravator. Affected joints are painful and often "creak" or grate as the person moves about.

Chondroitin sulfate—alone or in combination with glucosamine sulfate—is bringing relief to many patients with osteoarthritis. In fact, according to Jason Theodosakis, M.D., in *The Arthritis Cure,* "The one-two punch of glucosamine and chondroitin sulfates can actually halt the disease process in its tracks and help the body to heal itself."[1]

In a 1986 study in France, Theodosakis reported that 50 patients suffering from osteoarthritis of the knee were given oral doses of either 800 to 1,200 mg of chondroitin sulfates, or 500 mg of a pain medication. Cartilage samples were taken at the beginning of the study. After three months of therapy, the damaged cartilage in the chondroitin group had repaired itself to a significant degree.

The author also discussed a 1987 study in Buenos Aires, Argentina, which compared the effects of chondroitin sulfates to those of a placebo. Thirty-four patients with severe osteoarthritis of the knee were divided into two groups of 17 each. One group was given a daily injection of 150 mg of chondroitin sulfates plus 500 mg of aspirin three times daily for 20 weeks. The control group received a placebo injection and the same amount of aspirin. After 20 weeks, 13 of the 17 patients receiving chondroitin injections experienced pain relief, while only 2 of the 17 in the placebo group were pain free.

In a one-year, double-blind study, researchers at the University Hospital in Geneva, Switzerland, observed 42 volunteers between the ages of 35 and 38 who were diagnosed with symptomatic knee osteo-arthritis. The treatment group received 800 mg/day of chondroitin sulfate, while the controls were given a placebo. The supple-ment was well tolerated and brought reduced pain and increased overall mobility. Some of those receiving chondroitin noticed a stabilization of the medial femorotibial joint width, but joint space narrowing did not present with the placebo-treated patients. Metabolism of bone and joint sta-bilized in the treatment group, whereas it remained abnormal in those taking a placebo. Researchers concluded that oral chondroitin sulfate is a safe, slow-acting supplement for the treatment of knee osteoarthritis.[2]

In 127 patients with femorotibial knee arthritis at Salpetriere Hospital in Paris, researchers administered 1,200 mg/day of chondroitin sulfate oral gel, 400 mg of chon-droitin sulfate tablets, or a placebo three times daily for three months. The results—virtually identical with both dosages of chondroitin—indicate that chondroitin sulfate favors the improvement of subjec-tive symptoms, specifically improving joint mobility.[3]

At the University of Pisa, researchers evaluated 24 osteoarthritis patients who were given 0.8 g of chondroitin sulfate or a placebo for 10 days. The researchers found that oral supplements of chondroitin sulfate reach synovial fluid and cartilage and modify some pharmacologic and biochemical mark-ers in experimental animals and osteoarthri-tis patients. The substance may affect anti-inflammatory activity at the cellular level, but does not provide the unwanted side effects brought on by nonsteroidal anti-inflamma-tory drugs (NSAIDs).[4]

In evaluating 80 patients with osteo-arthritis of the knee between the ages of 39 and 83, researchers at Sammelweis Medical University in Budapest began the treat-ment with 400 mg capsules of chondroitin sulfate or a placebo twice daily. The walk-ing time of the patients, which was defined as how long it took them to complete 20 meters, showed a statistically significant reduction only in the chondroitin sulfate group. No significant side effects were reported by either group. The data strongly suggest that chondroitin sulfate acts as a symptomatic, slow-acting drug in patients with osteoarthritis of the knee.[5]

An unexpected application of chon-droitin sulfate was recorded at Erasme Hospital in Brussels when a chondroitin sul-fate solution was placed in each nostril of seven people who snored. They ranged in age from 41 to 57. The researchers con-cluded that chondroitin sulfate, as a long-lasting tissue-coating agent, has considerable potential for reducing snoring.[6]

If you are suffering from osteoarthritis, ask your doctor about chondroitin sulfate. If your physician is not familiar with the lit-erature, refer him to the references below.

Additional information is given in the entry on glucosamine sulfate in this book.

References

1. Theodosakis, Jason, et al., *The Arthritis Cure* (New York: St. Martin's Press, 1997), 29ff.
2. Ubelhart, D., et al., "Effects of Oral Chondroitin Sulfate on the Progression of Knee Osteoarthritis: A Pilot Study," *Osteoarthritis and Cartilage* 6(Suppl. A): 39–46, 1998.
3. Bourgeois, P., et al., "Efficacy and Tolerability of Chondroitin Sulfate 1,200 mg/day vs. Chondroitin Sulfate 3 × 400 mg/day vs. Placebo," *Osteoarthritis and Cartilage* 6(Suppl. A): 25–30, 1998.
4. Ronca, F., et al., "Anti-inflammatory Activity of Chondroitin Sulfate," *Osteoarthritis and Cartilage* 6(Suppl. A): 14–21, 1998.
5. Busci, L., and G. Poor, "Efficacy and Tolerability of Oral Chondroitin Sulfate as a Symptomatic Slow-Acting Drug for Osteoarthritis in the Treatment of Knee Osteoarthritis," *Osteoarthritis and Cartilage* 6(Suppl. A): 31–36, 1998.
6. Lenclud, Christine, et al., "Effects of Chondroitin Sulfate on Snoring Characteristics: A Pilot Study," *Current Therapeutic Research* 59(4): 234–43, April 1998.

16

Chromium

Of the 12 to 14 million Americans with diabetes, 5 percent (700,000) have insulin-dependent diabetes mellitus, or Type 1 diabetes, and 95 percent have non-insulin-dependent diabetes mellitus, or Type 2 diabetes. About half of the 11 to 13 million Americans who have Type 2 diabetes are not aware they have the disease, since the symptoms are subtle.[1]

Diabetes mellitus is characterized by an abnormally high level of glucose (sugar) in the blood. In healthy people, the concentration of glucose in a blood specimen should not exceed 140 mg/dl (milligrams of glucose per deciliter of blood). When concentrations are extreme (200 mg/dl or more) and the individual becomes hyperglycemic, the following characteristic symptoms usually present: excessive urination (polyuria), excessive thirst (polydipsia), and excessive eating (polyphagia).

People in China with Type 2 diabetes had specific reductions in their blood sugar and insulin levels following two to four months of chromium picolinate supplements, according to a study headed by the U.S. Department of Agriculture. Even those receiving 200 mcg of chromium daily improved in several indices of diabetes. Richard Anderson, Ph.D., of the USDA's Agricultural Research Service, explained that Americans with diabetes would need more than 200 mcg/day of chromium to respond as well as the Chinese did, since Americans tend to be larger than the Chinese and eat more fat and sugar.[2, 3]

For the Chinese study, Anderson and physicians Nanzheng Cheng and Nanping Cheng recruited 180 people with Type 2 diabetes from three Beijing hospitals and assigned them to three groups of 60 volunteers each. One group was given 100 mcg of chromium picolinate twice daily, while another group received 500 mcg twice daily. Dividing the supplement into two doses allows the body to absorb more of the mineral. The third group was given look-alike supplements or a placebo.

The patients getting 1,000 mcg/day (1 mg) improved significantly compared to the placebo group after only two months. In four months, their average hemoglobin A1C was 6.6 percent, compared to 8.5 percent in the placebo group. A normal level is usually less than 6.2 percent. This measure indicates how much hemoglobin (the oxygen-carrying pigment in red blood cells) has sugar bound to it, and is said to be the gold standard for diabetes tests.

In the diabetics receiving 200 mcg/day, hemoglobin A1C levels registered 7.5 percent, considerably lower than that of the placebo group. However, there was no significant difference in blood glucose between the two groups.

In those getting the higher amounts of the mineral, blood glucose after an overnight fast was down to 129 mg/dl, versus 160 mg/dl in the placebo group. The levels averaged 190 mg/dl two hours after a meal versus 223 mg/dl in the placebo group.

Commenting on the study, Lois Jovanovic-Peterson, M.D., a specialist in diabetes at the Sansum Medical Research Foundation in Santa Barbara, California, said that in nondiabetic people blood glucose is around 100 mg/dl after fasting and 120 mg/dl after eating. "These are improvements to the level of good control. It's as good as what we currently have available—oral hypoglycemic agents, diet, and exercise. If further research confirms these numbers, chromium supplements should be an add-on therapy to current treatments to further lower blood glucose."

The high-chromium group also experienced a significant drop in total cholesterol. Both high- and low-chromium volunteers had a significant drop in blood insulin two months into the therapy, with a further drop after four months. Those with Type 2 diabetes produce more insulin than normal in the early stages of the disease, because the hormone is less efficient at clearing glucose from the blood. Chromium seems to make the hormone more efficient, Anderson noted. The researchers controlled diabetes with a nutrient given at higher levels than can be achieved through diet. People with Type 2 diabetes absorb more chromium, but they also excrete more, resulting in lower tissue levels. This indicates that the body has difficulty using what it absorbs.

Writing in *Regulatory Toxicology and Pharmacology,* Anderson stated that the estimated safe and adequate dietary level for chromium is between 50 and 200 mcg, although most diets contain less than 60 percent of the minimum suggested intake. However, as demonstrated in the Chinese study, supplements up to 1,000 mcg/day have been given without toxicity. Deficiencies of the mineral are related to acute and chronic exercise, high-sugar diets, lactation, and physical trauma. As for lactation, the baby is perhaps ingesting much of the mother's chromium. Signs of a chromium deficiency include impaired glucose tolerance, hypoglycemia (low blood sugar), abnormal sugar in the urine, abnormal nitrogen balance, elevated circulating insulin, decreased lean body mass, and other conditions.[4]

Since chromium competes with another mineral, iron, for binding to transferrin (a globulin in blood plasma that binds and transports iron in the body), it had been speculated that high-dose supplementation might adversely affect iron status and cause an iron deficiency. In one study, researchers recruited 18 men, aged 56 to 69, and gave them either 924 mcg/day of chromium picolinate or a low-chromium placebo for 12 weeks. During that time the men engaged in a series of repetition exercises. The results showed that supplementing these older men with chromium picolinate at about 4.5 times the upper limit of the estimated safe and adequate daily dietary intake of chromium did not significantly affect any changes in iron transport during the resistive-training period. There was no indication that the volunteers would develop iron-deficiency anemia.[5]

In another study researchers gave 42 adults, 60 years of age or older, 150 mcg/day of chromium to determine its impact on cholesterol. Total and LDL cholesterol (the bad kind) were lower in some individuals, while HDL cholesterol (the good kind), triglycerides, and glucose were unchanged in those with the highest cholesterol. However, there was a significant decrease in apolipoprotein B, which has been found to be elevated in those with a family history of abnormal cholesterol levels, putting them at risk for ischemic heart disease.[6]

Researchers at Shaare Zedek Medical Center in Jerusalem found that chromium supplements reduce and regress plaque that leads to hardening of the arteries, independent of changes in blood lipids or lipoproteins. The study involved rabbits that were fed a high-cholesterol diet, followed by varying amounts of chromium and potassium chromate.[7]

Chromium picolinate may stimulate weight loss. In a double-blind study, researchers gave 122 volunteers either 400 mcg/day of chromium picolinate or a placebo. Those getting the supplement lost considerably more weight (7.79 kg versus 1.81 kg, respectively) and fat mass (7.71 kg versus 1.53 kg, respectively). The chromium takers also had a greater reduction in percent of body fat (6.3 percent versus 1.2 percent, respectively).[8]

Another form of chromium, chromium polynicotinate (chromium bound to vitamin B_3), may prevent some instances of high blood pressure and slow aging, according to Harry Preuss, M.D., of Georgetown University Medical Center in Washington, D.C. In animal experiments, he said, "We found that sugar-induced high blood pressure was significantly decreased when chromium bound to niacin, the B vitamin, was added to the diet."[9]

Preuss indicated that the average American diet contains about 18 percent of calories from sugars such as sucrose, fructose, and glucose, which are known to increase blood pressure in susceptible people. By enhancing insulin function, chromium helps to control blood sugar levels and prevent high blood pressure.

The National Research Council has pointed out that chromium is an essential trace mineral necessary for proper insulin function. In addition, studies at the Department of Agriculture have shown that diets high in sugar can deplete the body of its chromium stores and thus impair insulin function. "Hypertension in humans is often related to disturbances in the insulin system," Preuss added. "We believe that chromium supplements may prove beneficial for millions of people whose lives might otherwise be lost or impaired as a result of sugar-induced high blood pressure."

Niacin-bound chromium was superior to chromium picolinate in treating 43 healthy, sedentary, obese females. The women were assigned to one of four treatment groups: 400 mcg/day of chromium picolinate without exercise; 400 mcg/day of chromium picolinate with exercise training; 400 mcg/day of niacin-bound chromium with exercise training; or exercise training with a placebo. The exercise training consisted of aerobic dance for one hour twice a week and 30 minutes of cycling twice a week. Resistance training was also practiced twice a week.[10]

The researchers reported that chromium picolinate supplements brought a significant gain in weight in these individuals, while exercise combined with chromium nicotinate resulted in a significant weight loss. It was concluded that exercise combined with niacin-bound chromium may be more beneficial than exercise training alone in those patients who are at risk for coronary artery disease and Type 2 diabetes.

A controversy has been brewing over the safety of chromium picolinate. Concern arose when a study found that high levels of chromium picolinate damaged Chinese hamster ovary cells in a test tube. In a study at the Department of Agriculture, however, no toxicity was observed in a detailed analysis of blood and tissue samples from rats who were fed high amounts of chromium picolinate. The dosages were 0, 5, 25, 50, or 100 mg of chromium picolinate or chromium chloride per kg of diet.[11]

Following a four-year study, Gary W. Evans, Ph.D., reported that rats given chromium picolinate throughout their lives, and allowed to eat as often as they wanted, had a median life span of 45 months. This contrasted with 33 months for rats receiving less effective forms of chromium. At a meeting of the American Aging Association and the American College of Gerontology on October 19, 1992, in San Francisco, Evans said that this represents a 12-month or 36 percent increase in life span. Although the implications for human longevity remain to be seen, Evans suggested that this finding would be equivalent to extending human life from the current age of 75 to about 102.[12]

The best sources of chromium are brewer's yeast, wheat germ, bran, beef, poultry, whole-grain cereals, and cheese.

References

1. Crofford, Oscar B., "Diabetes," *Medical and Health Annual* (Chicago: Encyclopedia Britannica, 1995), 258ff.

2. McBride, Judy, "Chromium Supplements May Be Beneficial for Diabetics," *USDA Background Information,* Aug. 28, 1996.

3. Anderson, Richard A., et al., "Elevated Intakes of Supplemental Chromium Improve Glucose and Insulin Variables in Individuals with Type 2 Diabetes," *Diabetes* 46: 1786–91, 1997.

4. Anderson, Richard A., "Chromium as an Essential Nutrient for Humans," *Regulatory Toxicology and Pharmacology* 26: S35–S41, 1997.

5. Campbell, Wayne W., et al., "Chromium Picolinate Supplementation and Resistive Training by Older Men: Effects on Iron-Status and Hematologic Indexes," *American Journal of Clinical Nutrition* 66: 944–99, 1997.

6. Hermann, J., et al., "Chromium Reduces Serum Cholesterol in the Elderly," *Nutrition Report,* July 1994, 54.

7. Abraham, A., et al., "Chromium and Cholesterol-Induced Atherosclerosis in Rabbits," *Annals of Nutrition Metabolism* 35: 203–7, 1991.

8. Kaats, Gilbert R., et al., "A Randomized, Double-Masked, Placebo-Controlled Study of the Effects of Chromium Picolinate Supplementation on Body Composition: A Replication and Extension of a Previous Study," *Current Therapeutic Research* 59(6): 379–88, June 1998.

9. Preuss, Harry, "Study Shows Chromium Supplement May Prevent High Blood Pressure and Slow Aging," paper presented at the American College of Nutrition annual meeting, Washington, D.C., Oct. 14, 1995.

10. Grant, Kristen E., et al., "Chromium and Exercise Training: Effect on Obese Women," *Medicine and Science in Sports and Exercise* 29(8): 992–98, 1997.

11. Anderson, R. A., et al., "Lack of Toxicity of Chromium Chloride and Chromium Picolinate in Rats," *Journal of the American College of Nutrition* 16: 273–79, 1997.

12. Murray, Frank, *The Big Family Guide to All the Minerals* (New Canaan, Conn.: Keats Publishing, 1995), 256.

17

Cis-9-Cetyl Myristoleate (CMO)

Cetyl myristoleate, the common name for cis-9-cetyl myristoleate, is a natural substance found in certain animals and is being touted as another natural treatment for arthritis. On the one hand, cetyl myristoleate can reprogram faulty memory T-cells, the cause of arthritis, according to Chuck Cochran, D.C. On the other hand, the substance appears to normalize hyperimmune responses, providing favorable results for treating autoimmune conditions such as rheumatoid arthritis and systemic lupus erythematosus, another form of arthritis. It also seems to work as a lubricant and a powerful anti-inflammatory agent.[1]

Cetyl myristoleate capsules and topical cream have been found effective in treating rheumatoid arthritis, osteoarthritis, gout, ankylosing spondylitis, Reiter's syndrome, Sjogren's syndrome, and psoriasis.

It may also be useful in treating back pain that is arthritis related. If a joint can be moved only slightly, this therapy may improve joint mobility, assuming the bones have not fused.

Recommended dosages are taken according to weight. For example, one manufacturer produces 760-mg capsules. For those under 125 pounds, the recommended treatment is about 10 capsules daily. Another manufacturer provides 75-mg capsules. For larger people, the recommended dosage is 24 capsules daily. A third manufacturer produces several cetyl myristoleate products, including liquid and hard and soft gel capsules. Since most of these products are rather expensive, review your options with a health care practitioner.

Researchers at the Medical College of Virginia at Richmond reported that cetyl myristoleate provided good protection against arthritic states in rats. The substance was given by injection, and the injection site was important as to whether the cetyl myristoleate was reaching the part of the animal that needed protection.[2]

The developer of cetyl myristoleate, when applying for a patent, reported that a 250-pound, 75-year-old male diagnosed with osteoarthritis received four 1-cc capsules of cetyl myristoleate twice, with a two-month interval between dosages. There was a 75 percent alleviation of pain in the affected joints, the manufacturer reported.[3]

In another anecdotal case, a woman suffering severe back pain due to osteoarthritis applied a 10 percent solution of cetyl myristoleate in dimethyl sulfoxide topically twice daily until 11 cc had been used. She reported almost 90 percent of the back pain was relieved in about a week.

A 72-year-old male with osteoarthritis took three capsules, each containing 1 cc of cetyl myristoleate, followed five months later by four more capsules. He was able to discontinue other arthritis medication and to resume playing the guitar.

A research team in Baja California and Pamorski, Poland, conducted a randomized clinical trial involving three treatment groups, including a control group. It reported that cetyl myristoleate and cetyl myristoleate–supporting formulas (including glucosamine, sea cucumber, and other substances) appear to be beneficial in the treatment of a wide range of arthritic conditions, including long-standing and refractive cases.[4]

Since much of the research concerning cetyl myristoleate is anecdotal or involves animals, more research needs to be conducted. The results look promising, however, and those with various forms of arthritis should confer with their healthcare providers to see if this substance may be useful.

References

1. Cochran, Chuck, *Cetyl Myristoleate (CMO)* (New York: Healing Wisdom Publications, 1997).
2. Diehl, Harry W., and Everette L. May, "Cetyl Myristoleate Isolated from Swiss Albino Mice: An Apparent Protective Agent Against Adjuvant Arthritis in Rats," *Journal of Pharmaceutical Sciences* 83(3): 296–99, March 1994.
3. Diehl, Harry W., "Method for the Treatment of Osteoarthritis," United States Patent No. 5, 569, 676, Oct. 29, 1996.
4. Siemandi, H., et al., "The Effect of Cis-9-Cetyl Myristoleate (CMO) and Adjunctive Therapy on the Course of Arthritic Episodes in Patients with Various Autoimmune Diseases Characterized by the Common Terminology 'Arthritis' and 'Psoriasis,'" 1997, unpublished.

18

Conjugated Linoleic Acid (CLA)

Obesity, a chronic disease that affects over one-third of the adult population in the United States, is not a single disease per se, but rather a syndrome or collection of diseases. Approximately one-half of all Americans are on a diet at any given time, spending between $30 billion and $50 billion annually on diet aids, most of which are unsuccessful. Obesity is defined as weight that is more than 20 percent over desirable weight, as spelled out in the 1983 Metropolitan Life Insurance tables, or as weight more than 30 percent over the "ideal" body weight as listed in the original 1959 Metropolitan Life Insurance tables. Most of the definitions are flawed because they do not measure excess body fat, only excess weight.[1]

A relatively new approach to obesity is conjugated linoleic acid (CLA), which was isolated at the University of Wisconsin at Madison. CLA is a polyunsaturated fatty acid normally found in lamb, beef, veal, butter, milk, yogurt, cheese, and other foods. As a therapeutic agent, it needs to be obtained in larger amounts than are found in foods. A commercial product is now available over the counter, converted from the linoleic acid in sunflower and other oils.

At a conference sponsored by Scandinavian Clinical Research in Norway, a number of researchers reviewed some of the research on CLA:

- Annika Smedman, M.Sci., discussed a double-blind study in Sweden in 1998 involving 53 patients ranging in age from 23 to 63. They were pretreated with a placebo for two weeks, then given daily 4.2 g of CLA or a placebo for 12 weeks and were told not to change their regular diet or exercise habits. Upon completion of the study, there was a significant reduction in body fat in the CLA group.

- In Norway in 1997, a study involved 10 males and 10 females recruited at a fitness studio. After receiving 3 g of CLA daily for three months, they reported a significant decrease in body fat, according to Erling Thom, Ph.D.
- Two studies in Norway using CLA were recapped by Ola Gudmudsen, Dr. Philos. In the first study, 60 moderately obese volunteers were given either 3.4 g of CLA or 4.5 g of olive oil as a placebo for 12 weeks. None of the usual parameters, such as blood pressure, changed significantly during the trial, but the CLA group registered a significant weight loss. In the second study, 60 moderately obese people were given daily 0, 1.8, 3.6, 5.4, or 7.2 g of CLA for 12 weeks. All of the treatment groups had a significant reduction in body fat compared to the placebo group.[2]

At the University of Wisconsin at Madison, Michael Pariza, Ph.D., and colleagues fed mice, rats, and chicks a diet containing corn oil or corn oil plus CLA for four to eight weeks. The CLA-fed mice, rats, and chicks exhibited significant body fat reductions of 57 to 70 percent, 23 percent, and 22 percent, respectively. In another study, adult rats were given for four weeks diets containing tallow, corn oil, or coconut oil plus CLA. The CLA-supplemented animals exhibited significantly reduced body fat accumulation and increased lean body mass. The researchers concluded that CLA is a potent regulator of body fat accumulation and retention.[3]

Also at the University of Wisconsin, Yeonhwa Park et al. reported that mice fed a CLA-supplemented diet exhibited 57 percent and 60 percent lower body fat and 5 percent and 14 percent increased lean body mass than the controls.[4]

Martha Ann Belury, Ph.D., R.D., reviewed the literature on CLA and reported that it has a number of unique chemoprotective qualities that might protect humans from cancer.[5]

Preliminary studies indicate that CLA is a powerful anticarcinogen in the rat breast tumor model, according to Clement Ip., Ph.D. CLA shows that fats from meat and dairy products contain some component that has an attribute in cancer protection. CLA-enriched food products may act as a prototype of new designer foods that may appeal to those who are unwilling to change their eating habits but still want alternative food choices for cancer prevention.[6] In another article, Ip wrote that CLA is by far the most powerful naturally occurring fatty acid known to modulate tumor formation.[7]

Other researchers have found that cow's milk contains CLA, which is manufactured by bacteria in the animal's stomach and has been shown to protect against melanoma (skin cancer) and leukemia, as well as breast, colon, ovarian, and prostate cancers. CLA seems to work like a sponge, soaking up oxidants that can cause cancerous mutations in cells. However, a 154-pound individual would have to consume 3.5 g of CLA daily to derive any benefit. Most Americans consume only about 1 g of CLA daily.[8]

Rabbits fed CLA were found to have less cholesterol deposits that might contribute to hardening of the arteries. The animals' diets contained 0.1 percent cholesterol, or the cholesterol-laced diet and 1 percent CLA for 22 weeks. Fat deposition was considerably lower in the aortas of the CLA-fed animals.[9]

Jan Wadstein et al. of Oslo, Norway, wrote to the editor of *The Lancet* suggesting that CLA has been shown in animal studies to prevent or regulate diabetes in the Zucker diabetic rat. In January 1998, researchers enrolled in a CLA safety study a patient who had had Type 2 (adult-onset) diabetes since 1994. He was treated with 3 g of CLA daily for 12 weeks. This therapy reduced plasma levels of triglycerides, cholesterol, LDL cholesterol, and other parameters. At the same time, body fat was reduced from 27.6 to 26.0, and total body weight decreased from 101.2 to 99.2 kg. The researchers said that, to their knowledge, the patient was the first to illustrate a possible beneficial use of CLA in Type 2 diabetes.[10]

Although most of the CLA studies have been performed on animals, the research is stimulating enough to bode well for human benefits, including for obesity, cancer, atherosclerosis, and diabetes.

CLA is available in over-the-counter 500-mg capsules. Suggested dosage is two capsules before each meal as a dietary supplement. If you wish to use CLA for a health problem, consult your alternative medicine practitioner, since a larger dosage may be required.

References

1. Atkinson, Richard L., "Obesity," *Medical and Health Annual* (Chicago: Encyclopedia Britannica, 1995), 337ff.

2. Papers read at the Round Table Conference, Grand Hotel, Oslo, Norway, Feb. 25, 1999.

3. Pariza, M., et al., "Conjugated Linoleic Acid Reduces Body Fat," *FASEB Journal,* Washington, D.C., April 14–17, 1996.

4. Park, Yeonhwa, et al., "Effect of Conjugated Linoleic Acid on Body Composition in Mice," *Lipids* 32(8): 853–58, 1997.

5. Belury, Martha Ann, "Conjugated Dienoic Linoleate: A Polyunsaturated Fatty Acid with Unique Chemoprotective Properties," *Nutrition Reviews* 53(4): 83–89, April 1995.

6. Ip, Clement, et al., "Conjugated Linoleic Acid: A Powerful Anticarcinogen from Animal Fat Sources," *Cancer* 74: 1050–54, 1994.

7. Ip, Clement, et al., "Conjugated Linoleic Acid Suppresses Mammary Carcinogenesis and Proliferative Activity of the Mammary Gland in the Rat," *Cancer Research* 54: 1212–15, March 1, 1994.

8. "Cancer and Conjugated Linoleic Acid," *Nutrition Week* 27(2): 7, Jan. 10, 1997.

9. Lee, Kisun N., et al., "Conjugated Linoleic Acid and Atherosclerosis in Rabbits," *Atherosclerosis* 108: 19–25, 1994.

10. Wadstein, Jan, et al., "Can CLA Regulate Diabetes Type 2?" Research letter to the editor of *The Lancet,* January 13, 1999, unpublished.

19

Copper

Although there is no recommended dietary allowance (RDA) for copper, a deficiency in the mineral can lead to anemia, skeletal defects, demyelination and degeneration of the nervous system, defects in hair pigmentation and structure, reproductive failure, and elevated cholesterol levels. Copper and some vitamins are used in the body's metabolism of iron, and too much cadmium, calcium, iron, lead, molybdenum, sulfur, silver, and zinc in the diet inhibits this use of copper. Wilson's disease, a genetically determined inborn error of metabolism, is related to excessive deposits of copper in the liver, brain, and other organs, leading to hepatitis, kidney malfunction, and neurologic damage. The condition is reversible by controlling dietary copper intake and giving chelating agents to bind the copper and excrete it in the urine.[1]

The body has a defense system of protective enzymes and circulating chemicals called antioxidants to protect cells from harmful oxidation and limit free radical damage. Some of these chemicals are manufactured inside the body, while others, such as copper, come from food sources. Other dietary antioxidants include vitamins A, C, and E, carotenoids, bioflavonoids, selenium, manganese, zinc, and sulfur. Some antioxidants inhibit free radical damage and are destroyed in the process. Other antioxidants attack indirectly by activating enzymes that convert the free radicals to less destructive compounds.[2]

Patients who are given prolonged, forced tubal feeding are at risk of developing copper deficiency anemia. Intravenous administration of copper usually corrects the problem.[3]

Copper and especially ceruloplasmin (a copper-containing protein) are elevated by estrogens, causing the levels of both to rise during pregnancy, according to Carl C. Pfeiffer, Ph.D., M.D. Blood levels of copper are about 115 mcg % at the time of conception and reach a mean level of 260 mcg % at term. After the birth, it takes between two and three months before the mother's original serum copper level is reached. While more research is needed, the high postpartum copper level may be a factor in postpartum depression and psychosis. Postpartum psychosis is thought to be greater when the woman delivers a boy.[4]

Pfeiffer, who did landmark nutrition studies at the Brain Bio Center in New Jersey prior to his death, found that elevated blood or tissue copper levels may also contribute to paranoid and hallucinatory schizophrenia, high blood pressure, stuttering, autism, childhood hyperactivity, preeclampsia, premenstrual syndrome, psychiatric depression, insomnia, senility, and possibly functional low blood sugar.

A copper-zinc ratio is related to some forms of antisocial behavior. H. Ronald Isaacson, Ph.D., of the Health Research Institute in Naperville, Illinois, conducted a study of incarcerated young males who were dubbed either type A or type B. Type A were those chemically characterized by elevated copper/zinc ratios; elevated lead, cadmium, and magnesium; and a deficiency in sodium, potassium, and manganese. Type As, which have a history of episodic violence followed by remorse, also have a high incidence of learning disabilities, allergies, and acne.[5] Type Bs have depressed copper/zinc ratios; elevated levels of sodium, potassium, lead, calcium, and magnesium; and abnormal levels of manganese. This pattern is found in criminals who have a history of violent acts without remorse.

Researchers in Turkey evaluated 40 women suffering from premenstrual syndrome and 20 controls without PMS. Magnesium and zinc/copper ratios were significantly lower in those with PMS. Plasma levels of magnesium and zinc were significantly reduced during the luteal (egg-releasing) phase of the menstrual cycle.[6]

Since copper is a key nutrient in a special enzyme (lysl oxidase), which intertwines the tough, elastic fibers of collagen and elastin—two main connective tissue proteins in the body—the mineral plays an active role in repairing tissue following burns. Researchers at Charing Cross Hospital in London recommended that severe burn patients be supplemented with copper, zinc, and selenium as soon as possible after being admitted to the hospital. Their study involved a 48-year-old woman with diabetes who had severe burns to 60 percent of her body. Her copper and ceruloplasmin levels were undetectable, and her plasma copper levels remained low for several weeks in spite of copper supplementation. After three months, zinc concentrations increased to a normal range. The researchers suggested that burn patients should be supplemented with the three minerals at amounts considerably above the daily requirement to enhance healing and recovery.[7]

Another study reported that burn patients experience fewer hospital stays and lung infections when they are given these three supplements. Twenty patients with an average age of 40 were burned over 48 percent of their bodies. After studying the patients for 30 days, the researchers found that the number of infections per patient was significantly lower in the supplemented group, compared to the controls.[8]

A review of recent studies demonstrating that in vitro (test tube) activities of T cells are compromised by marginal copper deficiency in both adult rats and healthy human tissue suggests that suboptimal intakes of this mineral have the potential to weaken resistance to infectious diseases.[9]

Although vegetarian diets for adults often carry an adequate amount of trace minerals, these diets may put children at risk, since youngsters require large amounts of zinc for growth. A Canadian research team found that high amounts of phytic acid and dietary fiber in plant-based diets—and the low amounts of animal foods in many vegetarian diets—reduce the bioavailability of copper and zinc and possibly manganese and selenium.[10]

A copper deficiency can induce defects in the heart or large blood vessels. In addition, dietary copper is necessary for several microvascular control mechanisms which affect inflammation, circulation, and the regulation of peripheral blood flow.[11]

Excessive amounts of copper in the body have pro-oxidant or harmful effects, but data are accumulating that indicate that oxidant stress is associated with copper deficiency, and that copper is an antioxidant with important beneficial anti-inflammatory and cardioprotective properties.[12]

Cardiac abnormalities have been reported in animals given low-copper diets. Such diets tend to elevate blood levels of cholesterol. Lipid droplets increase in the myocardium, the middle muscular layer of the heart wall, leading to cardiomyopathies or abnormalities in the heart muscle.[13]

At Albany Medical College in New York, patients with rheumatoid arthritis were found deficient with regard to the RDA for vitamin B_6, magnesium, and zinc, and their copper and folic acid levels were found deficient when compared to the typical American diet. Researchers concluded that dietary supplementation with these nutrients is appropriate for both men and women who have rheumatoid arthritis.[14]

The age-old habit of wearing copper bracelets to alleviate arthritis pain has been well publicized. Robert M. Giller, M.D., indicates the mineral is more potent than aspirin as an anti-inflammatory agent. In arthritics, who are thought to have a copper deficiency, copper has been found to reduce morning stiffness and aid joint mobility, sometimes eliminating the need for other medication. Giller recommends 2 mg/day of copper salicylate with meals, along with 50 mg of zinc twice a day with meals. If there is no improvement within six weeks, discontinue the therapy.[15]

Supplementation with certain minerals slows or halts bone loss in postmenopausal women. A study involved 57 healthy post-menopausal women who were evaluated over a two-year period. Spinal bone loss was halted in the women getting 1,000 mg of calcium citrate malate, 15 mg of zinc, 5 mg of manganese, and 2.5 mg of copper daily. The placebo group lost significantly greater amounts of bone.[16]

A copper deficiency is associated with difficulty in regulating blood sugar, especially for Type 2 diabetics. When these people eat sugar, a substance called sorbitol, derived from glucose, is believed to accumulate in the tissues. Sorbitol draws water into the cells and forces important molecules out, promoting the development of cataracts, retinopathy (degenerative disease of the retina), diabetic neuropathy, and other complications associated with diabetes. For those with a copper deficiency, a dosage of 2 to 4 mg/day is recommended.[17]

The main food sources of copper include liver, lobster, oysters, canned crab, nuts, curry powder, soybeans, mushrooms, wheat bran, wheat germ, chocolate, molasses, cocoa powder, tea, yeast, and gelatin.

There are two faces of copper. On the one hand, it contributes to good health. On the other hand, it can be harmful in excessive amounts, especially if its ratio with zinc is compromised. Consult a holistic doctor for more information.

References

1. Ensminger, A., et al., *Foods and Nutrition Encyclopedia* (Clovis, Calif.: Pegus Press, 1983), 478ff.

2. Galland, Leo, *The Four Pillars of Healing* (New York: Random House, 1997), 205.

3. Masugi, Jiro, et al., "Copper Deficiency Anemia and Prolonged Enteral Feeding," *Annals of Internal Medicine* 121(5): 386, Sept. 1, 1994.

4. Pfeiffer, Carl C., *Mental and Elemental Nutrients* (New Canaan, Conn.: Keats Publishing, 1975), 325ff.

5. Hamilton, Kirk. "Violence and Copper/Zinc Ratio," *Clinical Pearls with The Experts Speak* (Sacramento, Calif.: Health Associates Medical Group, 1997), 336. Also, Isaacson, H. Ronald, "Elevated Blood Copper/Zinc Ratios in Assaultive Young Males," *Physiology and Behavior* 62(2): 327–29, 1997.

6. Posaci, Cemal, et al., "Plasma Copper, Zinc, and Magnesium Levels in Patients with Premenstrual Tension Syndrome," *Acta Obstetrics and Gynecology Scandinavia* 73: 452–55, 1994.

7. Sampson, B., et al., "Severe Hypocupraemia in a Patient with Extensive Burn Injuries," *Annals of Clinical Biochemistry* 33: 462–64, 1996.

8. Berger, M. M., et al., "Trace Element Supplementation Modulates Pulmonary Infection Rates After Major Burns: A Double-Blind, Placebo-Controlled Trial," *American Journal of Clinical Nutrition* 68: 365–71, 1998.

9. Failla, Mark L., and Robin G. Hopkins, "Is Low Copper Status Immuno-suppressive?" *Nutrition Reviews* 56(1): S59–S64, Jan. 1998.

10. Gibson, Rosalind S., "Content and Bioavailability of Trace Elements in Vegetarian Diets," *American Journal of Clinical Nutrition* 59: 1223S–32S, 1994.

11. Schuschke, Dale A., "Dietary Copper in the Physiology of the Microcirculation," *Journal of Nutrition* 127: 2274–81, 1997.

12. Strain, J. J., et al., "Trace Elements and Cardiovascular Disease, Role of Trace Elements and Cardiovascular Disease," *Role of Trace Elements for Health Promotion and Disease Prevention* 54:127–40, 1998.

13. Medeiros, Denis M., "Copper and Its Possible Role in Cardiomyopathies," *The Nutrition Report,* Dec. 1993, 89, 96.

14. Kremer, Joel M., and Jean Bigaouetts, "Nutrient Intake of Patients with Rheumatoid Arthritis Is Deficient in Pyriodoxine, Zinc, Copper, and Magnesium," *Journal of Rheumatology* 23(6): 990–94, 1994.

15. Giller, Robert M., and Kathy Matthews, *Natural Prescriptions* (New York: Carol Southern Books, 1994), 299ff.

16. Strause, L., et al., "Spinal Bone Loss in Postmenopausal Women Supplemented with Calcium and Trace Minerals," *Journal of Nutrition* 124: 1060–64, July 1994.

17. Werbach, Melvyn, *Healing with Food* (New York: HarperPerennial, 1993), 116–117.

20

CoQ10

Coenzyme Q10 (CoQ10) is a naturally occurring nutrient in beef muscle, beef heart, and eggs, and occurs in lesser amounts in spinach, grains, beans, and certain oils. As we age, however, the body becomes less effective at assimilating and synthesizing CoQ10 from foods. Since food sources normally do not provide enough of the nutrient for medicinal purposes, researchers usually recommend CoQ10 supplements as the preferred source.[1]

A research team at the University of Texas at Austin studied eight aging patients who were given CoQ10 for heart and blood vessel disease, diabetes, and cancer. Seven of the eight patients showed an elevation in antibody levels. Similar findings were demonstrated by researchers at Osaka University School of Medicine in Japan. Cancer and heart disease patients are often found to have alarmingly low levels of CoQ10.

At his Institute of Science and Medicine in California, Linus Pauling, Ph.D., reported that CoQ10 supplements strengthen the heart, even without exercise; normalize blood pressure; elevate energy levels; and contribute to life extension.

According to Debasis Bagchi, Ph.D., CoQ10 has profound beneficial effects: It acts as a novel antioxidant; enhances stamina, endurance, and energy levels; helps to reduce body weight; normalizes blood pressure; attenuates immune function; protects against cardiovascular dysfunction; reverses periodontal disease; and increases the effectiveness of various chemotherapeutic agents and antimalarial drugs.

Also called ubiquinone, CoQ10 is an important component of the mitochondria, where it plays a significant role in energy production, reported Michael T. Murray, N.D. A deficiency in the substance can be attributed to impaired CoQ10 synthesis related to nutritional deficiencies, a genetic or acquired defect in CoQ10 synthesis, or increased tissue needs. Increased levels of CoQ10 are beneficial in treating chest pains, high blood pressure, mitral valve prolapse, congestive heart failure, and a deterioration of the immune system in the elderly. In fact, biopsies of diseased heart tissue show a CoQ10 deficiency in 50 to 75 percent of the cases.[2]

In one study, Murray reported, 12 patients with angina pectoris were given 150 mg/day of CoQ10 for four weeks in a double-blind crossover study. Compared to placebo, CoQ10 brought a reduction in the frequency of chest pain attacks by 53 percent.

Stephen T. Sinatra, M.D., indicated that CoQ10 could represent one of the major medicinal advances in the 20th century in the treatment of heart disease. The tragedy is that it is still virtually ignored by the majority of physicians as well as by the conventional medical establishment. Therefore, many patients who have not responded to conventional treatment could achieve a higher quality of life with CoQ10.[3] Sinatra said that there have been 10 international symposia on the biomedical and clinical aspects of CoQ10 from 1976 through 1998, and these meetings have involved more than 450 papers presented by 250 physicians and scientists from 18 countries. The majority of these clinical studies have demonstrated CoQ10's positive impact on heart disease.

"Although some patients may respond to an initial dose of 30 to 60 mg of CoQ10 three times daily, many will not," Sinatra said. "For 'therapeutic failures,' CoQ10 levels should be obtained. If this serum evaluation is not possible, increasing the dosage of CoQ10 according to the clinical symptoms must be considered."

Robert M. Giller, M.D., wrote that CoQ10 has been of significant help to his patients with angina because it prevents the accumulation of fatty acids in the heart muscle. CoQ10 reduces angina pain and increases the ability to exert oneself without discomfort. He recommends 30 to 60 mg of CoQ10 three times daily. Results should manifest in one to three weeks.[4]

The supplement improves the function of the blood vessel wall and thus helps regulate blood pressure. In one 10-week trial, hypertensive patients taking CoQ10 found a mean systolic (beating) and diastolic (resting) pressure reduction of 10.6 and 7.7 mmHg, respectively, during the treatment period. There was no change in the placebo group.

Since CoQ10 increases exercise tolerance and also strengthens the heart, it is helpful for people with mitral valve prolapse, Giller added. The mitral valve controls the flow of blood in the heart between the left atrium and the left ventricle. When the valve prolapses, it billows back toward the atrium as the ventricle contracts, causing blood to leak across the valve. Although generally benign, this condition can be life threatening if the leak is substantial.

Giller went on to say that CoQ10 shows considerable promise in treating periodontal disease. Tests in Japan and the United States have found that CoQ10 supplements are remarkably effective in reversing this gum disorder, both in its early and later stages and in growing new tissue. Dramatic improvements have been found in patients who were no longer able to eat solid food until they were given CoQ10.

Researchers in India have found, in a double-blind trial involving patients getting antihypertensive drugs, that CoQ10 decreases blood pressure apparently by decreasing oxidative stress and insulin response. The dosage used was 60 mg twice daily.[5] The same team, headed by Ram B. Singh, M.D., reported that the same dosage decreased lipoprotein-a concentrations in patients with acute coronary disease. HDL cholesterol—the beneficial kind—showed a significant increase without affecting total cholesterol. Blood glucose levels decreased significantly in the CoQ10 volunteers. During the 28-day trial, CoQ10 brought a reduction of serum lipoprotein-a of 31.0 percent, compared to an 8.2 percent drop in the placebo group, or a net reduction of 22.6 percent attributed to CoQ10. Blood levels of lipoprotein-a are raised in those with early impairment of kidney function, and are associated with a greater prevalence of cardiovascular disease.[6]

Singh said that CoQ10 is more effective than vitamins in controlling arrhythmias, angina, and left ventricular failure in patients with myocardial infarction. The supplement can decrease hyperinsulinemia and also possibly lipoprotein-a, thought to be a genetic risk factor for coronary disease.[7]

For patients undergoing elective coronary artery bypass surgery, pretreatment with CoQ10 may play a protective role during routine coronary bypass grafting by reducing peroxidative damage and reperfusion arrhythmias. In an Italian study involving 40 patients, those getting CoQ10 had a lower incidence of ventricular arrhythmias during the recovery period.[8]

In Taiwan, researchers evaluated 12 patients in a double-blind study in which the treatment group was given between 150 and 200 mg/day of CoQ10 for five to seven days before their cardiovascular surgery. Those pretreated with CoQ10 had a reduced incidence of low cardiac output, as well as a wider pulse pressure. CoQ10 is an antioxidant that may possibly prevent reperfusion injury in the myocardium.[9]

Although preliminary studies suggest that CoQ10 has valuable therapeutic actions, including enhanced immunity, most of the interest has focused on its possible impact on cardiovascular disease, according to Sheldon Saul Hendler, M.D., Ph.D. Researchers at the Methodist Hospital in Indianapolis and the Institute for Bio-Medical Research at the University of Texas have had considerable success in treating heart failure patients. CoQ10 seems to enhance the pumping capacity of the heart and eliminate the major side effects associated with conventional heart failure drugs. Patients were said to have a deficiency in CoQ10 in the heart, and supplements are thought to increase production of energy in the heart muscle cells. About 91 percent of the patients improved within 30 days of getting the supplement. Also, there is a direct relationship between CoQ10 and vitamin E.[10]

As an antioxidant, CoQ10 plays an essential role in the movement of sperm, which helps protect the sperm cell membranes from oxidative damage, according to researchers at Catholic University in Rome. This was revealed after the research team evaluated seminal fluid in 77 men. The data suggest a strong pathophysiological effect on CoQ10 in human seminal fluid and a possible molecular defect in varicocele patients. They added that CoQ10 measurements could be an important way of examining infertile men and provide a rationale for the possible treatment with CoQ10 in patients with irregular sperm.[11] Varicocele, which refers to abnormally distended veins, essentially varicose veins, is a rather common condition that affects the left testis in about 10 to 15 percent of males. The condition is usually harmless but can cause discomfort in the scrotum.

In evaluating 48 chronic hemodialysis patients, CoQ10 levels were found to be abnormally low in 62 percent of the patients. Reduced levels of CoQ10 may contribute to the defective serum antioxidant activity and increase the risk of per-oxidative damage in uremic patients on chronic hemodialysis.[12]

In a clinical protocol in Denmark, 32 patients with high-risk breast cancer were treated with antioxidants, fatty acids, and 90 mg/day of CoQ10. Six of the patients showed partial regression of their tumors. One patient's dosage was increased to 390 mg/day. After one month, the tumor was no longer visible, and in another month, mammography confirmed that the tumor had disappeared. Another patient, who had a verified residual tumor following non-radical surgery, was treated with 300 mg/day of CoQ10. After three months, the patient was in excellent health and no residual tumor tissue was detected.[13]

Karl Folkers, Ph.D., and colleagues at the University of Texas at Austin reported that patients with Duchenne disease, Becker disease, Charcot-Marie-Tooth disease, and Welander disease, and others suffering from muscle dystrophies should be treated with CoQ10 indefinitely. Their studies showed that while 100 g/day of CoQ10 was probably too low, it was effective and safe.[14]

Since the amount of CoQ10 in the diet is probably not enough to protect against the various disorders discussed here, a CoQ10 supplement would be good health insurance.

References

1. Bagchi, Debasis, "Coenzyme Q10: A Novel Cardiac Antioxidant," *Journal of*

Orthomolecular Medicine 12(1): 4–10, 1997.

2. Murray, Michael T., "Important Considerations in Angina," *Natural Medicine Journal* 2(2): 5, Feb. 1999.

3. Sinatra, Stephen T., "CoEnzyme Q10—A Cardiologist's Commentary," ibid., 9–15.

4. Giller, Robert M., and Kathy Matthews, *Natural Prescriptions* (New York: Ballantine Books, 1994), 14, 88, 199, 253ff., 274.

5. Singh, R. B., et al., "Effect of Hydrosoluble Coenzyme Q10 on Blood Pressure and Insulin Resistance in Hypertensive Patients with Coronary Artery Disease," *Journal of Human Hypertension* 13: 203–8, March 1999.

6. Singh, R. B., et al., "Serum Concentration of Lipoprotein-a Decreases on Treatment with Hydro-soluble Coenzyme Q10 in Patients with Coronary Artery Disease: Discovery of a New Role," *International Journal of Cardiology* 68: 23–29, January 1999.

7. Hamilton, Kirk, "Acute Myocardial Infarction and Antioxidants," *Clinical Pearls with The Experts Speak* (Sacramento, Calif.: Health Associates Medical Group, 1998), 17–18. Also, Ram B. Singh, "Intervention Therapy with Mega Dose of Antioxidant Vitamins in Patients with Acute Myocardial Infarction: Could We Throw Caution to the Wind?" *American Journal of Cardiology* 80: 823–24, Sept. 15, 1997.

8. Chello, Massimo, et al., "Protection by Coenzyme Q10 from Myocardial Reperfusion Injury During Coronary Artery Bypass Grafting," *Annals of Thoracic Surgery* 58: 1427–32, Nov. 15, 1994.

9. Chen, Yang-Fu, et al., "Effectiveness of Coenzyme Q10 on Myocardial Preservation During Hypothermic Cardioplegic Arrest," *Journal of Thoracic Cardiovascular Surgery* 107(1): 242–47, 1994.

10. Hendler, Sheldon Saul, *The Doctors' Vitamin and Mineral Encyclopedia* (New York: Simon and Schuster, 1990), 341.

11. Mancini, Antonio, et al., "Coenzyme Q10 Concentrations in Normal and Pathological Human Seminal Fluid," *Journal of Andrology* 15(6): 591–94, Nov.–Dec. 1994.

12. Triolo, Luigi, et al., "Serum Coenzyme Q10 and Uremic Patients and Chronic Hemodialysis," *Nephron* 66: 153–56, 1994.

13. Lockwood, K., et al., "Partial and Complete Regression of Breast Cancer in Patients in Relation to Dosage of Coenzyme Q10," *Biochemical and Biophysical Research Communication* 199: 1504–08, March 30, 1994.

14. Folkers, K., and R. Simonsen, "Two Successful Double-Blind Trials with Coenzyme Q10 (Vitamin Q10) on Muscular Dystrophies and Neurogenic Atrophies," *Biochemical and Biophysical Acta* 1271: 281–86, May 24, 1995.

21

Cranberry

Cystitis, an inflammation of the inner lining of the bladder, is one of the most common disorders affecting women. Approximately one-half of all women will have a bladder infection at some point in their lives, and an estimated 20 percent will have these infections repeatedly. Repeated treatments with antibiotics can increase the likelihood of an infection, making a natural approach to the problem an ideal choice.[1]

A bladder infection results when bacteria—which usually migrate from the bowel—travel a short distance to the urethra and then up into the bladder. The individual feels a frequent need to urinate, accompanied by pain and/or burning upon urinating. Fever, low back pain, and/or blood in the urine may indicate a kidney infection, which should be screened by a doctor.

Women are more susceptible to cystitis than men because the anus is so close to

the urethra, making it easier for bacteria to reach the bladder. Even women who are not sexually active can develop infections by wiping from back to front after a bowel movement, which drags bacteria into the genital area. Cystitis also develops in women who delay urination, since urine held in the bladder gives bacteria—which double in density every 20 minutes—more time to multiply. Feminine hygiene sprays, douches, and bubble baths are other causes.

In evaluating 604 causes of urinary tract infection (UTI) compared to 629 controls, researchers at the Veterans Affairs Medical Center in Seattle said that the odds ratio for a UTI increased with frequency of condom exposure from 0.91 for weekly use or less during the previous month, to 2.11 for more than once a week. Prophylactics coated with spermicide created a higher risk of infection, with an odds ratio ranging from 1.09 for weekly use or less, to 3.05 for more than one use per week. In fact, spermicide-coated condoms were responsible for 42 percent of the UTIs among women who were exposed to these products. The researchers evaluated a spermicide called nonoxynol-9.[2]

At Weber State University in Ogden, Utah, a cranberry concentrate was more effective than a placebo in reducing the occurrence of UTI. In the double-blind study, 10 women ages 18 to 45 were given 400-mg cranberry capsules or a dicalcium phosphate placebo. During the trial, 21 UTIs were recorded. While ingesting the cranberry capsules, as opposed to placebo, 7 of the 10 women reported fewer UTIs; two had the same number of UTIs; and one volunteer had more UTIs than the others. During the three months of taking cranberry, only six UTIs were recorded among the cranberry users. There were 15 UTIs among the women on placebo.[3]

Researchers at Brigham and Women's Hospital in Boston evaluated 153 elderly women who were given either 300 ml/day of a cranberry beverage or a synthetic placebo drink. The results confirmed the belief that the use of a cranberry beverage reduces the frequency of bacteria and pus in the urine of older women.[4]

Cranberries (Vaccinium macrocarpon) are effective in treating UTIs because they contain, among other things, a unique blend of quinic acid, malic acid, and citric acid. In the Boston study above, bacteria and pyuria (pus) were observed in 28 percent of the women in the placebo group, whereas bacteria and pyuria was found in only 15 percent of the cranberry-beverage group.[5]

In his book *Natural Prescriptions,* Robert M. Giller, M.D., recommends cranberry juice concentrate or cranberry concentrate capsules for cystitis. The suggested dosage is one capsule three times daily with an 8-ounce glass of water. He also recommends 500 mg of buffered vitamin C every four hours during the infection, reduced to 1,000 to 1,500 mg daily postinfection as a maintenance dose. In addition, Giller suggests 1 g/day of bioflavonoids, 25,000 IU/day of vitamin A during the infection, and 50 mg/day of zinc.[6]

References

1. Giller, Robert M., and Kathy Matthews, *Natural Prescriptions* (New York: Ballantine Books, 1994), 100ff.
2. Fihn, Stephan D., et al., "Association Between Use of Spermicide-Coated Condoms and *Escherichia coli* Urinary Tract Infection of Young Women," *American Journal of Epidemiology* 144(5): 512–20, 1996.
3. Walker, Edward B., et al., "Cranberry Concentrate: UTI Prophylaxis," *Journal of Family Practice* 45(2): 167–68, 1997.
4. Avorn, Jerry, et al., "Reduction of Bacteriuria and Pyuria After Ingestion of Cranberry Juice," *Journal of the American Medical Association* 271(10): 751–54, March 9, 1994.
5. Kuzminski, L. N., "Cranberry Juice and Urinary Tract Infections: Is There a Beneficial Relationship?" *Nutrition Reviews* II: S87–S90, Nov. 1996.
6. See note 1 above.

22

Creatine

Most people consume between 1 and 2 g of creatine in their daily diets. Those who eat red meat ingest more; vegetarians consume less. Creatine is also synthesized in the liver, pancreas, and kidneys. After biosynthesis or ingestion, creatine is transported into skeletal muscle from plasma against a concentration gradient that may approach 200:1. To achieve ergogenic effects, some researchers recommend loading doses of 20 g/day for five days, followed by maintenance doses of 5 to 10 g/day.[1]

For patients with congestive heart failure, creatine supplementation can benefit the Krebs cycle, a sequence of enzymes that oxidize the major fuels in the body to produce energy. In one group of patients, there was an increased number of muscle contractions after creatine supplementation. Whether increased muscle endurance and improved metabolism—which results from creatine supplementation—will improve symptoms of patients with heart failure has yet to be determined. In some patients, however, creatine supplementation may improve symptoms. It is believed that only those with low levels of muscle creatine may benefit from this therapy.[2] In muscles, glycogen stores are broken down into glucose and then into molecules called pyruvate. Some of the pyruvate is used by the muscles for energy, and some is converted to alanine, an amino acid, and transported to the liver, where it is converted into glucose. Creatine makes the body's usage of pyruvate more efficient.

At University Hospital in Nottingham, England, 22 male patients who had had chronic heart failure were observed for at least three months. Using a handgrip exercise, the researchers evaluated forearm muscle metabolism. During the test, the patients were given either 20 g/day of creatine or a matching placebo for five days. Contractions until exhaustion at 75 percent of maximum contraction increased following creatine therapy. There was no effect from the placebo. Creatine supplementation seems to enhance skeletal muscle endurance and attenuates the abnormal skeletal muscle metabolism response to exercise in patients with chronic heart failure.[3]

Researchers at the University of Oxford, England, reported that intercellular creatine is in short supply in patients with heart disease. It has been shown that 20 g/day of creatine for 10 days in patients with congestive heart failure improved exercise performance by 10 to 20 percent. In addition, phosphocreatine may be beneficial for patients with acute myocardial infarction.[4]

Creatine may improve the muscle strength of patients with muscular dystrophy according to a study at McMaster University, Ontario, Canada. Although relatively small, the study involved 81 patients with various neuromuscular diseases who were given 10 g/day of creatine for five days and 5 g/day for an additional week. Muscle strength increased about 10 percent.[5]

Creatine may be useful in treating patients with neuromuscular diseases such as amyotrophic lateral sclerosis (ALS), or Lou Gehrig's disease. ALS, which killed the famous New York Yankees baseball player, is characterized by weakness in the arms and hands and wasting of muscles.

The disorder usually affects people over age 50, and more men than women.[6]

In a study published in *Natural Medicine,* creatine improved endurance in mice who had an animal form of ALS, and also extended their lives. Creatine was twice as effective as riluzole, the approved drug for ALS. With further studies, creatine may eventually prove useful in treating patients with Parkinson's and Alzheimer's diseases, as well as inhibiting muscle loss in the elderly.

Supplementation with creatine is a common practice among competitive athletes. Tennis star Mary Pierce and baseball players Sammy Sosa of the Chicago Cubs and Mark McGwire of the St. Louis Cardinals have acknowledged taking creatine for additional power, the *New York Post* reported. Pierce uses creatine as part of a nutritional routine designed by food scientists, said her trainer, Mark Verstegen. McGwire has been quoted as saying, "Everything I've done is natural. Everybody I know in the game of baseball uses the same stuff that I use."[7]

Studies have shown that 20 to 30 g/day of creatine for a week or more can enhance the performance of short-term strenuous exercise. Creatine exists in muscle as creatine phosphate, which provides high-energy phosphates for adenosine diphosphate to restore adenosine triphosphate (ATP) levels quickly.[8] ATP, which contains high-energy phosphate bonds, contains chemical energy, which must be constantly replenished and recycled within the cells.

As an ergogenic agent, creatine increases muscle creatine and phosphocreatine concentrations, which leads to a higher rate of ATP resynthesis. This not only delays the onset of muscular fatigue, but it also aids recovery during repeated bouts of high-intensity exercise. Daily ingestion of about 20 g of creatine for five or six days can significantly increase resting total muscle creatine concentration in sedentary individuals and moderately active athletes.[9]

Studies in Scotland have shown that creatine at 20 g/day for five days can increase total creatine and phosphocreatine content in the muscle. Vegetarians often show the largest increase because of their low dietary intake of the substance. Creatine supplementation can increase performance in high-intensity exercise such as repeated sprints. The transfer of the phosphate group from creatine phosphate to adenosine diphosphate helps restore ATP, which is the immediate energy source of muscle contraction. When high doses were given for four to six days, the muscle creatine content remained elevated for several weeks. Creatine, which has not been found to be harmful in doses up to 30 g/day, improves the muscles' ability to maintain power output during high-intensity exercise. This is especially useful during energy bouts with short recovery periods.[10]

Creatine ingestion at four 5-g doses a day for five days prior to exercise will increase intramuscular creatine and phosphocreatine concentrations and will enhance phosphocreatine resynthesis during recovery from exercise, especially in those who had low creatine prior to the supplement. Creatine may allow athletes to train without fatigue at a higher intensity than they are accustomed to. About 60 percent of creatine content in the muscle is phosphocreatine.[11]

In a one-week study involving 11 competitive swimmers who were taking high levels of creatine, creatine was found to be an efficient performance-enhancing supplement for short-term endurance athletes.[12]

Creatine was discovered almost 160 years ago, according to researchers at Karolinska Institute, Stockholm, Sweden. It helps increase body mass by 1 or 2 kg and has a positive effect on high-intensity intermittent exercise. The benefit may be due to increased recovery between exercise sprints, which delays the onset of fatigue.[13]

In a single-blind, controlled study, nine male athletes with a mean age of 25.7 years performed five 15-second bouts of maximum cycling after seven days of placebo and again after 5 g of creatine plus 1 g of glucose five times a day for seven days, with a 2-week intervention period. Six of the nine athletes completed five 1-minute bouts of maximal exercise after an additional two days of placebo and creatine therapy. Creatine ingestion resulted in a significant increase in work performed during each 15-second bout of maximal exercise compared to placebo trials.[14]

In a double-blind trial at Pennsylvania State University at University Park, 14 men were divided into two groups. Seven were given 25 g/day of creatine monohydrate and the other seven got a placebo. Treatment with creatine significantly improved peak power output, particularly in jump-squats and the bench press. The researchers suggested that one week of creatine supplementation at 25 g/day enhances muscle performance during repeated sets of bench press and jump-squat exercises.[15]

Researchers in Estonia evaluated sprinters and jumpers during creatine monohydrate supplementation at 20 g/day for five days. They found that creatine, compared to placebo, in a double-blind trial, led to a significant enhancement of performance capacity in jumping tests by 7 percent during the first 15 seconds, and by 12 percent during the second 15 seconds. However, this positive effect was not seen in the last third of the continuous jumping exercise, when the contribution of anaerobic metabolism was decreasing. But the time of intensive running to exhaustion improved by 13 percent. These data show that creatine supplementation helps to prolong the time during which the maximal rate of power output can be maintained. Supplementing with 20 g/day for five days showed a statistically significant improvement in continuous jumping and exhaustive running tests.[16]

A study at the Pierre et Marie Curie University in France found that creatine is safe even in relatively high doses. Through urinary analysis and blood tests, researchers monitored volunteers for five days, nine weeks, and finally two years, giving each person dosages of up to 21 g/day. Creatine is not responsible for muscular cramps, even in high doses, and no liver or kidney damage was observed in the participants. In a healthy individual, creatine increases lean muscle tissue, improves performance in athletes, and delays the onset of fatigue during high-intensity exercise.[17]

With such glowing testimonials, it is easy to see why many athletes are turning to creatine. The supplement has great promise in treating neuromuscular disorders, such as ALS, muscular dystrophy, Parkinson's disease, and Alzheimer's disease, as well as chronic heart disease.

References

1. Toler, Steven M., "Creatine Is an Ergogen for Anaerobic Exercise," *Nutrition Reviews* 55(1): 21–24, Jan. 1997.

2. Schaufelberger, M., and K. Swedberg, "Is Creatine Supplementation Helpful for Patients with Chronic Heart Failure?" *European Heart Journal* 19: 533–34, 1998.

3. Andrews, R. L., et al., "The Effect of Dietary Creatine Supplementation on Skeletal Muscle Metabolism in Congestive Heart Failure," *European Heart Journal* 19: 617–22, 1998.

4. Field, M. L., "Creatine Supplementation in Congestive Heart Failure," *Cardiovascular Research* 31: 174–75, 1996.

5. "Creatine May Benefit MD Patients," *Nutritional Outlook,* May 1999, 56.

6. "A Weapon Against Lou Gehrig's Disease," *Newsweek,* March 22, 1999, 65.

7. Tung, Jennifer, "How 'The Body' Turned into 'The Hulk,'" *New York Post,* May 11, 1999, 22–23.

8. Clarkson, Priscilla M., "Nutrition for Improved Sports Performance: Current Issues on Ergogenic Aids," *Sports Medicine* 21(6): 339–41, June 1996.

9. Mujika, I., and S. Padilla, "Creatine Supplementation as an Ergogenic Aid for Sports Performance in Highly Trained Athletes: A Critical Review," *International Journal of Sports Medicine* 18: 491–96, 1997.

10. Maughan, Ronald J., "Creatine Supplementation and Exercise Performance," *International Journal of Sports Medicine* 5: 94–101, 1995.

11. Greenhaff, Paul L., "Creatine and Its Applications as an Ergogenic Aid," *International Journal of Sports Nutrition* 5: S100–S110, 1995.

12. Hotke, V., et al., "The Development of Endurance Capacity of Elite Level Swimmers After One Week of Creatine Supplementation," *International Journal of Sports Medicine* 19: S48, 1998.

13. Ekblom, Ejorn, "Effects of Creatine Supplementation on Performance," *American Journal of Sports Medicine* 24(6): S38–S39, 1996.

14. Schneider, Donald A., et al., "Creatine Supplementation and the Total Work Performed During 15-Second and 1-Minute Bouts of Maximal Cycling," *Australian Journal of Science and Medicine in Sport* 29(3): 65–68, 1997.

15. Volek, Jeff S., et al., "Creatine Supplementation Enhances Muscular Performance During High-Intensity Resistance Exercise," *Journal of the American Dietetic Association* 97: 765–70, 1997.

16. Bosco, C., et al., "Effect of Oral Creatine Supplementation on Jumping and Running Performance," *International Journal of Sports Medicine* 18: 369–72, 1997.

17. "Creatine 'Safe in High Doses,'" *Health Food Business* (England), Nov. 1999, 13.

23

Curcumin

A constituent in turmeric *(Curcuma longa)*, curcumin has been shown to be as effective as cortisone and the anti-inflammatory drug phenylbutazone in decreasing inflammation. Similar to cayenne, curcumin contains pain relievers that keep the neurotransmitter substance P from sending pain signals to the brain. It also decreases inflammation by lowering prostaglandin activity. Curcumin apparently increases cortisone's anti-inflammation action by making the body more sensitive to the hormone.[1]

In trials involving patients with rheumatoid arthritis, curcumin has been found to have beneficial effects comparable to those achieved with standard drugs. One double-blind study involved patients with RA, who were given either 1,200 mg/day of curcumin or 300 mg/day of phenylbutazone. While similar improvements in duration of morning stiffness, walking time, and joint swelling were observed in both groups, phenylbutazone is associated with significant adverse effects. Curcumin does not produce any side effects when taken at the recommended dosage. The recommended dosage for curcumin as an anti-inflammatory is 400 to 600 mg three times daily.[2]

A study in Bombay, India, evaluated 40 patients ages 15 to 68 who had had a hernia or hydrocele operation. Following the operations, the patients experienced spermatic cord swelling and tenderness due to the handling of the cord during surgery. Group A was given 400 mg of curcumin; Group B, 250 mg of lactose powder as a placebo; and Group C, 100 mg of phenylbutazone. The capsules were given three times daily for five days, and the patients were also given ampicillin.[3]

Twenty-four hours after surgery, all patients developed inflammation. A significant reduction in pain on day 6 was observed only in the curcumin and phenylbutazone groups, but curcumin was found to be effective in reducing all four parameters of inflammation. Phenylbutazone was effective in reducing pain at the site, cord swelling, and cord tenderness. The placebo reduced pain at the site of the surgery and cord tenderness but had no effect on cord edema.

Curcumin reduced cord edema and cord tenderness significantly, when compared to placebo and the drug. Since it has a different chemical structure from nonsteroidal, anti-inflammatory drugs, curcumin may act differently than inhibition of prostaglandin synthesis. In addition, curcumin is less likely to cause an ulcer than a dose of phenylbutazone is. Curcumin has been found safe in this short-term study, and it and its analogs deserve further evaluation in inflammatory and rheumatic disorders such as rheumatoid arthritis.

In a study at the Pharmaceutical Institute, Tohoku University, Sendai, Japan, curcumin was found to show strong preventive activity against liver injury from carbon tetrachloride in both humans and in laboratory glassware. Researchers believe the liver-protecting effects are due to such analogs as ferulic acid. The spice has long been used in Eastern medicine for stomach disorders, as a diuretic, and for jaundice.[4]

A research team at Rutgers University, Piscataway, New Jersey, found that curcumin was more effective than ascorbyl palmitate (vitamin C) in reducing colon cancer in laboratory mice.[5] In two colon cancer cell lines, curcumin reduced the proliferation rate of both cell lines, which brought a decrease of 96 percent within 48 hours. Researchers suggest that curcumin inhibits colon cancer cell proliferation in lab glassware. This effect is independent of its ability to inhibit prostaglandin synthesis.[6]

At the University of Texas Medical Branch at Galveston, laboratory animals were given either 75 mg/kg of curcumin in corn oil daily or corn oil alone for 14 days. The lenses of the curcumin-treated animals were much more resistant to opacification than the lenses of the control animals. The protective effect of curcumin may be related through the induction of glutathione S-transferase, and therefore may be effective in protecting against cataract damage induced by lipid peroxidation.[7]

Using a mouse model, researchers gave the animals a standard diet or a diet containing 1 percent curcumin. They then applied DMBA, a tumor initiator, and TPA, a tumor promoter, to the animals' skin. The curcumin significantly inhibited the number of tumors per animal, as well as the size of the tumors.[8]

At King/Drew Medical Center in Los Angeles, Wibert C. Jordan, M.D., reported that curcumin inhibits HIV transmission. In three case reports of HIV-positive men over 20 years of age, 1 g of curcumin was given three times daily. Eight weeks later there was a dramatic reduction in polymerase chain reaction/ribonucleic acid (PCR/RNA) levels, suggesting a strong anti-HIV effect.[9]

Researchers at Tufts University School of Medicine in Boston induced human breast cancer cells using the estrogenic activity of an endosulfane/chlordane/DDT mixture or 17-beta estradiol. When curcumin from turmeric and genistein from soybeans were added, a synergistic effect inhibited the induction of the cells. The researchers suggested that the inclusion of turmeric and soybeans in the diet might help to prevent hormone-related cancers.[10]

For more information on *Curcuma longa,* see the entry on Turmeric in this book.

References

1. Keville, Kathi, *Herbs for Health and Healing* (Emmaus, Pa.: Rodale Press, 1996), 47.

2. Murray, Michael, and Joseph Pizzorno, *Encyclopedia of Natural Medicine,* rev. 2nd ed. (Rocklin, Calif.: Prima Publishing, 1998), 783–84.

3. Satoskar, R. R., et al., "Evaluation of Anti-inflammatory Property of Curcumin (Diferuloyl Methane) in Patients with Postoperative Inflammation," *International Journal of Clinical Pharmacology, Therapy, and Toxicology* 24(12): 651–54, 1986.

4. Kiso, Yoshinobu, et al., "Antihepatotoxic Principals of *Curcuma Longa* Rhizomes," *Journal of Medicinal Plant Research* 49: 185–87, 1983.

5. Huang, M. T., et al., "Effect of Dietary Curcumin and Ascorbyl Palmitate on Azoxymethanol-Induced Colonic Epithelial Cell Proliferation in Focal Areas of Dysplasia," *Cancer Letters* 64: 117–21, 1992.

6. Hanif, Rashid, "Curcumin, a Natural Plant Phenolic Food Additive, Inhibits Cell Proliferation and Induces Cell Cycle Changes in Colon Adenocarcinoma Cell Lines by a Prostaglandin-Independent Pathway," *Journal of Laboratory and Clinical Medicine* 130: 576–84, 1997.

7. Awasthi, Sanjay, et al., "Curcumin Protects Against Hydroxy-2-Trans-Nonenal-Induced Cataract Formation in Rat Lenses," *American Journal of Clinical Nutrition* 64: 761–66, 1996.

8. Limtrakul, P., et al., "Inhibitory Effect of Dietary Curcumin on Skin Carcinogenesis in Mice," *Cancer Letters* 116: 197–203, 1997.

9. Jordan, Wilbert C., "Curcumin—A Natural Herb with Anti-HIV Activity," monograph, 1996, 1–3.

10. Verma, Surendra P., et al., "Curcumin and Genistein, Plant Natural Products, Show Synergistic Inhibitory Effects on the Growth of Human Breast Cancer MCF-7 Cells Induced by Estrogenic Pesticides," *Biochemical and Biophysical Research Communications* 233: 692–96, 1997.

24

DHEA

A steroid produced by the adrenal glands, dehydroepiandrosterone (DHEA) is formed from cholesterol and released into the bloodstream. Unlike other steroid hormones, however, DHEA peaks in the body between the ages of 25 and 30 and declines as we age. By the age of 70, we have only about 20 percent of the hormone as we did at age 25.[1]

The amount of DHEA circulating in the blood is a combination of free-formed DHEA and DHEA sulfate (DHEA-S), which is DHEA with a sulfur molecule attached to it. While most researchers consider the two forms to be virtually equal, clinical studies use both forms in oral supplements and injections.[2]

Although clinical research on DHEA is in its infancy, it has been reported that the lowest blood levels of the hormone are found in elderly patients with the greatest

physiological evidence of senescence—that is, frailty and apparent impairment of heart, lung, kidneys, and other major organs. DHEA is believed to have a regulatory influence on the immune system. Researchers at the University of Utah at Salt Lake City said that DHEA-S restored the ability of T cells to produce their normal patterns of interleukins and other immune-modulating substances following activation. Older animals treated with DHEA-S were found to generate exuberant antibody responses after receiving shots of the hormone. The modified form of DHEA has tremendous potential for clinical use in the enhancement of age-reduced immune function.[3]

Each year, many older people are urged to get flu shots, since influenza viruses are a major cause of death and hospitalization among this age group. However, the injections are not all that effective, especially for those living in nursing homes. Several studies have suggested that DHEA, which seems to enhance the activity of white blood cells, might boost the effectiveness of the shots. In one instance, DHEA injections or a placebo was given to a group of 78 volunteers whose average age was 78, and 20 volunteers under the age of 40. The hormone enhanced the antibody response to the flu shot with a very positive effect. The volunteers received either a flu shot or 3.6 to 5.6 mg of the hormone.[4]

In a study using DHEA supplements, volunteers were given 50 mg of the hormone before the flu shot and 24 mg after. Again, the hormone enhanced the immune system response to the vaccine and should be considered by health professionals when prescribing the shots to the elderly.[5]

The debate over DHEA continues. Two physicians writing in *Family Practice News* expressed differing opinions. Per Gunnar Brolinson, M.D., said that blood levels of DHEA are markedly reduced in many acute and chronic diseases, such as obesity, diabetes, high blood pressure, coronary artery disease, many cancers, immune deficiency, and autoimmune diseases. In a 1986 study involving 242 middle-aged men given 100 mg/day of DHEA for 12 years, there was a 48 percent decrease in cardiovascular disease deaths and a 36 percent decrease in mortality from other diseases. In a study of obese patients, there was a 31 percent decrease in body fat with DHEA supplements. He added that DHEA is beneficial for treating rheumatoid arthritis, lupus, scleroderma, polyneuropathy (the noninflammatory degeneration of many of the peripheral nerves), amyotrophic lateral sclerosis (Lou Gehrig's disease), and multiple sclerosis. DHEA is also beneficial for fatigue, anxiety, depression, and pain associated with osteoporosis. Brolinson would consider DHEA supplementation for those with low levels of the hormone and certain diseases such as HIV or autoimmune disease, medically significant obesity, and stress-related problems. He thinks a DHEA supplement would be useful for patients with elevated cardiovascular disease risk.

Taking an opposing view is E. Lee Rice, M.D., who stated that according to epidemiologic data, populations with low DHEA levels live longer. He added that most of the DHEA studies have been relatively small and that there is no clear-cut evidence that the hormone enhances bone status or well-being.[6]

A 12-month study using DHEA replacement therapy on 14 postmenopausal women between the ages of 60 and 70 found that bone mineral density increased in the hip from 0.744 to 0.759 g/cm. Eighty percent of the women reported increased energy and well-being. This double-blind study utilized a cream containing 10 percent DHEA, and the dosage was adjusted to the amount of the hormone in the patient's blood. Admittedly a small study, but the hormone shows promise in treating a variety of postmenopausal conditions.[7]

At the University of California School of Medicine at La Jolla, researchers conducted a double-blind study in which 13 men and

17 women were given 50 mg/day of DHEA for six months. Their ages ranged from 40 to 70, and it was found that DHEA and DHEA-S serum levels were restored to those found in young adults within two weeks of supplementation. The supplements brought a remarkable increase in physical and psychological well-being for most of the men and women, with no change in libido.[8]

In *Miracles Do Happen,* C. Norman Shealy, M.D., Ph.D., wrote that at least half of depressed patients are deficient in DHEA. Not one of the more than 1,000 depressed patients tested at the Shealy Institute in Springfield, Missouri, has had optimal levels of DHEA (550 nanogram/ deciliter or higher in women; 750 ng/dl or higher in men). A nanogram is one-billionth of a gram. Most chronically ill people who are often depressed are also deficient in this critical hormone. In fact, 99 percent of chronically depressed patients have DHEA levels far below the optimal amounts.[9]

DHEA holds promise as a new treatment for mild to moderate systemic lupus erythematosus (SLE). A study at Stanford University concerned 10 patients with mild to moderate SLE and other disorders who were given 200 mg/day of DHEA-S for three to six months. Indices for overall SLE activity were improved and cortico-steroid requirements were decreased. Of three patients with significant proteinuria (excess protein in the urine), two showed marked reduction in protein excretion, with a modest reduction in the third. DHEA was well tolerated by the patients;

the only notable side effect was a mild form of dermatitis.[10]

Clinical studies have shown that low levels of DHEA are associated with obesity, as reported in the book *Stopping the Clock*. A 1964 study revealed that DHEA was not found in urine samples of 32 elderly obese diabetics. Obese people seem to excrete less DHEA. DHEA behaves somewhat like thyroid hormone by indirectly enhancing thermogenesis, or the burning of heat by the body. It is believed that DHEA's antiobesity effects are due to its ability to block a certain enzyme called glucose-6-phosphate-dehydrogenase. By inhibiting G6PD, DHEA seems to block the body's ability to store and produce fat.[11]

In a small study conducted in 1988, five male volunteers of normal weight were given 1,600 mg/day of DHEA. Following 28 days of treatment, four of them experienced an average body fat decrease of 31 percent, although there was no change in their overall weight. The fat loss had been equaled by a gain in muscle mass. In addition, levels of low-density lipoprotein cholesterol (LDL, the so-called bad kind) had decreased 7.5 percent, thereby protecting the men against cardiovascular disease.

New York physician Ronald L. Hoffman, M.D., has measured DHEA blood and urine levels in some of his patients. He reported that DHEA has been found to help rheumatoid arthritis and lupus and is widely prescribed in Europe to extend longevity, boost the immune system, and combat nervousness and exhaustion. Those who suspect their adrenal function is low can ask their doctors to measure their DHEA levels, he recommended. DHEA is a potent hormone, however, and megadosing may lead to mood changes, excess body hair in women, scalp-hair recession or acne, or increased thyroid hormone activity.[12]

Although there is little documentation to support the claim, DHEA is being used for patients with AIDS to reduce muscle loss in the wasting syndrome. Dosages for treatment range from 750 to 1,500 mg/day. In evaluating a group of patients who were HIV-positive, HIV-negative, or with full-blown AIDS, the 10 patients with AIDS had the lowest DHEA-S readings, while 8 HIV-positive and 9 HIV-negative patients had higher concentrations.[13]

In his book, *Dr. Whitaker's Guide to Natural Healing,* Julian Whitaker, M.D., examined one study that looked at a 47-year-old woman with a lifelong learning and memory disturbance who had not been helped with conventional therapies. Her blood levels of DHEA were abnormally low. DHEA supplements brought a marked improvement, and she is now operating her own business.[14]

In another study, the blood levels of DHEA in Alzheimer's patients were lowering, by 48 percent, the body's ability to respond normally to stimuli. The level of DHEA required to improve brain power appears to be 25 to 100 mg/day, Whitaker said. Human and animal studies have found the hormone to be exceptionally safe; however, in dosages greater than 90 mg/day, masculinization has been reported in a few

women (facial hair and a deeper voice). The side effects cease with a reduction in the dosage.

The vasodilative effects of DHEA-S might be beneficial in the treatment of preeclampsia. Preeclampsia, which develops in late pregnancy, is a toxic condition associated by a rise in blood pressure, excessive weight gain, severe headache, generalized edema or swelling, and other conditions. In a study, pregnant women were given 200 mg of DHEA dissolved in dextrose. There was no effect on blood pressure, heart rate, or other variables, but the hormone vasodilates the ophthalmic artery, thus increasing blood flow. Similar changes may occur in other cerebral vessels.[15]

In *Vanity Fair,* Gail Sheehy wrote of several well-known DHEA researchers who take the supplement. William Regelson, M.D., of the Medical College of Virginia at Richmond, said: "I take DHEA because I'm trying to delay aging as a physiological event in my life." Samuel Yen, M.D., one of the nation's leading DHEA researchers, added that DHEA steadily increases muscle strength and physical mobility in most men and women, while making bodies leaner. Like melatonin, the hormone promotes deeper, more restorative sleep. Yen said that the greatest benefits of the hormone are usually psychological and very subtle. Norman Orentreich, M.D., a renowned New York dermatologist and researcher, has done studies on DHEA for the National Institute of Aging and also takes the hormone. Like Yen, he is concerned about hormone overkill and that consumers will overdose without a careful monitoring of the hormone levels in their blood.[16]

DHEA is found in small amounts in Mexican wild yam. Suggested supplement doses range from 5 to 50 mg/day, with a maximum dose for women at 25 mg/day and 50 mg/day for men. See your health-care practitioner. To learn about another form of DHEA, see the entry on 7-keto DHEA.

References

1. Ebeling, Pertti, and Veikko Kolvisto, "Physiological Importance of Dehydroepiandrosterone," *The Lancet* 343: 1479–81, 1994.

2. Shealy, C. Norman, *DHEA: The Youth and Health Hormone* (New Canaan, Conn.: Keats Publishing, 1996).

3. Ershler, William B., *Intriguing Insights into Longevity* (Chicago: Encyclopaedia Britannica, 1993), 395.

4. Degelau, J., et al., "The Effect of DHEAs on Influenza Vaccination in Aging Adults," *Journal of the American Geriatrics Society* 45: 747–51, 1997.

5. Evans, T. G., et al., "The Use of Oral Dehydroepiandrosterone Sulfate as an Adjuvant in Tetanus and Influenza Vaccination of the Elderly," *Vaccine* 14(16): 1531–37, 1996.

6. Brolinson, Per Gunnar, and E. Lee Rice, "Is DHEA Useful to Help Prevent and Treat Certain Illnesses?" *Family Practice News*, March 1, 1998, Vol. 17.

7. Labrie, F., et al., "Effect of 12-Month Dehydroepiandrosterone Replacement Therapy on Bone, Vagina, and Endometrium in Postmenopausal Women," *Journal of Clinical Endocrinology Metabolism* 82: 3498–505, 1997.

8. Morales, Arlene, et al., "Effects of Replacement Dose of Dehydroepiandrosterone in Men and Women of Advancing Age," *Journal of Clinical Endocrinology and Metabolism* 78: 1360–67, 1994.

9. Shealy, C. Norman, *Miracles Do Happen* (Rockport, Mass.: Element, 1995), 193.

10. Van Vollenhoven, Ronald, "An Open Study of Dehydroepiandrosterone in Systemic Lupus Erythematosus," *Arthritis and Rheumatism* 37(9): 1305–10, Sept. 1994.

11. Klatz, Ronald, and Robert Goldman, *Stopping the Clock* (New Canaan, Conn.: Keats Publishing, 1996), 57ff.

12. Hoffman, Ronald L., *Intelligent Medicine* (New York: Simon & Schuster, 1997), 101.

13. Centurelli, Maria A., and Marie A. Abate, "The Role of Dehydroepiandrosterone in AIDS," *Annals of Pharmacotherapy* 31: 639–42, May 1997.

14. Whitaker, Julian, *Dr. Whitaker's Guide to Natural Healing* (Rocklin, Calif.: Prima Publishing, 1995), 97–98.

15. Hata, Toshiyuki, et al., "Effect of Dehydroepiandrosterone Sulfate on Ophthalmic Artery Flow Velocity Wave Forms in Full-Term Pregnant Women," *American Journal of Perinatology* 12(2): 135–37, March 1995.

16. Sheehy, Gail, "Endless Youth," *Vanity Fair*, June 1996, 76ff.

25

DLPA

L-phenylalanine is an essential amino acid that plays a part in a number of biochemical processes concerning the synthesis of neurotransmitters such as dopamine, norepinephrine, and epinephrine in the brain. Researchers have concluded that L-phenylalanine can increase mental alertness, help control addictive substance abuse, promote sexual arousal, and release hormones that can curb appetite. D-phenylalanine is a nonnutrient amino acid that breaks down opiatelike substances known as enkephalins in the brain. Consequently, D-phenylalanine is said to help alleviate chronic pain.[1]

DL-phenylalanine (DLPA), available over the counter, is an equal mixture of D-phenylalanine and L-phenylalanine and reportedly is effective in treating chronic pain related to arthritis, fibrositis, and other complaints.

In 1972, Candace Pert, M.D., and Solomon Snyder, M.D., of the Johns Hopkins University School of Medicine at Baltimore discovered receptors for morphine in human brain tissue. They theorized that the brain apparently produces its own variety of morphine. In 1975, the first of these morphinelike substances was discovered and named endorphin—a contraction of endogenous (made by the body) and morphine.[2]

Since then, researchers have found that endorphins can block certain types of chronic pain and depression. In fact, one of these endorphins, beta endorphin, is 18 to 50 times more powerful than morphine. Another, dynorphin, is over 500 times more powerful.

DLPA keeps endorphin levels high by interfering with endorphin-engulfing enzymes made by the body. Therefore,

DLPA enables endorphin levels to build up sufficiently to reduce many forms of chronic pain and depression. Arnold Fox, M.D., prescribes DLPA for most of his patients with these complaints. He recommends 750 mg at breakfast and again at lunch. Beneficial results have been achieved in about 80 percent of his patients.

Unlike L-phenylalanine, DLPA is less likely to raise blood pressure and may be useful as an adjunctive treatment for depression, according to Andrew Weil, M.D.[3] If you have high blood pressure and want to use phenylalanine for depression or increased energy, Weil recommends 1,000 to 1,500 mg of DLPA on an empty stomach early in the morning, and 100 mg of vitamin B_6, 500 mg of vitamin C, and a piece of fruit or glass of fruit juice later in the day. Monitor your intake for any change in arousal, energy, or mood. For those with high blood pressure, Weil suggests starting with 100 mg of DLPA and gradually raising the dose over a few weeks, monitoring your blood pressure regularly.

DLPA has been found useful in alleviating acute or chronic pain that athletes experience after injury. The theory is that the substance protects the endorphins in the body from destruction, thereby allowing them to distribute their morphinelike relief throughout the injured area. Recommended dosages range from 500 to 1,500 mg/day. People with phenylketonuria should not take any form of phenylalanine since they cannot properly metabolize this amino acid.[4]

While there is limited research for DLPA, the use of this important nutrient apparently is being neglected. This is another natural substance that deserves more attention for pain relief, depression, and other health problems.

References

1. Hendler, Sheldon Saul, *The Doctor's Vitamin and Mineral Encyclopedia* (New York: Simon and Schuster, 1990), 225–26.

2. Fox, Arnold, "Real Pain Relief," *Let's Live,* Nov. 1998,32–35.

3. Weil, Andrew, *Natural Health, Natural Medicine* (Boston: Houghton Mifflin, 1990), 222–23.

4. Gastelu, Daniel, and Fred Hatfield, *Dynamic Nutrition for Maximum Performance* (Garden City Park, N.Y.: Avery Publishing Group, 1997), 42.

26

Echinacea

Echinacea was introduced into Western medicine by a doctor named H.C.F. Meyer, of Pawnee City, Nebraska, who learned about the herb's therapeutic value from Native Americans around 1871. Nine species of echinacea grow in North America, although *E. purpurea, E. angustifolia,* and *E. pallida* are the most common. Ironically, most of the clinical studies on echinacea have been conducted in Europe, where the North American varieties were taken for study.[1]

David Taylor reported that 80 percent of the world's population relies on traditional medicine and not on Western medicine to treat disease. He mentioned an article in the *New England Journal of Medicine* in 1993, which stated that in more than 350 studies, echinacea has been shown to stimulate growth and development of immune cells and to exhibit interferon-like, antiviral activity. Interferon is a group of antiviral glycoproteins that the body produces to counteract parasites, bacteria, and so forth.[2]

Echinacea is by far the most popular antiviral herb, according to James A. Duke, Ph.D. Containing caffeic acid, chicoric acid, and echinacin, echinacea is an immune stimulant that helps the body defend itself more effectively. Echinacea may increase the body's level of properdin, a compound that activates a specific part of the immune system called the complementary pathway. It is responsible for sending disease-fighting white blood cells into infected areas to battle viruses and bacteria. Duke also recommends the herb for athlete's foot, Lyme disease, yeast infections, laryngitis, and other health problems. Combined with goldenseal, it is an ideal treatment for bladder infections. If you taste an extract of echinacea, your tongue may tingle or feel slightly numb, but this effect is harmless.[3] In fact, it indicates that the echinacea is of good quality.

At Elisabeth Hospital, Uppsala, Sweden, researchers conducted a placebo-controlled study to investigate the efficacy of several echinacea preparations in the treatment of the common cold. In the study, 246 of 559 healthy volunteers caught a cold and took two tablets three times daily of Echinaforce, an *E. purpurea* preparation, or an *E. purpurea* concentrate. These preparations were more effective than a special echinacea extract or placebo. The researchers concluded that echinacea concentrate, as well as Echinaforce, represent a low-risk and effective alternative treatment for the common cold.[4]

Thirty-two double-blind studies suggest that echinacea can combat colds and flu, according to Harold H. Bloomfield, M.D. To fight a cold or flu, he recommends using standardized concentrations of echinacea and following the label directions. Check to ensure that the product is standardized for echinacoside, the active compound in the herb, and that it contains *E. purpurea* and/or *E. angustifolia*. Take the preparation at the first sign of a cold or flu and continue the therapy for one week. Echinacea has been known to trigger watery eyes in those allergic to daisies, since it is a member of the daisy family. The herb is so safe that it can be used by six-month-old babies to fight viral respiratory infections.[5]

E. angustifolia and *E. purpurea* are recommended for acute treatment (10 to 14 days) of colds and flu, reported Leo Galland, M.D., a New York physician. The dose needed is 900 mg/day, and he prefers *E. purpurea* in capsules or extracts.[6]

"Some people with chronic or recurrent infections benefit from taking echinacea for prolonged periods, especially during the winter," Galland said. "I recommend you take it continuously for eight weeks at a time, then stop for a week or two between each eight-week period to avoid tolerance."

In a short-term study at the University of Florida at Gainesville, Susan Percival has shown that *E. purpurea* can stimulate the immune system. Ten male college students were given 150 mg/day of active ingredients in echinacea, known as echinosides, for four days. On the first and last days of the trial, Percival drew blood and segregated the neutrophils. These white blood cells react to infectious agents by generating superoxide anion, a highly reactive and biologically damaging oxidant. Neutrophils collected after the herbal treatment produced three times the amount of superoxide anion as those taken at the beginning of the study.[7]

In human and animal experiments, *E. purpurea* preparations have produced immune effects, and the number of white blood cells and spleen cells are increased. The capacity for phagocytosis is activated. Phagocytes are white blood cells that destroy foreign particles that enter the body. The herb provides supportive therapy for colds and chronic infections of the respiratory and lower urinary tract. For external use, *E. purpurea* is said to be useful for healing wounds and chronic ulcerations. Allergic reactions may surface in susceptible individuals.[8]

Mixed results were found when researchers at Ludwig-Maximilians-Universitat in Munich tested five echinacea preparations for boosting the immune system. In two studies, phagocytic activity was significantly enhanced compared with placebo, but in two other studies no significant effects were observed. There were no side effects with any of the preparations. The study reported an immune system boost from echinacea in two preparations, with negative results in two other trials. However, the research team admitted that three studies were difficult to interpret due to the different methods of measuring phagocytosis, the relevant changes in phagocytic activity within most placebo and treatment groups, and the small sample size. Future trials should be performed on ill patients rather than on healthy volunteers.[9]

Researchers at Technische Universitat in Munich stated that a prophylactic effect of echinacea extracts could not be found, but based on this and two other studies, they agreed that echinacea products might reduce infections by between 10 and 20 percent.

In a study in Australia, a 37-year-old woman experienced anaphylactic shock after ingesting echinacea and other substances and had to be transported to the hospital. It was suggested that those with an inherited disposition to asthma, hay fever, and hives should consult a physician before taking echinacea. Anaphylactic shock is a severe and sometimes fatal reaction to a specific antigen (food, wasp venom, penicillin, plants, etc.). It produces respiratory symptoms, fainting, and itching.[11]

If you are susceptible to colds, flu, and other infections, consider echinacea instead of the various over-the-counter preparations that do not strengthen the immune system to fight the infection naturally.

References

1. Foster, Steven, and Varro E. Tyler, *Tyler's Honest Herbal* (New York: Haworth Herbal Press, 1999), 143ff.
2. Taylor, David, "Herbal Medicine at the Crossroads," *Environmental Health Perspectives* 104(9): 924–28, 1996.
3. Duke, James A., *The Green Pharmacy* (Emmaus, Pa.: Rodale Press, 1997), 69, 83, 306, 314, 449–50.
4. Brinkeborn, R. M., et al., "Echinaforce and Other Echinacea Fresh Plant Preparations in the Treatment of the Common Cold: A Randomized, Placebo-Controlled, Double-Blind Clinical Trial," *Phytomedicine* 6: 1–6, March 1999.
5. Bloomfield, Harold H., *Healing Anxiety with Herbs* (New York: HarperCollins, 1998), 61–62.

6. Galland, Leo, *The Four Pillars of Healing* (New York: Random House, 1997), 244.

7. Raloff, Janet, "New Support for Echinacea's Benefits," *Science News* 155(13): 207, March 27, 1999.

8. Blumenthal, Mark, senior ed., *The Complete German Commission E Monographs* (Boston: Integrative Medicine Communications, 1998), 122–23. Also, American Botanical Council, Austin, Texas.

9. Melchart, D., et al., "Results of Five Randomized Studies on the Immuno- modulatory Activity of Preparations of Echinacea," *Journal of Alternative Complementary Medicine* 1: 145–60, Summer 1995.

10. Melchart, D., et al., "Echinacea Root Extracts for the Prevention of Upper Respiratory Tract Infections: A Double-Blind, Placebo-Controlled Randomized Trial," *Archives of Family Medicine* 7: 541–45, Nov.–Dec. 1998.

11. Mullins, Raymond J., "Echinacea-Associated Anaphylaxis," *Medical Journal of Australia* 168: 170–71, Feb. 16, 1998.

27

Ester-C

Ascorbic acid (vitamin C) has been a favorite nutrient of researchers ever since Albert Szent-Gyorgyi, Ph.D., a Hungarian-American, was awarded the Nobel Prize for isolating the vitamin in 1937.

While vitamin C is commonly used in the prevention and treatment of the common cold, some forms of cancer, gum disease, backache, male infertility, heart disease, cataracts, and certain forms of mental illness, some consumers are unable to take ascorbic acid because of its acidity to the stomach. Many have found a reliable substitute in Ester-C, a polyascorbate that contains various derivatives of vitamin C without the acidity. Ester-C is nonacidic, has a neutral pH of 7.0 (the same as distilled water), and therefore does not cause the acidic reactions, flatulence, and diarrhea that some people experience with ascorbic acid.

As the name *polyascorbate* implies, Ester-C is a mixture of several forms of vitamin C, including calcium ascorbate; ascorbate and dehydroascorbate (the form that vitamin C assumes in the cells); various metabolites of vitamin C, such as aldonic acids; calcium carbonate; water; and a small amount of lecithin.

Anthony J. Verlangieri, Ph.D., and Marilyn J. Bush, Ph.D., reported that Ester-C is absorbed more readily than ascorbic acid. In addition, it is more fat soluble (ascorbic acid is water soluble) and passes through the mucosal barriers more rapidly than regular vitamin C. Ascorbic acid was found in the urine of ascorbate-treated animals twice as early as those given Ester-C, suggesting a more rapid excretion of vitamin C.[1]

The researchers added, "If the unique structure of Ester-C promotes more rapid absorption and delayed excretion of ascorbic acid compared to the salt or acid form of the vitamin, as the results of our experiments clearly imply, it may be advantageous in increasing circulating ascorbic acid concentration and promoting rapid tissue saturation."

Verlangieri recommends 1,000 to 2,000 mg/day of vitamin C to prevent cardiovascular disease in nondiabetics and to possibly even reverse accelerated cardiovascular disease in diabetics. Since vitamin C may cause a false-positive urine test for glucose, he also recommends blood testing. He has also demonstrated in his research that a lack of vitamins C and E contributes to hardening of the arteries, and that therapy using these vitamins slows the progress of atherosclerosis and may even reverse it.[2]

Ester-C products were originally developed to provide a form of vitamin C that does not have the disadvantages of having to supplement with large amounts of ascorbic acid. Therefore, the pH-neutral form of vitamin C (Ester-C) presented an attractive alternative.[3] These products allow dietary supplementation of the mineral ion used in the preparation of the neutral ascorbate salt; for example, calcium, magnesium, and zinc. In addition, neutralization during the manufacture of Ester-C prevents gas (carbon dioxide) from being generated in the stomach. Gas bloating and discomfort can occur after taking products containing a dry blend of ascorbic acid and calcium carbonate powders.

In a clinical study, Jonathan V. Wright, M.D., evaluated 12 men ranging in age from 27 to 45 to see how long Ester-C remained in their blood. For one week prior to the study, the volunteers were instructed not to eat citrus products or large amounts of green leafy vegetables. The men were divided into three groups. The first group was given Ester-C; the second, ascorbic acid; and the third, citric acid.[4]

Blood samples were taken at the beginning of the study and at intervals of 4, 8, and 24 hours after beginning the supplements. After 24 hours, urine and oxalate levels were studied. Two days into the study, the men were asked to switch to another supplement. The Ester-C group took citric acid; the citrate group, ascorbic acid; and the ascorbate group, Ester-C. The results demonstrated that Ester-C increased ascorbate levels in the white blood cells four times more than regular ascorbic acid, and there was only one-third as much of the substance lost in urine without being utilized. Some researchers have indicated that between 78 and 88 percent of regular ascorbic acid passes through the body without being absorbed and utilized.

If you are satisfied with the vitamin C that you are now taking, continue with that formula. If ascorbic acid upsets your stomach, however, you may wish to switch to Ester-C. Your health food store has a variety of Ester-C formulas, including regular Ester-C, Ester-C with bioflavonoids,

Ester-C with mineral polyascorbates (calcium, magnesium, and zinc), Ester-C in skin-care products, and other formulas.

References

1. Bush, Marilyn J., and Anthony J. Verlangieri, "An Acute Study on the Relative Gastro-Intestinal Absorption of a Novel Form of Calcium Ascorbate," *Research Communications in Chemical Pathology and Pharmacology* 57: 1, July 1987.

2. Evans, Susan, and Barbara Lago, "Hardening of the Arteries," *Pharmacy Report,* Spring and Summer, 1988.

3. Brunzie, Gerald F., "Ascorbic Acid Metabolites Play a Role in Vitamin C-Supplementation," *International Clinical Nutrition Review* 10: 1, Jan. 1990.

4. Wright, Jonathan V., and Raymond M. Suen, "A Human Clinical Study of Ester-C vs L-Ascorbic Acid," 1987, unpublished.

28

Evening Primrose Oil

In his New York City practice, Leo Galland, M.D., estimates that 15 percent of his patients are unable to metabolize omega-6 essential fatty acids (EFAs). For these patients with dry skin, dry or unruly hair, dandruff, brittle nails, menstrual cramps, premenstrual breast tenderness, and other complaints, he usually prescribes evening primrose oil, borage oil, or black currant seed oil, all of which contain the EFA gamma-linolenic acid (GLA). Omega-6s are also found in corn, sunflower, safflower, and other oils, but a deficiency in these EFAs, which cannot be synthesized by the body but must come from the diet, can cause impairment of growth and fertility, hormonal disturbances, and immunologic abnormalities. Galland recommends four to six capsules of evening primrose oil; two or three capsules of borage oil; or three or

four capsules of black currant seed oil daily, assuming that each capsule contains 500 mg of oil.[1]

Galland generally reserves GLA supplements for those whose dry skin does not respond to omega-3 (fish oil) supplements. Since the omega-3 and omega-6 EFAs compete with one another in the body, giving fish oil to a person who needs GLA may actually increase that person's omega-6 deficit.

"An increase in these symptoms with omega-3 supplements is almost surely a sign to switch to GLA," Galland added. "Controlled studies have demonstrated therapeutic benefits for people suffering from arthritis, eczema, and premenstrual syndrome. EFA therapy does not treat disease, it improves cellular function."

According to David F. Horrobin, Ph.D., who has been researching EFAs in diabetics for 13 years, linolenic acid is the major essential fatty acid in the diet. However, it is not the acid itself but rather its metabolites—GLA, dihomogammalinolenic acid, and arachidonic acid—that are required for normal function of neurons and nerve microcirculation. In diabetes, the conversion of linoleic acid to GLA is impaired, and therefore the neurons are deprived of the metabolites they need. Clinical trials have used 480 mg/day of GLA in the form of evening primrose oil to treat diabetic neuropathy.[2] In an animal study at the University of Cincinnati Medical Center in Ohio, researchers found that evening primrose oil, as well as linoleic acid from safflower oil, also provided protection against diabetic neuropathy, one of the most crippling complications of diabetes, since it damages nerve fibers.[3]

At the Metropolitan Geriatric Hospital in Tokyo, 4 g of evening primrose oil, 2.4 g of sardine oil, and 200 mg of vitamin E all were useful in improving abnormal fat and thromboxane A2 metabolism in diabetic patients. Thromboxanes are a series of substances that cause constriction of vascular and bronchial smooth muscle and promote blood coagulation.[4]

A London study evaluated 111 patients with diabetic neuropathy at seven treatment centers with a double-blind, placebo-controlled study. The volunteers were given 12 capsules daily of evening primrose oil—equal to 480 mg/day of gamma-linolenic acid—or a placebo. During the one-year trial, the supplements brought a significant improvement to the patients receiving it. It was concluded that GLA beneficially affected the course of diabetic neuropathy and may impede deterioration in mild cases. Neither treatment group experienced any significant side effects.[5]

Another study in England evaluated 40 patients with rheumatoid arthritis and upper gastrointestinal lesions due to NSAIDs. Nineteen patients were given 5 g/day of evening primrose oil (equal to 540 mg/day of GLA), and 21 volunteers received a placebo of 6 g/day of olive oil. A significant reduction in morning stiffness with GLA was noted at three months, and a reduction in pain and articular index was observed at six months with olive oil. The researchers recommend evening primrose oil for mild rheumatoid arthritis only. Since olive oil can be useful in treating rheumatoid arthritis, it should no longer be used as a placebo, but should be investigated on its own as a treatment for arthritis symptoms.[6]

Although borage seed oil was the source of GLA in this study with rheumatoid arthritis patients, the researchers said that evening primrose oil is also a good source of GLA. In a study at Massachusetts Medical Center in Worcester, 19 patients with rheumatoid arthritis were given 1.4 g daily of GLA, while 18 others received cottonseed oil as a placebo. GLA reduced the number of tender joints by 36 percent; the tender joint score by 45 percent; swollen joint count by 28 percent; and swollen joint score by 41 percent. There was no improvement in the placebo group. None of the patients withdrew from the treatment group, even though they were being given a very high dose of GLA.[7]

In *Natural Prescriptions,* Robert M. Giller, M.D., wrote that evening primrose oil has been helpful in lessening some of the symptoms associated with PMS, such as cramping, irritability, breast discomfort, anxiety, tiredness, and swollen fingers and ankles. One study found that while women had a significant decrease in symptoms after their first cycle, the best results came after the fifth cycle. He recommended four 500-mg capsules of evening primrose oil in the morning and four in the evening. If no relief comes after five cycles, discontinue the therapy. People with eczema have a problem digesting essential fatty acids, and evening primrose oil brings relief to about half of the sufferers when taken as a supplement or used topically. For eczema, Giller suggests 1,000 mg three times daily. As symptoms subside, reduce the dose to 500 mg daily. The oil can be rubbed on the skin twice daily.[8]

In a general review article on the role of diet and nutrients on skin problems, S. C. Rackett et al. said that fish oil, evening primrose oil, and Chinese herbal teas may be useful therapy for atopic dermatitis (eczema, etc.). The authors also discussed vitamins A, B_6, C, D, E, and the minerals selenium and zinc.[9]

In nine double-blind studies, evening primrose oil has been found to be an effective treatment for eczema, and was especially useful in reducing itching, according to Melvyn Werbach, M.D., in *Healing with Food.* He recommends 1 to 2 g three times daily. Evening primrose oil has been shown to benefit some women with PMS, even those with treatment-resistant symptoms. In one case, a woman who complained of irritability or depression several days prior to menses was relieved of all symptoms with evening primrose oil and vitamin B_6, which is necessary for metabolizing the oil. Progesterone was ineffective in relieving the woman's symptoms. The suggested dosage of evening primrose oil for PMS is 1.5 g twice daily.[10]

If you are suffering from one of the disorders related to an EFA, ask your holistic physician for guidelines.

References

1. Galland, Leo, *The Four Pillars of Healing* (New York: Random House, 1997), 127, 144–47.

2. Hamilton, Kirk, "Diabetes Mellitus and Essential Fatty Acids," *Clinical Pearls with The Experts Speak* (Sacramento, Calif.: Health Associates Medical Group, 1998), 39. Also, David F. Horrobin, "Essential Fatty Acids in the Management of Inspired Nerve Function in Diabetes," *Diabetes* 46 (Suppl. 2): S90–S93, 1997.

3. Barcelli, Uno O., et al., "High Linoleic Acid Diets Ameliorate Diabetic Neuropathy in Rats," *American Journal of Kidney Diseases* 16(3): 244–51, 1990.

4. Takahashi, R., et al., "Evening Primrose Oil and Fish Oil in Non-Insulin-Dependent Diabetes," *Prostaglandins, Leukotrienes, and Essential Fatty Acids* 49: 569–71, 1993.

5. Keen, Harry, et al., "Treatment of Diabetic Neuropathy with Gamma-Linolenic Acid," *Diabetes Care* 16(1): 8–15, Jan. 1993.

6. Brzeski, M., et al., "Evening Primrose Oil in Patients with Rheumatoid Arthritis and Side-Effects of Non-Steroidal Anti-inflammatory Drugs," *British Journal of Rheumatology* 30: 370–72, 1991.

7. Leventhal, Lawrence J., et al., "Treatment of Rheumatoid Arthritis with Gamma-Linolenic Acid," *Annals of Internal Medicine* 119(9): 867–73, Nov. 1, 1993.

8. Giller, Robert M., and Kathy Matthews, *Natural Prescriptions* (New York: Carol Southern Books, 1994), 133, 279.

9. Rackett, S. C., et al., "Dermatol: The Role of Dietary Manipulation in the Prevention and Treatment of Cutaneous Disorders," *Journal of the American Academy of Dermatology* 29: 447–61, 1993.

10. Werbach, Melvyn, *Healing with Food* (New York: HarperPerennial, 1993), 125, 330.

29

Feverfew

Nine out of 10 Americans experience at least one headache a year, and the cause of this painful condition remains elusive. Headache is the main cause of absenteeism in the workplace, with 150 million lost workdays and productivity losses estimated at $15 billion annually.[1]

Tension headaches, which result in the tightening of the muscles in the face, neck, and scalp, are often caused by stress or poor posture. Migraines are severe, incapacitating headaches often accompanied by visual and/or stomach disturbances. Cluster headaches bring intense pain behind one eye and can last for weeks or months.[2] Some of the causes of headache include hangover, irregular meals (which disrupt blood sugar levels), prolonged travel, poor posture, a noisy or stuffy work area, excessive sleep, certain foods (cheese, chocolate, red wine), food additives, sinusi-

tis, toothache, an ear infection, head injury, and cervical osteoarthritis.

Feverfew *(Tanacetum parthenium)* has been used since the time of Dioscorides (A.D. 78) to reduce the frequency and severity of migraine, as well as migraine associated with nausea and vomiting. The beneficial constituent in the plant is said to be parthenolide, a sesquiterpene lactone whose concentration varies from plant to plant. Canadian researchers have suggested that a quality feverfew product should contain a minimum concentration of 0.2 percent parthenolide.[3] Feverfew is a popular migraine remedy in Europe. It has some of the same anti-inflammatory effects as aspirin without the side effects. However, it usually must be taken for several weeks before its effects are felt.[4]

In a four-month double-blind trial in England, information was evaluated on 59 of 60 patients, each suffering from a migraine headache. Treatment with feverfew brought a reduction in the number and severity of migraine attacks during each two-month test period; there was also less vomiting. The 82-mg feverfew capsules contained the equivalent of about two medium-size feverfew leaves. Little relief was felt among the placebo volunteers, who were given capsules containing dried cabbage leaves.[5]

Painful symptoms of migraine and arthritis can often be alleviated with feverfew, especially in patients unable to obtain relief from conventional therapies. The plant's pharmacology inhibits prostaglandin 2, lessens platelet aggregation, and inhibits platelet deposition. It is now known that the parthenolides in feverfew inhibit prostaglandins and leukotrienes, two of the most important inflammatory substances in the human body. They also inhibit the production of arachidonic acid (a precursor of prostaglandins) on the surface of blood platelets. Consumption of these parthenolide phytochemicals reduces the inflammation associated with migraines and arthritis. By stopping platelet aggregation and its deposition on collagen (a constituent of connective tissue), hardening of the arteries, stroke, and other conditions are also indirectly influenced.[6]

At the University of London, 17 patients with migraines participated in a double-blind study. Eight were given capsules containing freeze-dried feverfew powder, and nine received a look-alike capsule. The placebo patients had a significant increase in the frequency and severity of headache, nausea, and vomiting during the early months of the therapy. The study provides evidence that feverfew, taken prophylactically, prevents attacks of migraines. Further studies are warranted, preferably with a formulation controlled for its sesquiterpene lactone content. Given the variation in sesquiterpene lactone content between feverfew plants, the researchers suggested that commercial preparations be standardized to ensure efficacy.[7]

A 1983 survey found that 70 percent of 270 migraine sufferers who had ingested feverfew daily for prolonged periods claimed that the herb decreased the frequency and/or intensity of their attacks. This improvement prompted two clinical investigations of the therapeutic and preventive effects of feverfew in migraine treatment. In one of these trials, feverfew was clearly demonstrated to treat migraine attacks. Follow-up studies have shown that the herb works by inhibiting the release of blood-vessel-dilating substances from platelets, by inhibiting the production of inflammatory substances, and by reestablishing proper blood vessel tone. In one of the studies, 82 mg of powdered leaves were effective in preventing an attack, but a higher dose (1 or 2 g) is necessary during an acute attack.[8]

Feverfew is well tolerated and no serious side effects have been reported with its use. However, chewing the leaves may cause ulcers in the mouth and swelling of the lips and tongue.

References

1. National Cancer Institute, press release, 7th International Headache Congress, Toronto, Ontario, Canada, September 15–20, 1995.
2. Clayman, Charles B., ed., *The American Medical Association Home Medical Encyclopedia* (New York: Random House, 1989), 507.
3. Robbers, James E., and Varro E. Tyler, *Tyler's Herbs of Choice* (New York: Haworth Herbal Press, 1999), 173–74.
4. Giller, Robert M., and Kathy Matthews, *Natural Prescriptions* (New York: Carol Southern Books, 1994), 251.
5. Murphy, J. J., et al., "Randomized Double-Blind Placebo-Controlled Trial of Feverfew in Migraine Prevention," *The Lancet,* July 23, 1998, 189–92.
6. Grauds, Constance, "Treating Migraine and Arthritis with Feverfew," *Pharmacy Times,* July 1995, 32–33.
7. Johnson, E. S., et al., "Efficacy of Feverfew as Prophylactic Treatment of Migraine," *British Medical Journal* 291: 569–73, Aug. 31, 1985.
8. Murray, Michael T., *Natural Alternatives to Over-the-Counter and Prescription Drugs* (New York: William Morrow and Co., 1994), 193ff.

30

Fiber

The term *fiber* indicates the complex of carbohydrates and other substances found mainly in the cell walls of food plants. These substances include cellulose, hemicelluloses, gums, mucilages, pectic substances, and lignin. Because they are poorly digested, these substances have little nutritional value but play a major role in keeping us healthy. Other terms for fiber include nonnutritive fiber, crude fiber, bulk, roughage, undigestible residue, and others.[1]

During the Middle Ages, when food was scarce, Europeans often extended cereal flours with flourlike materials made from ground acorns, bark, beans, nuts, peas, and twigs. Early American colonists gained fiber from beans, unrefined corn, cornmeal, fruits, and vegetables. Throughout the 1800s, health and religious concerns promoted the advantages of diets based mainly on whole grains, vegetables, and fruits. This concern was motivated by the high consumption of alcoholic beverages during the 1820s and 1830s. Sailors and laborers were often given part of their wages in liquor, and children were encouraged to drink hard cider, which actually was safer than the drinking water.

A former Presbyterian minister, Sylvester Graham (1794–1851), after whom graham crackers and graham flour were named, began promoting vegetarianism, abstinence from alcoholic beverages, and the use of coarse, unbolted flour for making high-fiber breads. Mother Ellen Harmon White, a leader of the Seventh-Day Adventists, was influenced by Graham and introduced whole grains into the diets of patients at the famous Battle Creek Sanitarium in Michigan, which she founded and which was managed by Dr.

John Harvey Kellogg and his brother, Will.

Interest in whole-grain breads and vegetarianism gradually waned until the 1960s, when a number of British physicians, notably Denis Burkitt, Peter Cleave, Neil Painter, and Hugh Trowell, reported that certain African people who consumed high-fiber diets had much lower rates of various gastrointestinal diseases than people in England and the United States. Many high-fiber products began appearing in the marketplace.

In the June 9, 1973, issue of *The Lancet,* Drs. R. F. Harvey, E. W. Pomare, and K. W. Heaton of the Bristol Royal Infirmary in England described an experiment in which they gave 20 people bran while evaluating their regular diet of refined carbohydrates (white bread, noodles, spaghetti, etc.). On the refined-food diet, the transit time for stools was 3.8 days. In other words, food eaten at one meal did not appear in stools until almost four days later, indicating a very slow passage of time and hence considerable constipation. After the volunteers were given 30 g/day of bran, the transit time was reduced to 2.4 days.[2]

Fiber is divided into two categories: soluble and insoluble. Soluble fibers dissolve in water and become sticky. These include pectin, found in fruits, nuts, legumes, and some vegetables; guar; carrageenan; other gums found in seaweed and algae; and mucilages, found in plant seeds and some plant secretions. Insoluble fibers do not dissolve and therefore pass through the digestive tract relatively unchanged. These include cellulose, found in bran, whole grains, and vegetables; hemicellulose, found in fruits, nuts, whole grains, and vegetables; and lignin, found in bran, nuts, whole grains, and the skins of fruits.[3]

A fact sheet from the *American Family Physician,* Kansas City, Missouri, recommends eating five servings of fruits and vegetables daily. Fruits and vegetables that contain high amounts of fiber include apples, oranges, broccoli, cauliflower, berries, pears, brussels sprouts, lettuce, figs, prunes, carrots, and potatoes. It is also recommended that white bread be replaced with whole-grain breads and cereals, and white rice with brown rice. Other high-fiber foods include bran muffins, oatmeal, popcorn, and multigrain cereals, both cooked and dry. Dry bran cereal should be eaten for breakfast, and one-fourth cup of wheat bran should be added to cooked cereal, applesauce, or meat loaf each week. Cooked beans should be consumed once a week.[4]

Researchers in Boston found that in evaluating 43,881 male health professionals between the ages of 40 and 75, insoluble fiber intake was inversely associated with the risk of diverticular disease. The association was especially strong for cellulose.[5] Diverticular disease is characterized by the formation of small sacs called diverticula in weakened segments of the large intestine. In 10 to 25 percent of the cases, diverticula become filled with feces and the pouches become inflamed, causing abdominal pain, nausea, vomiting, diarrhea, and/or constipation. Blood may be seen in the stools. The main cause of the disease seems to be highly processed, low-fiber diets.

In a double-blind, crossover trial for two consecutive four-week periods, Italian researchers evaluated 24 patients who were given 20 g of bran or a placebo during a 24-hour period. Bran was more effective than placebo in improving bowel frequency and transit time. During the bran treatment, transit time became normal only in the patients with slow colonic transit. The placebo treatment consisted of saccharose, cocoa powder, and maltose.[6]

In a study involving 698 male and 494 female Japanese, Caucasian, Filipino, Hawaiian, and Chinese patients with adenocarcinoma of the colon or rectum, compared with 1,192 controls, a strong dose-dependent inverse association was seen in both sexes with fiber intake measured as crude fiber, dietary fiber, and nonstarch polysaccharides. However, the protective effect of fiber was limited to fiber from vegetable sources. There was the same magnitude of association for soluble and insoluble vegetable fiber.[7]

In a rat model, dietary wheat-bran fiber was protective against colon cancer. Fiber products in the gut can produce compounds such as butyric acid, which may have a protective effect on colonic and fecal pH.[8]

At the Arizona Cancer Center at Tucson, a research team evaluated a randomized, double-blind trial of wheat-bran fiber at 2.0 and 13.5 g/day in the form of cereal and supplemented with calcium carbonate at 250 to 1,500 mg/day. High-dose wheat-bran fiber and calcium supplements, given for nine months, are associated with statistically significant reductions in both total and secondary fecal bile acid concentrations and excretion rates in patients with colon cancer.[9]

A plant-based diet low in calories from fat, high in fiber, and rich in legumes (especially soybeans), whole-grain foods, vegetables, and fruits was found to reduce the risk of endometrial cancer in a study involving 332 patients with endometrial cancer and 511 controls.[10]

Researchers at the Thomas Hospital in London reviewed the rationale for the role of dietary fiber in reducing the risk of breast cancer. Their conclusions: (1) A high-fiber diet reduces circulating estrogens; (2) many plants and vegetables contain isoflavones and lignins, which are capable of being converted into weak estrogens in the bowel that may compete with estrogen binding sites; (3) a high-fiber diet is generally not associated with obesity, a risk factor for breast cancer; (4) a high-fiber diet usually has a lower content of fat and a higher content of antioxidant vitamins which may protect against breast cancer; and (5) diets rich in fiber and complex carbohydrates can improve insulin sensitivity with associated reduction in circulating estrogen levels.[11]

Different types of fiber may be beneficial for irritable bowel syndrome, diverticulosis, colorectal cancer, diabetes, high cholesterol levels, and obesity. The fiber of choice for irritable bowel syndrome is methylcellulose or polycarbophil; for diverticulosis, psyllium, pectin, or guar gum; for diabetes, any fiber supplement; for high cholesterol levels, psyllium, pectin, or guar gum; for obesity, any fiber supplement that is tolerated. Methylcellulose is a variety of gummy products that swell in water and are used as bulk laxatives. Polycarbophils are used as a gastrointestinal absorbent.[12]

Fifty-nine patients with moderately high cholesterol levels were given 20 g/day of fiber for 36 weeks. The fiber consisted of guar gum, pectin, soy, and pea and corn bran. Levels of total cholesterol and LDL cholesterol as well as the LDL/HDL ratio were considerably reduced. Following 51 weeks of treatment, there was a 5 percent reduction in total cholesterol, 9 percent in LDL cholesterol, and 11 percent for the LDL/HDL ratio. Reductions were apparent after three weeks, with maximum reductions occurring by the 15th week.[13]

At Iowa State University at Ames, seven healthy women consumed 15 g/day of dietary fiber or a wheat-fiber supplement containing 40 g dietary fiber as part of a crossover study. Both treatment and control groups were given 0.6 mg of isoflavones (from tofu or texturized protein) per kg of body weight. The fiber-rich diet brought a 55 percent lower plasma genistein level at 24 hours and a 20 percent reduction in genistein in the urine. It was concluded that high-fiber diets can reduce the absorption of isoflavones, which may affect the biological function of isoflavones.[14]

In a study of 22,000 Finnish men between the ages of 50 and 69, those who consumed more than 10 g/day of fiber over a six-year period reduced their risk for coronary artery disease by 17 percent. Soluble fiber was more beneficial than insoluble fiber in lowering cholesterol and blood pressure levels. The men typically consumed 25 g/day of fiber, much more than American men ingest. Rye grain may be an ideal weapon against heart disease since it contains both water-soluble and insoluble fiber.[15]

Dietary fiber in conjunction with fish oil supplements may be beneficial in treating diabetic patients, according to researchers at the North Coast Institute of Diabetes and Endocrinology, West Lake, Ohio. Their study involved 15 non-insulin-dependent diabetics who were observed for eight weeks. The patients received 20 g/day of fish oil, and their dietary fiber intake was increased with a 15-g pectin supplement at the midpoint of the trial. Fish oil lowered levels of triglyceride and very low density lipoprotein (VLDL) cholesterol by 41 and 36 percent, respectively. When fiber was increased, total and LDL cholesterol decreased significantly with the fish oil treatment. Plasma triglyceride levels decreased further by 44 percent, and diabetic control was maintained during the study course of treatment.[16]

In a study involving 15 healthy males with a mean age of 25, sugar beet fiber was found to reduce blood glucose levels, serum insulin response, and other parameters compared to a formula without fiber. Sugar beet fiber may be a useful addition to tube-feeding nutrition because it may reduce high amounts of sugar in the blood.[17]

Twenty-eight children with cystic fibrosis were given 7 g/day of fiber compared to 14.6 g/day for the control group. Fiber intake in patients with abdominal symptoms was significantly lower in those with less or no symptoms. Cystic fibrosis patients often have low-fiber diets, which may be related to their gastrointestinal complaints.[18]

If you are unable to eat five or more servings of fruits and vegetables a day, or to consume bran and other high-fiber products, consider the fiber products available in the marketplace. Fiber provides protection against a number of serious illnesses. One cup of bran contains about 100 g.

References

1. Ensminger, A., et al., *Foods and Nutrition Encyclopedia* (Clovis, Calif.: Pegus Press, 1983), 709ff.

2. Adams, Ruth, and Frank Murray, *The Good Seeds, the Rich Grains, the Hardy Nuts for a Healthier, Happier Life* (New York: Larchmont Books, 1977), 270ff.

3. Weiss, Suzanne E., ed., *Foods That Harm, Foods That Heal* (Pleasantville, N.Y.: Reader's Digest Association, 1997), 146.

4. "How to Increase the Amount of Fiber in Your Diet," *AFP Journal,* Feb. 1995.

5. Aldoori, Walid H., et al., "A Prospective Study of Dietary Fiber Types and Symptomatic Diverticular Disease in Men," *Journal of Nutrition* 128: 714–19, 1998.

6. Badiali, Danilo, et al., "Effect of Wheat Bran in the Treatment of Chronic, Nonorganic Constipation: A Double-Blind Controlled Trial," *Digestive Diseases and Sciences* 40(2): 349–56, Feb. 1995.

7. Le Marchand, Loic, et al., "Dietary Fiber and Colorectal Cancer Risk," *Epidemiology* 8(6): 658–65, 1997.

8. Kritchevsky, D., "Dietary Fiber and Cancer," *European Journal of Cancer Prevention* 6: 435–41, 1997.

9. Alberts, David S., et al., "Randomized, Double-Blind, Placebo-Controlled Study of Effect of Wheat Bran Fiber and Calcium on Fecal Bile Acids in Patients with Resected Adenomatous Colon Polyps," *Journal of the National Cancer Institute* 88(2): 81–91, Jan. 17, 1996.

10. Goodman, Marc T., et al., "Association of Soy and Fiber Consumption with the Risk of Endometrial Cancer," *American Journal of Epidemiology* 146(4): 294–306, 1997.

11. Stoll, B., et al., "Can Supplementary Dietary Fiber Support Breast Cancer Growth?" *British Journal of Cancer* 73: 557–59, 1996.

12. Bennett, William G., and James J. Cerda, "Benefits of Dietary Fiber: Myth or Medicine?" *Postgraduate Medicine* 99(2): 153–72, Feb. 1996.

13. Hunninghake, Donald B., "Long-Term Treatment of Hypercholesterolemia with Dietary Fiber," *American Journal of Medicine* 97: 504–8, Dec. 1994.

14. Twe, Bee-Yen, et al., "A Diet High in Wheat Fiber Decreases the Bioavailability of Soybean Isoflavones in a Single Meal Fed to Women," *Journal of Nutrition* 126: 871–77, 1996.

15. "Heart Disease and Rye Grain," *Nutrition Week* 27(1): 7, Jan. 3, 1997.

16. Sheehan, John P., et al., "Effect of High Fiber Intake in Fish Oil–Treated Patients with Non-Insulin-Dependent Diabetes Mellitus," *American Journal of Clinical Nutrition* 66: 1183–87, 1997.

17. Thorsdottir, L., et al., "Sugar Beet Fiber in Formula Diet Reduces Postprandial Blood Glucose, Serum Insulin, and Serum Hydroxyproline," *European Journal of Clinical Nutrition* 52: 155–56, 1998.

18. Gavin, J., et al., "Dietary Fiber and the Occurrence of Gut Symptoms in Cystic Fibrosis," *Archives of Disabilities in Children* 76: 35–37, 1997.

31

Fish Oil

Several decades ago, researchers working in the Arctic reported that the Inuit (Eskimo) people who inhabited the area rarely developed coronary artery disease, even though their diet, which consisted primarily of whale meat, seal meat, and fish, was high in fat and cholesterol. Epidemiological studies confirmed that coronary heart disease rates in Greenland Inuits are much lower than those in Western countries. The difference isn't due to the amount of fat in the diet, since the amount of total fat in the Inuit diet is similar to that of a Western-type diet. The difference is the *source* of fats. Inuits get their fat mostly from marine mammals and fish, whereas Westerners get their fat from land animals and plants (omega-6s).[1]

"These early observations prompted extensive investigations of the possibility that some component of seafood might be protective against coronary heart disease," wrote William Harris, Ph.D. "Most of the research has focused on omega-3 polyunsaturated fatty acids, a distinctive type of fatty acid that is found in substantial amounts of fish oils. The most prominent long-chain omega-3s in fish oils are eicosapentaenoic acid (EPA) and docosahexaenoic acid (DHA). The richest sources of EPA and DHA are fatty fish such as mackerel, herring, and salmon. Lean white fish such as cod and flounder have only small amounts of omega-3s."

Researchers at Northwestern Medical School in Chicago and various institutions collaborated on a study with data taken from the Chicago Western Electric Study. They analyzed the association between fish consumption and the risk of death from myocardial infarction, coronary heart disease, and cardiovascular disease. A 42 percent lower death rate from nonsudden myocardial infarction was found among men who consumed 35 g or more of fish per day compared to nonfish eaters. Long-chain omega-3 polyunsaturated fatty acids found in fish may be the mitigating factor in providing protection, since omega-3s have been shown in clinical trials to lower the risk of cardiac arrhythmias, prevent restenosis, and decrease abnormally high triglyceride levels. Coronary restenosis is the recurrence of blocked arteries as well as chest pain within six months of a successful angioplasty, a procedure that dilates or expands a blocked coronary artery.[2]

A monthlong trial evaluated natural fish oil and a sunflower oil placebo in the diet of 47 healthy males between the ages of 29 and 60. The fish oil was given at 4 g/day, equivalent to 0.91 g of omega-3 fatty acids, or one or two weekly servings of fatty fish. The fish oil brought a 30 percent decline in plasma triglycerides, which may be the main mechanism by which fish oils contribute to the prevention of ischemic heart disease.[3]

In Denmark, researchers evaluated 55 patients who had had a myocardial infarction before 75 years of age. The volunteers were given either 5.2 g of omega-3 fatty acids or olive oil daily for 12 weeks. Findings showed that fish oils may increase heart rate variability in survivors of a heart attack, and this may increase ventricular fibrillation and protect the myocardium against ventricular arrhythmias.[4]

An Italian study involved 11,324 patients who had suffered a myocardial infarction in the previous three months. Researchers gave 1 g/day of fish oil capsules, which cut the risk of these patients for further fatal or nonfatal episodes by 10 to 15 percent over a 3.5-year follow-up. It was suggested that approximately 20 lives could be saved per 1,000 heart attack patients treated with fish oil supplements.[5]

At the Medical Hospital and Research Center, Moradabad, India, a group studied 122 patients who were supplemented with fish oil at 1.08 g/day; 120 who received mustard oil at 2.9 g/day; and 118 who were given a placebo. Following one year of therapy, total cardiac events were significantly lower in the fish oil and mustard oil groups compared with the controls, at 24.5 and 28 percent, respectively, and 34.7 percent in the controls. Nonfatal myocardial infarctions were also significantly less in the fish oil and mustard oil groups compared with placebo, at 13.0, 15.0, and 25.4 percent, respectively. The fish oil and mustard oil patients showed a significant reduction in total cardiac arrhythmias, left ventricular enlargement, and angina pectoris (chest pain), compared with the controls.[6]

In Tromso, Norway, 78 volunteers with untreated high blood pressure were given 4 g/day of EPA and DHA or corn oil at 4 g/day for 16 weeks. The fish oil lowered blood pressure, triglycerides, and LDL cholesterol. Blood sugar levels were unchanged.[7]

Fish oil does not appear to have a harmful effect on glucose tolerance, but it has beneficial effects on blood pressure and blood lipids, especially triglycerides, according to researchers at Oregon Health Sciences University at Portland. Fish or fish oil may be beneficial in the prevention of vascular disease in diabetics.[8]

Epidemiological data show that those who eat fish (30 to 35 g/day), compared to those who don't, have a reduced rate of death from cardiovascular disease, according to the Center for Genetics in Washington, D.C. For example, the ingestion of omega-3 fatty acids following a heart attack appears to reduce the rate of cardiac death. In the secondary prevention of coronary heart disease, 300 g of fatty fish providing 2.5 g of EPA from fish or fish oil per week decreased the risk of sudden death by 29 percent. A dose of 4 g/day of fish oil concentrate prevented occlusions following coronary artery bypass grafting. When giving omega-3 fatty acid to help prevent restenosis, the supplements should be administered at least three weeks prior to surgery and angioplasty.[9]

At the North Coast Institute of Diabetes and Endocrinology in West Lake, Ohio, 15 non-insulin-dependent diabetics were given 20 g/day of fish oil, and their usual dietary fiber intake was increased with a 15-g pectin supplement at the midpoint of the study. The trial lasted eight weeks. Fish oil lowered triglyceride and very low density lipoprotein cholesterol (VLDL) by 41 and 36 percent, respectively. There was no change in other cholesterol parameters. When the amount of fiber was increased, total and LDL-cholesterol concentrations decreased significantly with the fish oil treatment. Plasma triglycerides decreased an additional 44 percent. Researchers concluded that a high-fiber diet may be beneficial when treating diabetic patients with fish oil supplements.[10]

Joseph P. Grande, M.D., Ph.D., and colleagues at the Mayo Foundation in Rochester, Minnesota, reported that recent studies provide support that supplementation with omega-3 fatty acids can retard kidney disease progression in high-risk patients with IgA nephropathy, or Berger's disease. In one study of 106 patients with the disorder, only 6 percent of the patients given a fish oil supplement developed severe kidney disease. Thirty-three percent in the control group experienced kidney problems. Normally, between 20 and 40 percent of these patients will develop kidney failure between 5 and 25 years after diagnosis.[11]

One study involved 38 volunteers with Crohn's disease in remission who were given either a diet rich in cold-water fish or a control diet for two years. It was found that only 20 percent of those on the fish diet had relapses, compared to 58 percent of the controls. In a 12-month study involving fish oil in the maintenance of 78 patients with Crohn's disease in remission, ranging in age from 18 to 75, enteric-coated fish oil was given at a daily dose of 1.8 g of EPA and 0.9 g of DHA. After one year, 59 percent in the fish oil group were in remission, compared to 26 percent of the controls. Gastrointestinal side effects and the fish odor, which are largely eliminated with enteric-coated supplements, make fish oil an ideal maintenance therapy. Fish oil is also a promising agent for other inflammatory conditions, high blood pressure, coronary artery disease, and cancer.[12]

German researchers suggested that fish oil may provide protection against colon cancer. They evaluated 24 healthy volunteers who consumed a low- or high-fat diet while getting 4.4 g/day of fish oil or corn oil. The daily excretion of potential cancer-causing carcinogens was significantly lower in the fish oil group than in the controls.[13]

Rheumatoid arthritis patients in a study at Albany Medical College in New York were able to halt their NSAID dosage without experiencing a flare-up in their disease. The study involved 66 patients who took 130 mg/kg per day of fish oil, compared to nine capsules a day of corn oil given to the controls. The patients were also taking the NSAID diclofenac ophthalmic at 75 mg twice daily. A placebo replaced the drug at 18 or 22 weeks into the study, and fish oil supplements were continued for eight weeks. In the fish oil group there was a significant decrease in mean number of tender joints, duration of morning stiffness, and evaluation of pain. No changes were observed in the corn oil controls. In the patients taking fish oil supplements, there was a decrease in the number of tender joints for eight weeks after the drug was stopped.[14]

A fish oil supplement helps stabilize the volatile moods of those suffering from manic depression, also known as bipolar disorder, according to researchers at McLean Hospital in Belmont, Massachusetts. The study involved 30 patients who were receiving drugs for manic depression. During four months of therapy, 14 were also given daily doses of omega-3 fatty acids containing fish oil concentrate. The rest were the controls. Eleven of the volunteers receiving fish oil improved or maintained their emotional status during the study, compared with 6 of 16 controls.[15] Recent studies have shown that depressed patients often have low levels of omega-3 fatty acids, especially DHA. Increasing omega-3 fatty acids in the diet can improve bouts of depression.[16]

People with depression have lower levels of omega-3s. It is now known that during pregnancy the fetus takes omega-3 from the mother to make brain and nervous tissue, causing some pregnant women to suffer from postpartum depression, according to Lucy Puryear, M.D., of the Baylor College of Medicine in Houston. Those who suffer from this disorder experience sleep difficulties, excessive crying, loss of energy and appetite, and lack of interest in activities. The condition usually begins within the first month after delivery but can occur up to four to six months afterward.[17]

Omega-3 fatty acids are found in cell membranes throughout the body, Puryear explained. But over the years the American diet has had a decrease in omega-3s. At the same time, omega-6 fatty acids, also found in cell membranes, have increased. "We think this shift is affecting brain chemical receptors and impacting the brain's levels of serotonin, which is thought to be linked to depression," she continued. "Women with a history of postpartum depression have a 50-to-80 percent chance of getting it again."

Puryear has begun a study involving 20 pregnant women with past histories of postpartum depression. They will receive fish oil capsules starting in the 34th week of pregnancy and will continue until four months after delivery. Fish oil capsules do not harm the fetus, and some studies have shown that omega-3s might enhance the baby's cognitive and visual development.

One study involved six volunteers who were fed a control diet for three weeks. Ten to 12 weeks later, 6 g/day of fish oil replaced the 6 g/day of visible fat in the control diet. The volunteers were observed for another three weeks. Although energy intake was unchanged, body fat mass decreased with the substitution of the fish oil. The researchers concluded that dietary fish oil reduces body fat mass and stimulates lipid oxidation in healthy adults.[18]

At the University of Liverpool, 13 patients with photosensitivity to ultraviolet radiation were evaluated. They were given five capsules twice daily containing 1 g of MaxEPA (fish oil), which contained 18 percent EPA and 12 percent DHA. The trial lasted three months. The researchers increased ultraviolet-B irradiation, but the UVA provocation test was reduced in nine of the patients. The study provides evidence that dietary fish oil protects against UV provocation in those with a photosensitive disorder. Some protective properties may be mediated partially by reduced prostaglandin-2 levels. PGE-2 may play a role in the growth of skin cancers, and a diet rich in omega-3 fatty acids may inhibit the UV-induced carcinogenesis process on the skin.[19]

It has been said that many Americans are ingesting larger amounts of omega-6 fatty acids (vegetable oils) but neglecting the omega-3s. This could lead to health problems down the road. You may want to consider eating more cold-water fish and adding fish oil supplements to your regimen.

References

1. Harris, William, "Fish Oils, Omega-3 Polyunsaturated Fatty Acids, and Coronary Heart Disease," *PUFA Information Backgrounder* 2(1), July 1997.

2. Daviglus, Martha L., et al., "Fish Consumption and the 30-Year Risk of Fatal Myocardial Infarction," *New England Journal of Medicine* 336: 1046–53, April 10, 1997.

3. Marckmann, Peter, et al., "Dietary Fish Oil (4 g Daily) and Cardiovascular Risk Markers in Healthy Men," *Arteriosclerosis, Thrombosis, and Vascular Biology* 17: 3384–91, 1997.

4. Christensen, Jeppe Hagstrup, et al., "Effect of Fish Oil on Heart Rate Variability in Survivors of Myocardial

Infarction: A Double-Blind, Randomized, Controlled Trial," *British Medical Journal* 312: 677–78, 1996.

5. Norton, Amy, "Fish Oil Supplements Benefit MI Patients," *Medical Tribune,* April 8, 1999, 7.

6. Singh, Ram B., et al., "Randomized, Double-Blind, Placebo-Controlled Trial of Fish Oil and Mustard Oil in Patients with Suspected Acute Myocardial Infarction: The Indian Experiment of Infarct Survival-4," *Cardiovascular Drugs and Therapy* 11: 483–89, 1997.

7. Toft, Ingrid, et al., "Effects of Omega-3 Polyunsaturated Fatty Acids on Glucose Homeostasis and Blood Pressure in Essential Hypertension: A Randomized, Controlled Trial," *Annals of Internal Medicine* 123(12): 911–18, Dec. 15, 1995.

8. Connor, William E., "Diabetes, Fish Oil, and Vascular Disease," *Annals of Internal Medicine* 123(12): 950–51, Dec. 15, 1995.

9. Simopoulos, Artemis P., "Omega-3 Fatty Acids in the Prevention-Management of Cardiovascular Disease," *Canadian Journal of Physiology and Pharmacology* 75: 234–39, 1997.

10. Sheehan, John P., et al., "Effect of High Fiber Intake in Fish Oil–Treated Patients with Non-Insulin-Dependent Diabetes Mellitus," *American Journal of Clinical Nutrition* 66: 1183–87, 1997.

11. Grande, Joseph P., and James V. Donadio Jr., "Dietary Fish Oil Supplementation in IgA Nephropathy: A Therapy in Search of a Mechanism?" *Nutrition* 14(2): 240–42, 1998.

12. Kim, Young-In, "Can Fish Oil Maintain Crohn's Disease in Remission?" *Nutrition Reviews* 54(8): 248–57, Aug. 1996.

13. Bartram, Hans-Peter, et al., "Effects of Fish Oil on Fecal Bacterial Enzymes and Steroid Excretion in Healthy Volunteers: Implications for Colon Cancer Prevention," *Nutrition and Cancer* 25(1): 71–76, 1996.

14. Kremer, Joel M., et al., "Effects of High-Dose Fish Oil on Rheumatoid Arthritis After Stopping Non-Steroidal Anti-inflammatory Drugs," *Arthritis and Rheumatism* 38(8): 1107–14, Aug. 1995.

15. Bower, Bruce, "Feeling Better with Fish Oil," *Science News* 155: 362, June 5, 1999.

16. Peet, M., et al., "Depletion of Omega-3 Fatty Acid Levels in Red Blood Cell Membranes of Depressed Patients," *Biological Psychiatry* 43: 315–19, 1998.

17. Major, Kathy. "Fish Oil Studied As Method to Prevent Post-Partum Depression," *Baylor College of Medicine News,* March 26, 1999.

18. Couet, C., et al., "Effect of Dietary Fish Oil on Body Fat Mass and Basal Oxidation in Healthy Adults," *International Journal of Obesity* 21: 637–43, 1997.

19. Rhodes, Lesley E., et al., "Dietary Fish Oil Reduces Basal and Ultraviolet B–Generated PGE-2 Levels in Skin and Increases the Threshold to Provocation of Polymorphic Light Eruption," *Journal of Investigative Dermatology* 105: 532–35, 1995.

32

Flaxseed and Flaxseed Oil

Flax *(Linum usitatissimum)* is an herbaceous annual that originated in the Mediterranean region. The Abyssinians are said to be the first to use flax as a food by roasting and eating the shiny oval seeds. The mucilage obtained by infusing one-half ounce of flaxseed into a pint of boiling water is reportedly helpful in alleviating constipation, dysentery, catarrh, and other inflammatory disorders of the respiratory tract, intestines, and urinary passages.[1] The names flaxseed oil and linseed oil are used interchangeably.

In ancient times, flaxseed was a great delicacy and was believed to be a love potion. It was prescribed for respiratory ailments, and generations of Europeans used it to help poor elimination. "Today, flaxseed is again coming into its own," the late Gayelord Hauser wrote in *Mirror, Mirror on the Wall*. "I saw sugar bowls filled with ground flaxseed meal on every table in the dining room at the famous Buchinger Sanatorium in Uberlingen, Germany, to be sprinkled over food. It is as tasty as wheat germ and inexpensive. A particular value of flaxseed is its mild laxative quality. Flaxseed mixed with your morning cereal makes a natural 'bowel motor' for lazy intestines."[2]

In his book, *The Omega-3 Phenomenon*, Donald O. Rudin, M.D., explained that linseed oil contains 60 percent omega-3 fatty acids and is high in alpha-linolenic acid, making it ideal for cooking. Unlike fish oils, which are high in eicosapentaenoic acid (EPA) and docosahexaenoic acid (DHA), linseed oil is the only source of large amounts of alpha-linolenic acid. Since the body cannot make alpha-linolenic acid, this omega-3 essential fatty acid is the only one that affects certain enzymes in the production of specific types of prostaglandins. From alpha-linolenic acid, the body can make EPA and DHA.[3]

Rudin wrote that linseed/flaxseed oil brings relief from cystitis and enlarged prostate; cardiovascular disease; menopausal complaints, including headache; and irritable bowel syndrome, among others. He has worked out a daily formula based on a person's weight:

100 lb.	About 1 tbsp.
125 lb.	About 1–2 tbsp.
150 lb.	About 2–3 tbsp.
175 lb.	About 3 tbsp.
200 lb.	About 3–4 tbsp.

Those who are sensitive or allergic may begin with 1 teaspoon (about four capsules) a day and increase that dose gradually every four days. Results do not come quickly, so do not increase the dosage if immediate results are not achieved. One tablespoon of flaxseed oil contains about 100 calories.

"In my study," Rudin continued, "patients very often discovered a threshold dose was needed to achieve a therapeutic effect. For instance, there might be no tangible results from one teaspoon of linseed oil taken daily over many weeks or months. However, with an increase in dosage from one to two teaspoons, a complete remission of symptoms—of osteoarthritis, for example—might then be achieved in a few weeks. The smallest dose that worked for any subject was one-fourth teaspoon (one capsule) daily."

Flaxseed oil can be toxic in large doses. Some people may suffer diarrhea, insomnia, muscle aches, or skin deterioration. Monitor any changes daily.

Flaxseeds are the most abundant source of lignans, special compounds that are useful for reducing hot flashes in menopausal women, as well as for their anticancer, antibacterial, antifungal, and antiviral properties. Research shows that flaxseed lignans are changed by bacteria in the intestine into compounds that protect against cancer, especially breast cancer. As a treatment for rheumatoid arthritis, studies have shown positive results with EPA and GLA supplements at a dosage of 1.8 and 1.4 g, respectively.[4]

Flaxseed supplementation in healthy adults improves bowel movements, modestly reduces LDL, and raises polyunsaturated fatty acids in blood plasma, according to researchers at the University of Toronto in Canada. Ten volunteers were given 50 g of flaxseed, baked into muffins, daily for four weeks. A 30 percent increase in weekly bowel movements was noted.[5]

A research team at the Jordan Heart Fund, Montclair, New Jersey, evaluated 15 patients with high cholesterol levels. The volunteers received 800 IU/day of vitamin E along with three slices of flaxseed-containing bread and 15 g of ground flaxseed. This diet, rich in alpha-linolenic acid and fiber, significantly reduced total and LDL cholesterol in the blood during the three-month trial. However, HDL cholesterol, the beneficial kind, did not change. Thrombin-stimulated platelet aggregation, which might produce a blood clot, decreased during the study.[6]

For prostate problems, Robert M. Giller, M.D., recommends 1 or 2 tablespoons of cold-pressed flaxseed oil daily for several months. He also suggests adding sunflower oil or soy oil to the diet, along with other diet recommendations.[7]

At Royal Adelaide Hospital in Australia, 30 healthy male volunteers were given flaxseed, rich in alpha-linolenic acid and low in linoleic acid, and a control group of 15 were given a diet high in linoleic acid and low in alpha-linolenic acid, which is similar to the typical Western diet. These diets were analyzed for four weeks, followed by an additional four weeks in which the patients were supplemented with fish oil containing 1.62 g EPA daily and 1.08 g/day of DHA.[8]

The flaxseed oil diet brought a significant increase in alpha-linolenic acid concentrations in plasma phospholipid, cholesteryl ester and triglyceride fractions, and neutrophil phospholipids. EPA concentrations increased by 2.5-fold in the plasma lipid fractions and neutrophil phospholipids. Following fish oil supplementation, EPA amounts went down in both dietary groups but remained higher in the flaxseed group.

These results suggest that vegetables rich in alpha-linolenic acid can be used to enhance EPA levels in tissue concentrations similar to those associated with fish oil supplementation. Flaxseed oil may also be valuable in such inflammatory conditions as rheumatoid arthritis, psoriasis, and ulcerative colitis. It may be useful in conjunction with fish oil, since omega-3 fatty acids have been shown to improve these conditions.

A research team at the University of Sydney in Australia studied 11 healthy males who received either 40 g of flaxseed oil or sunflower oil daily for 23 days. In the flaxseed volunteers, the platelet EPA more than doubled but remained unchanged in the sunflower controls. However, the EPA-arachidonic acid ratio, a marker of thromboxane production and platelet aggregation potential, increased in the flaxseed group. (Thromboxanes are substances that constrict blood vessels and promote blood clots, which can lead to a heart attack or stroke.) Also, the aggregation response induced by collagen was reduced in those getting flaxseed oil. These data are further evidence that oils rich in alpha-linolenic acid may protect against cardiovascular disease over linoleic-rich oils through their ability to keep platelets from sticking together.[9]

Your local health food store should carry a variety of flaxseed and flaxseed oil supplements. Most of these products need to be refrigerated to keep the oil from turning rancid. Whole-food bakeries also sell various goods containing flaxseed.

References

1. Ensminger, A., et al., *Foods and Nutrition Encyclopedia* (Clovis, Calif.: Pegus Press, 1983), 765–66.
2. Hauser, Gayelord, *Mirror, Mirror on the Wall* (New York: Farrar, Straus and Cudahy, 1961), 94.

3. Rudin, Donald O., Clara Felix, and Constance Schrader, *The Omega-3 Phenomenon* (New York: Rawson Associates, 1987), 10–14, 23, 94–97.

4. Whitaker, Julian, *Dr. Whitaker's Guide to Natural Healing* (Rocklin, Calif.: Prima Publishing, 1995), 50–51.

5. Cunnane, Stephen C., et al., "Nutritional Attributes of Traditional Flaxseed in Healthy Young Adults," *American Journal of Clinical Nutrition* 61: 62–68, 1995.

6. Bierenbaum, Marvin L., et al., "Reducing Atherogenic Risk in Hyperlipidemic Humans with Flaxseed Supplementation: A Preliminary Report," *Journal of the American College of Nutrition* 12(5): 501–4, 1993.

7. Giller, Robert M., and Kathy Matthews, *Natural Prescriptions* (New York: Carol Southern Books, 1994), 287.

8. Mantzioris, Evandeline, et al., "Dietary Substitution with Alpha-Linolenic Acid-Rich Vegetable Oil Increases Eicosapentaenoic Acid Concentrations in Tissues," *American Journal of Clinical Nutrition* 59: 1304–9, 1994.

9. Allman, M. A., et al., "Supplementation with Flaxseed Oil versus Sunflower Oil in Healthy Young Men Consuming a Low-Fat Diet: Effects on Platelet Composition and Function," *European Journal of Clinical Nutrition* 49: 169–78, 1995.

33

Flower Pollen Extract

As men age, the prostate gland, located just below the bladder, often increases in size. The prostate produces the fluid that bathes sperm at the time of ejaculation. Enlargement of the gland is called benign prostatic hyperplasia (BPH) and often results in restricted urinary flow, difficulty in starting the flow, frequent urination, and the urgent need to urinate.

Researchers in Europe and Japan have found that flower pollen extracts often relieve the symptoms of BPH. Flower pollen extract is not to be confused with bee pollen. The microbiological extract of dried pollen, now available over the counter in supplement form, contains 21 amino acids, lipids, saccharides, phospholipids, enzymes, DNA, RNA, small amounts of estrogen, and vitamins and minerals. The eight pollen strains in the supplement are derived from timothy, corn, rye, hazel, sallow, aspen, oxeye daisy, and pine.[2]

As far back as 1960, E. Ask-Upmark, a Swedish researcher, reported that flower pollen was effective in treating prostatitis, or inflammation of the prostate gland. Although the mode of action is still being debated, it has been theorized that the pollen augments the production of interferon, a protein produced by cells as a defense against viruses. It may also stimulate the thymus gland, which plays an active role in the body's defense against infections.

Flower pollen extracts are usually either water-alcohol extracts or lipophilic (fatty acid) extracts. Since the protein fraction of pollen is usually what causes allergic reactions, pollen extracts can be made that are free of allergens. While no cases of serious toxic side effects have been reported in the literature, warnings concerning the possibility of allergic reactions are routinely published.[3]

For his patients with prostatitis, Ronald L. Hoffman, M.D., a New York physician, prescribes a flower pollen extract, which seems to have a positive effect on the inflammation.[4] "I think it's important to consider that this is not just an infection but rather an inflammatory disease," he said. "A chronic inflammatory process can still be churning away, even in the absence of any virus or bacteria. Prostatitis can sometimes be allergic, and a food allergy profile may be worth doing. If the prostate is already inflamed, and thereby predisposed, it could react to an allergen in the diet."

Researchers at University Hospital of Wales in Cardiff evaluated 53 men aged 56 to 89 who were awaiting surgery for an enlarged prostate. In the double-blind, placebo-controlled, six-month trial, the volunteers were given either two capsules twice a day of flower pollen extract or a placebo. The flower pollen extract brought a 69 percent improvement in the treatment group, compared to 29 percent in the controls.[5]

A study involving 96 patients with BPH was conducted in Hamburg, Germany. The men ranged in age from 42 to 85. During the 12-week study, the volunteers were given three capsules daily of flower pollen extract. The men in the treatment group made fewer trips to the bathroom than did those getting a placebo. The treatment group assessed the flower pollen treatment as "very good" or "good" more frequently than did those in the control group.[6]

In Tokyo, 25 men with enlarged prostates were given six tablets daily of flower pollen extract. The study lasted for three months. Symptom improvement was most striking for prolonged difficulty in urination (54 percent), nighttime urination (50 percent), reduced urine flow (47 percent), straining during urination (41 percent), and delayed urination (22 percent). The findings suggested that the extract removes the swelling of the urethral mucosal surface, improves urination, and alleviates the irritation found in the bladder neck. No side effects were observed.[7]

At Academic Hospital in Celle, Germany, beta-sitosterol was found to be an effective option in the treatment of benign prostatic hypertrophy. In the study at 13 different treatment centers, 130 mg/day of beta-sitosterol were given to 177 patients with BPH.[8] Sitosterols are widespread in plants (wheat germ, soybean oil, etc.), and beta-sitosterol is an effective cholesterol-lowering agent that also protects against colon cancer. It is not clear how this phytosterol protects against BPH.

An over-the-counter product for BPH contains flower pollen extract (378 mg in two tablets), beta-sitosterol, and standardized saw palmetto.

References

1. Hanno, Philip M., "Men's Health," *Medical and Health Annual* (Chicago: Encyclopaedia Britannica, 1994), 353ff.

2. Murray, Frank. "Flower Pollen Extract: A Natural Way to Ease Prostate Pain," *Let's Live,* June 1997, 75–76.

3. Clouatre, Dallas, *Pollen Extract for Prostate Health* (San Francisco: Pax Publishing, 1997), 10.

4. Hoffman, Ronald L., *Intelligent Medicine* (New York: Simon & Schuster, 1997), 248.

5. Buck, A. C., et al., "Treatment of Outflow Tract Obstruction Due to Benign Prostatic Hyperplasia with the Pollen Extract, Cernilton," *British Journal of Urology* 66: 398–404, 1990.

6. Becker, H., and L. Ebeling, "Conservative Treatment of Benign Prostatic Hyperplasia (BPH) with Cernilton-N," *Urologe B* 28: 301–6, 1988.

7. Takeuchi, H., et al., "Quantitative Evaluation on the Effectiveness of Cernilton on Benign Prostatic Hypertrophy," *Acta Urologica Japonica* 27: 317–27, 1981.

8. Klippel, K. F., et al., "A Multicentric, Placebo-Controlled, Double-Blind Clinical Trial of Beta-Sitosterol (Phytosterol) for the Treatment of Benign Prostate Hyperplasia," *British Journal of Urology* 80: 427–32, 1997.

34

Folic Acid

Consumers often use the terms *folic acid* and *folate* interchangeably, but there is an important distinction between the two, according to Lynn Bailey, Ph.D., of the University of Florida at Gainesville. *Folate* is a generic term that describes a complex chemical form, of which the simple form, folic acid, is readily available to the body. The body absorbs only 50 percent of the folate in foods, compared to 85 percent absorbed from supplements or fortified foods.[1]

Folic acid intakes are consistently low among the U.S. population, especially among women of childbearing age, Bailey said. A report from the Centers for Disease Control and Prevention (CDC) showed that only one-third of U.S. women of childbearing age consume 400 mcg/day of folate, the recommended amount. Because neural tube defects occur within the first

month of fetal development, regular intakes of at least 400 mcg of folic acid daily before conception are recommended to reduce the risk of birth defects. For this reason, and since 50 percent of pregnancies in the United States are unplanned, the FDA mandated the enrichment of grain products with folic acid to reduce the risk of birth defects. This may also lower the risk of cardiovascular disease.

When 251 pregnant women in Atlanta, Georgia, were interviewed, 57 percent had heard of folate, but 70 percent could not name one of its food sources, which include orange juice and leafy green vegetables.[2] In the United States, about 4,000 pregnancies are affected by neural tube defects annually, but 50 to 70 percent of these could be prevented with daily intakes of 400 mcg of folic acid throughout the periconception period, according to the CDC. In 1992, the Public Health Service suggested that all women capable of becoming pregnant should consume 400 mcg/day of folic acid throughout their childbearing years to reduce the risk of delivering a baby with a neural tube defect. In 1998, the Institute of Medicine recommended that all women of childbearing potential consume 400 mcg/day of synthetic folic acid from fortified foods and/or a supplement in addition to food folate from a varied diet.[3]

A neural tube defect is a developmental problem affecting the spinal cord and brain in the embryo. In the initial fetal development, there is a ridge of neural-like tissue along the back of the embryo. This material eventually develops into the spinal cord and body nerves at the lower end and the brain at the upper end. If anything goes wrong during this sequence, the result can be total lack of a brain (anencephaly) or spina bifida, in which the back bones do not form a complete ring to protect the spinal cord. Many of these children die at birth or in early infancy.[4]

Researchers have calculated that hospital charges related to three major health conditions could be reduced by almost $20 billion annually if large numbers of people regularly consumed vitamin and mineral supplements. The three disorders: folic acid and birth defects; multivitamins and minerals and low-birth-weight infants; and vitamin E and coronary heart disease.[5]

Folic acid supplements could reduce health care costs due to the prevention of many health problems. There is strong evidence that babies of pregnant women who take folic acid supplements before conception and during the early months of gestation experience a reduction in both occurrence and recurrence of neural tube defects, congenital heart defects, obstructive urinary tract problems, limb deficiencies, cleft palates, and other problems. For the mother, a folic acid deficiency is associated with preterm deliveries, intrauterine growth retardation, breakage in the placenta, and heart problems. In all adults, a folic acid deficiency is associated with cardiovascular disease and some forms of cancer.[6]

Studies show that 400 mcg/day of folic acid resulted in 72 percent fewer cases of neural tube defects. For women who are at risk for delivering one of these children, the recommendation is 800 mcg/day of folic acid, not to exceed 5 mg/day. Supplementation should begin before conception and continue for at least 10 to 12 weeks of pregnancy.[7]

The March of Dimes Birth Defects Foundation in Emeryville, California, reported that women who take multivitamins containing folic acid periconceptionally had a 25 to 50 percent reduction in the risk for offspring with a cleft palate compared to women who did not use the vitamins. Orofacial clefts cause feeding and speech problems as well as ear infections, not to mention psychological trauma. The estimated lifetime medical cost for children with these defects born each year in California is over $86 million.[8]

More than 30 years ago, Kilmer McCully, M.D., a researcher at Harvard

University, suggested a link between elevated levels of homocysteine, a breakdown product of protein metabolism, and the risk of coronary heart disease. Few people listened to his proposal, and he was ultimately dismissed from Harvard. Numerous studies have since confirmed that elevated homocysteine is a risk factor for hardening of the arteries, heart attack, stroke, and vascular disease.[9] McCully, who is now with the Providence VA Medical Center in Rhode Island, told an audience at a 1998 New York seminar that the Framingham Study, which has been monitoring the causes of heart disease for more than 50 years, has confirmed a strong correlation between blood levels of homocysteine and the development of stenosis (narrowing of arteries due to plaque buildup). Stenosis appeared in 58 percent of men with the highest levels of homocysteine, compared with 27 percent of men with the lowest levels. Almost two-thirds of all cases were associated with inadequate intakes of one or more of the B vitamins—folic acid, vitamin B_6, and vitamin B_{12}. The only source of homocysteine is the amino acid methionine, available from dietary proteins. During metabolism, methionine is converted to homocysteine and back to methionine. The three B vitamins are necessary for these conversions. Without proper metabolism, homocysteine can build up (homocysteinemia) and damage blood vessels. Other causes of homocysteinemia are genetics, aging, certain drugs, and hormones.

In an eight-week, placebo-controlled trial in the Netherlands and the United Kingdom, a dose of folic acid as low as 250 mcg/day significantly decreased plasma homocysteine concentrations in healthy young women. Homocysteine is normally processed by the body, but if there is an accumulation in the bloodstream, it is thought to increase the risk of stroke, heart attack, and blood clots in the legs and lungs.[10]

Researchers in Belfast, Northern Ireland; Dublin, Ireland; the University of Berne, Switzerland; and the University of Pennsylvania found that supplementing a group of Belfast volunteers with three B vitamins—folic acid, B_6, and B_{12}—in doses 2.5 to 10 times the RDA lowered homocysteine levels by about 32 percent.[11]

In 1996, the FDA issued a regulation, effective January 1, 1998, requiring that all enriched flour, rice, pasta, cornmeal, and other grain products contain 140 mcg of folic acid per 100 grams. That is in addition to the B_1, B_2, B_3, and iron already required in these foods. It was estimated that folic acid fortification at that level would provide an additional 80 to 100 mcg of folic acid daily to women of childbearing age and 70 to 120 mcg to the diet of middle-aged and older adults. The debate continues as to whether these amounts are sufficient.[12]

To test these amounts, researchers at the USDA Human Nutrition Research Center on Aging at Tufts University in Boston and other area facilities evaluated

350 volunteers who were studied after fortification began (which was before the 1998 FDA deadline), and 756 people who were studied before fortification began. Enriched grain products with folic acid were associated with a substantial improvement in folate status in middle-aged and older adults.

Fortifying cereal products with folic acid levels may not provide enough of the vitamin to prevent coronary heart disease, according to Manuel R. Manlinow, M.D., and colleagues at Oregon Health Sciences University in Portland. However, cereals providing 449 and 665 mcg/day of folic acid reduced homocysteine levels by 11 and 14 percent, respectively.[13]

A research team at Brigham and Women's Hospital and Harvard Medical School reported that among 88,756 women in the Nurses' Health Study, those who took folic acid in a multivitamin supplement for more than 15 years were 75 percent less likely to develop colon cancer than the women who did not take the supplements. Those who took multivitamins containing folic acid for 5 to 14 years were 20 percent less likely to develop colon cancer.[14]

An analysis of 16 epidemiological studies has reported overwhelming evidence that a folic acid deficiency is associated with colorectal cancer. The usual dosage in the studies was 5 mg/day.[15]

At the University of Calgary, Alberta, Canada, 1,171 people aged 65 and older were studied for folic acid stores in their blood. Those with the lowest folic acid status were more likely to suffer a stroke. Those with low levels of the vitamin were also likely to be demented, institutionalized, depressed, and prone to losing weight and lower body mass.[16]

While mortality rates from cervical cancer have dropped in recent years, the disorder kills thousands of women annually (4,400 in 1992). Risk factors for cervical cancer include multiple sex partners, partners who have had multiple sex partners, cigarette smoking, HIV, infection, and inadequate diet. One study found that the lowest blood levels of folic acid put many women at risk for developing the disease. For example, the odds of having cervical cancer were 10 times higher for those with the lowest levels of the vitamin, compared to those with the highest levels.[17]

Researchers have suggested that a *Helicobacter pylori* infection creates a folic acid deficiency, which could lead to coronary artery disease. *Helicobacter pylori* is a bacterium known to colonize the gastric mucosa, possibly leading to ulcers and heart problems.[18]

Vitiligo is a disorder characterized by white blotches on the skin. At University Hospital in Uppsala, Sweden, the spread of vitiligo stopped in 64 percent of the patients who were given 1 g of vitamin B_{12} and 5 mg twice daily of folic acid. They were also instructed to spend some time in the sun or under a sun lamp. During the three- to six-month treatment, repigmentation was observed in 52 patients, including 37 who exposed their skin to summer sun and six who used sun lamps in the winter. Repigmentation was most apparent in the sun-exposed areas, where 38 percent reported repigmentation. Total repigmentation was found in six patients.[19]

Folic acid supplements are readily available in stores. Fortified grains are another source of the vitamin, but since B vitamins lose their potency when exposed to light and heat, it is not known how much remains in the foods after processing.

References

1. Bailey, Lynn, "Folic Acid Improves Pregnancy Outcomes," paper presented at Beyond the Basics: Breakthroughs in B Vitamin Research," sponsored by the Vitamin Nutrition Information Service, New York, May 19, 1998.
2. Norton, Amy, "Women Unaware Folate Prevents Birth Defects," *Medical Tribune,* Feb. 4, 1999, 17.
3. "Knowledge of Use of Folic Acid by Women of Childbearing Age—United States, 1995 and 1998," *Morbidity and Mortality Weekly Report, Centers for Disease Control and Prevention* 48(16): 1–2, April 30, 1999.
4. Clayman, Charles B., ed., *The AMA Home Medical Encyclopedia* (New York: Random House, 1989), 722.
5. Benedich, A., et al., "Potential Health Economic Benefits of Vitamin Supplementation," *Western Journal of Medicine* 166: 306–12, 1997.
6. Hall, J., and F. Solehdin, "Folic Acid for the Prevention of Congenital Anomalies," *European Journal of Pediatrics* 157: 445–50, 1998.
7. Van Allen, Margot I., et al., "Recommendations on the Use of Folic Acid Supplementation to Prevent the Recurrence of Neural Tube Defects," *Canadian Medical Association Journal* 149(9): 1239, Nov. 1, 1993.
8. Shaw, Gary M., et al., "Risks of Orofacial Cleft in Children Born to Women Using Multi-Vitamins Containing Folic Acid Periconceptionally," *The Lancet* 346: 393–96, Aug. 12, 1995.
9. McCully, Kilmer, "Diminishing Heart Disease Risk: B Vitamins Offer Powerful Means of Defense," paper presented at Beyond the Basics: Breakthroughs in B Vitamin Research, sponsored by the Vitamin Nutrition Information Service, New York, May 19, 1998.
10. Brouwer, Ingeborg A., et al., "Low-Dose Folic Acid Supplementation Decreases Plasma Homocysteine Concentrations: A Randomized Trial," *American Journal of Clinical Nutrition* 69: 99–104, 1999.
11. Woodside, Jayne V., et al., "Effect of B-Group Vitamins and Antioxidant Vitamins on Hyperhomocysteinemia: A Double-Blind, Randomized, Factorial-Design, Controlled Trial," *American Journal of Clinical Nutrition* 67(5): 858–66, 1998.
12. Jacques, Paul F., et al., "The Effect of Folic Acid Fortification on Plasma Folate and Total Homocysteine Concentrations,"

New England Journal of Medicine 340: 1449–54, May 13, 1999.

13. Christensen, Damaris, "More Folate in Food Needed to Stave Off CHD, Data Suggest," *Medical Tribune,* May 21, 1998, 12.

14. Christensen, Damaris, "Folic Acid in Multivitamins May Lower Colon-Cancer Risk," *Medical Tribune,* Oct. 22, 1998, 1.

15. Mason, J. B., "Folate and Colon Cancer: A Fascinating Puzzle We Have Yet to Complete," *Clinical Nutrition* 17: 41–43, 1998.

16. Ebly, E. M., et al., "Folate Status, Vascular Disease, and Cognition in Elderly Canadians," *Age and Aging* 27: 485–91, 1998.

17. Van Eenwyk, Juliet, "The Role of Vitamins in the Development of Cervical Cancer," *Nutrition Report* 11(1): 1, 8, Jan. 1993.

18. Markle, H. V. "Coronary Artery Disease Associated with *Helicobacter Pylori* Infection Is at Least Partially Due to Inadequate Folate Status," *Medical Hypotheses* 49: 289–92, 1997.

19. Juhlin, Lennart, and Mats J. Olsson, "Improvement of Vitiligo After Oral Treatment with Vitamin B_{12} and Folic Acid and the Importance of Sun Exposure," *Acta Dermatologica Venerol* (Stockholm) 77: 460–62, 1997.

35

Fructooligosaccharides (FOS)

Fructooligosaccharides (FOS), which are naturally occurring sugars in foods, enhance the proliferation of "friendly bacteria"—acidophilus, bifidus, and faecium—into the gastrointestinal tract. They are also known as probiotics. *E. coli* and other pathogenic bacteria found in the gut, however, are unable to benefit from these sugars. In addition to stimulating beneficial bacteria, FOS reportedly reduce blood pressure in those with excessive fats in the blood; reduce carbohydrate and fat absorption, thus normalizing blood glucose and serum lipids; alter the metabolism of bile acids; and disrupt the metabolism of carbohydrates and fats in diabetics. Since FOS are not widely available in sufficient amounts from foods, supplements are often recommended by physicians for various health conditions such as diarrhea. FOS are available over the counter in indi-

vidual formulas and are incorporated into various probiotic formulas.

FOS act as food for *Lactobacillus bifidus* and acidophilus and are recommended as a treatment for constipation, diarrhea, foul-smelling stools and gas, bowel toxicity, and other conditions in which healthful lacto-bacillus bacteria are useful, according to Ralph Golan, M.D.[1] FOS can be synthesized and taken in powder or liquid form. Resistant to digestive enzymes, they are not absorbed and do not raise blood sugar levels. They can also be used as a sweetener. Golan suggests up to 8 g daily, or about 1 teaspoon twice daily. As a maintenance dose, he recommends 1 to 4 g daily. Megadoses may produce diarrhea. FOS assist in the normalization of bowel function and may in time lessen the need for lactobacilli supplements.

Colonic foods and FOS, such as oligo-fructose and inulin (not to be confused with insulin), a polysaccharide found in certain plants, are naturally occurring ingredients for which convincing experimental evidence in favor of a health-promoting effect is available, according to researchers at Catholic University of Louvain in Brussels. Thus, probiotics, prebiotics, and symbiotics in general and oligofructose and inulin in particular have properties of a health-enhancing functional food ingredient.[2]

FOS from food sources is only about 800 mg, which is not sufficient for diarrheal relief. The supplement dosage of FOS in this instance is 2,000 to 3,000 mg/day. This amount is said to be completely safe, with the only possible side effects being increased gas and abdominal distention in higher amounts. For children, the recommended dose is 100 mg/kg of body weight.[3]

The growth of bifidobacteria in the large bowel is dependent on a person's diet, according to Leo Galland, M.D. These sugars are concentrated in garlic, onion, artichoke, asparagus, and chicory root. Research in Japan, Europe, and the United States shows that adding FOS to the diet encourages the growth of healthful bifidobacteria and discourages the growth of undesirable organisms in the intestine. In fact, Galland said, 1 teaspoon daily of FOS lowers the concentration of toxic bacterial enzymes in the large intestine. These enzymes, called beta-glucaronidase and glycholate hydrolase, convert normal constituents to the stool, derived from either food or bile, into potential cancer-causing carcinogens. Therefore, regular consumption of foods rich in FOS may decrease the risk of colon cancer.[4]

Dutch researchers evaluated 30 men ranging in age from 33 to 64. Three times daily, the men consumed 12.5 ml of a test product containing milk fermented by yogurt starters and *Lactobacillus acidophilus* along with 2.5 percent FOS, 0.5 percent vegetable oil, and 0.5 percent milk fat, or they consumed a reference product that was a traditional yogurt containing milk fermented only by yogurt along with 1 percent milk fat. The test product significantly lowered total cholesterol, LDL cholesterol, and the LDL/HDL ratio by 4.4 percent, 5.4 percent, and 5.3 percent, respectively. However, blood levels of HDL cholesterol, triglycerides, and blood glucose were not significantly different after the two treatments.[5]

References

1. Golan, Ralph, *Optimal Wellness* (New York: Ballantine Books, 1995), 164, 229.
2. Gibson, Glenn, R., and Marcel B. Roberfroid, "Dietary Manipulation of Human Colonic Microbiota: Introducing the Concept of Prebiotics," *Journal of Nutrition* 125: 1401–12, 1995.
3. Oli, M. W., et al., "Evaluation of Fructooligosaccharide Supplementation of Oral Electrolyte Solutions for Treat-

ment of Diarrhea: Recovery of the Intestinal Bacteria," *Digestive Diseases and Sciences* 43: 138–47, 1998.

4. Galland, Leo, *The Four Pillars of Healing* (New York: Random House, 1997), 198–99.

5. Schaafsma, G., et al., "Effects of Milk Product, Fermented by Lactobacillus Acidophilus and with Fructo-Oligosaccharides Added, on Blood Lipids in Male Volunteers," *European Journal of Clinical Nutrition* 52: 436–40, 1998.

36

Garlic

The potential benefits of garlic have their origins in antiquity, where researchers have found one of the earliest documented examples of plants used for disease treatment and maintenance of health. Garlic cloves were found in the tomb of Tutankhamen (1370–52 B.C.), and the Egyptian medical volume *Ebers Codex* records the use of garlic in more than 20 health treatments. In the Bible, when the Jews departed Egypt, they regretted having to leave their garlic behind. The Greek physician Hippocrates prescribed garlic for a variety of health problems, and garlic was administered to Olympic athletes in Greece.[1] Garlic was used by the Romans, Chinese, and Indians, and was employed against the plague that struck London in the 17th century. Modern scientific research is now confirming many of the benefits of garlic in ancient medicine,

defining its mechanisms of action, and exploring garlic's potential in disease prevention and treatment.[1]

Over the centuries, garlic *(Allium sativum)*, often called the "stinking rose" and associated with bad breath and vampires, has been used as a treatment for cough, intestinal spasms, circulatory disorders, headaches, insect bites, wounds, worms, and tumors, reported Jerry Mason. Today, researchers are finding that many of these traditional uses have some value. A bulbous member of the lily family, garlic contains dozens of chemical compounds. One of these is the antibiotic allium, a sulfur-containing compound that, with its breakdown products, produces garlic's pungent odor.[2]

Mason also wrote of a study at Tagore Memorial College in Udaipur, India, in which more than 400 patients who had

had previous heart attacks were randomly divided into two groups. One took a garlic supplement, the other did not. The garlic-taking group had lower blood pressure and serum cholesterol levels, and after three years nearly twice as many patients in the control group had died of heart complications. Researchers at the Illinois Institute of Technology have shown that another of garlic's compounds, diallyl disulfide, is a strong anticancer agent. These findings have been confirmed by investigators at the University of Texas Health Science Center at Houston. Studies in China and Italy suggest that garlic is associated with low rates of stomach cancer, prompting William J. Blot, a statistician at the National Cancer Institute, to agree that these are impressive findings.

Writing in *Environmental Bulletin,* Catherine Golub, R.D., quoted Paul Lachance, Ph.D., of Rutgers University in New Brunswick, New Jersey, as saying, "Garlic is one of the most studied chemical compounds from a food source. Over 1,200 papers on garlic's health-protective effects have been published since the 1950s, with 500 of these appearing since the mid-1950's." F. Gilbert McMahon, M.D., and other researchers found a reduction of both cholesterol and LDL cholesterol in 12 weeks with 900 mg/day of powdered garlic tablets or the equivalent of 1½ cloves of garlic.[3]

A review of the literature shows that 300 to 900 mg of powdered garlic supplements daily can reduce cholesterol levels by about 12 percent, Golub added. She quoted Elise Malechi, Ph.D., a researcher at Penn State, as saying, "Garlic has demonstrated a protective effect in several epidemiological studies." The Iowa Women's Health Study found that of all foods studied, garlic showed the strongest association with a lowered risk of colon cancer. In China, areas with the highest garlic consumption have the lowest rates of stomach cancer.

Researchers at Memorial Hospital of Rhode Island in Pawtucket found that supplementation with aged garlic extract has beneficial effects on the lipid profile and blood pressure in people with moderately high levels of cholesterol. In the double-blind study, 41 men were started on 7.2 g/day of aged garlic extract or an equivalent placebo for six months. They were then switched to the other supplement for four months. A drop in total serum cholesterol of 6.1 or 7.0 percent occurred in comparison with the average concentrations during the placebo period. LDL dropped by 4.6 percent in the treatment group when compared to the controls, and there was also a 5.5 percent decrease in systolic (beating) blood pressure, along with a modest drop in diastolic (resting) blood pressure.[4]

The oxidation of LDL cholesterol is thought to be an important step in the development and progression of hardening of the arteries. In a study at Massey University at Palmerston North, New Zealand, volunteers were supplemented daily with one of three protocols: 6 g raw garlic, 2.4 g aged garlic extract, or 0.8 g vitamin E. The study lasted for seven days. LDL was significantly more resistant to oxidation when the volunteers were given aged garlic extract or vitamin E, but not raw garlic. If antioxidants are proven to be antiatherogenic, aged garlic extract may be useful in preventing atherosclerotic disease.[5]

At Kuwait University at Safat, a fresh clove of garlic was given daily to a group of male volunteers ranging in age from 40 to 50. This amounted to about 3 g of garlic a day. After 26 weeks, there was an approximately 20 percent reduction in blood cholesterol levels and about an 80 percent reduction in serum thromboxane, any of several substances that promote blood clotting. Small amounts of fresh garlic consumed over a long period may be beneficial in the prevention of thrombosis or the formation of a blood clot that could cause a heart attack or stroke.[6]

A double-blind study at Brown University and East Carolina University evaluated 75 men ranging in age from 32 to 68 who had elevated levels of cholesterol. They were given either 7 g/day of aged garlic extract or a placebo. After six months, the men were switched to the other protocol. It was found that aged garlic extract lowered blood cholesterol by 5 to 8 percent. While the garlic extract lowered LDL cholesterol, there was no effect on HDL cholesterol. The garlic brought a slight reduction in blood pressure.[7]

Although garlic had less potent antiatherosclerotic effects than various synthetic drugs, its broad-spectrum action, which affects all risk factors, gives it an important advantage over drugs. The herb has an indirect inhibitory effect on hardening of the arteries by reducing high cholesterol levels and high blood pressure, and by preventing the formation of clots and possibly diabetes.[8]

In India, 30 patients with coronary artery disease were given two garlic capsules twice daily. Each capsule contained garlic oil equivalent to 1 g of raw garlic. Thirty controls received a placebo. In the treatment group, there was a significant reduction in total serum cholesterol and triglycerides, and a significant increase in HDL cholesterol.[9]

At a meeting of the American Institute for Cancer Research held September 2–3, 1999, in Washington, D.C., Lenore Arab Kohlmeier, Ph.D., reviewed the literature from 1966 and presented an analysis of 19 case studies. There was strong evidence of garlic's effectiveness in reducing the risk and occurrence of various cancers, especially stomach and colorectal cancers.[10]

In evaluating 20 epidemiological trials, researchers at the University of Exeter in the United Kingdom reported that the majority concerned the consumption of onions and cancer, while eight studies evaluated garlic consumption and cancer. All of the studies except one suggested that *Allium* vegetables have a protective effect, especially on gastrointestinal tract cancers. The antibacterial and antimutagenic effects of the *Allium* family are probably the reason for its beneficial effects against cancer.[11]

In 1996, an estimated 53,000 cases of bladder cancer were diagnosed in the United States, and about 11,700 of these patients succumbed to the disease. Using laboratory mice, researchers at West Virginia University at Morgantown added 5, 50, and 500 mg of garlic per 100 ml to the animals' drinking water. The mice getting 50 mg had significant reductions in tumor volume, compared with the animals given a saline solution. However, the animals getting 500 mg had "significant reductions" in both bladder cancer tumor volume and mortality.[12]

Aged garlic extract dramatically diminished the growth of human prostate cancer cells in a laboratory experiment, reported Janet Raloff. In the study at Memorial Sloan-Kettering Cancer Center in New York, a research team used a group of cells that retain many of the features similar to those in a diseased prostate. For example, they multiply faster when exposed to testosterone or DHT, a potent analog that the body derives from testosterone.[13] When the cancer cells were exposed to S-allylmercaptocysteine (SAMC), a sulfur compound formed as garlic ages, the cancer cells broke down testosterone two to four times more quickly than normal. At concentrations that could develop in the blood of people taking aged garlic supplements, SAMC slowed the cancer cells'

growth by as much as 70 percent, compared to the rate in untreated cells.

In the paper from which the preceding material was taken, which was read at an April 1997 meeting of Experimental Biology, Richard S. Rivlin, M.D., said that it is unlikely that eating fresh garlic would obtain the same results.

At Bastyr University in Bothell, Washington, Gowsala Sivam, Ph.D., and colleagues stated that garlic has been used all over the world to fight bacterial infections. They have demonstrated in laboratory glassware that some antibiotic-resistant *Helicobacter pylori* strains are susceptible to garlic. *H. pylori* is a bacterium implicated in the cause of stomach cancer and ulcers.[14]

References

1. Rivlin, Richard, "Historical Perspective on the Use of Garlic," paper presented at the Garlic as a Supplement Conference, Nov. 14–17, 1998, Newport Beach, Calif.
2. Mason, Jerry, "Drugs: Some Do Grow on Trees," *Medical and Health Annual* (Chicago: Encyclopaedia Britannica, 1993), 148.
3. Golub, Catherine, "Pungent, Powerful Garlic May Help Fight Infection, Heart Disease," *Environmental Nutrition* 18(12): 1, 6, Dec. 1995.
4. Steiner, Manfred, et al., "A Double-Blind Crossover Study in Moderately Hypercholesterolemic Men That Compared the Effect of Aged Garlic Extract and Placebo Administration on Blood Lipids,"

American Journal of Clinical Nutrition 64: 866–70, Dec. 1996.

5. Munday, J. S., "Daily Supplementation with Aged Garlic Extract, But Not Raw Garlic, Protects Low-Density Lipoprotein Against In Vitro Oxidation," *Atherosclerosis* 143: 399–404, 1999.

6. Ali, M., and M. Thomson, "Consumption of a Garlic Clove a Day Could Be Beneficial in Preventing Thrombosis," *Prostaglandins, Leukotrienes, and Essential Fatty Acids* 53: 211–12, Sept. 1995.

7. "Cholesterol, Blood Pressure, and Garlic," *Nutrition Week* 27(20): 7, May 23, 1997.

8. Orekhov, Alexander N., and Jorg Grunwald, "Effects of Garlic on Atherosclerosis," *Nutrition* 13(7/8): 656–63, 1997.

9. Bordia, A., et al., "Effects of Garlic *(Allium sativum)* on Blood Lipids, Blood Sugar, Fibrinogen, and Fibrinolytic Activity in Patients with Coronary Artery Disease," *Prostaglandins, Leukotrienes, and Essential Fatty Acids* 58(4): 257–63, 1998.

10. "Botanicals Headline Cancer and Liver Disease Conference," *CRN News,* Oct. 1999, 2–3.

11. Ernst, E., "Can Allium Vegetables Prevent Cancer?" *Phytomedicine* 4(1): 79–83, 1997.

12. Riggs, Dale R., et al., "*Allium Sativum* (Garlic) Treatment of Murine Transitional Cell Carcinoma," *Cancer* 79: 1987–94, 1997.

13. Raloff, Janet, "Aged Garlic Could Slow Prostate Cancer," *Science News* 151(16): 239, April 19, 1997.

14. Sivam, G. P., et al., "Protection Against *Helicobacter pylori* and Other Bacterial Infections by Garlic," paper presented at the Garlic As a Supplement Conference, Nov. 14–17, 1998, Newport Beach, Calif.

37

Ginger

Since ancient times, doctors in China and India have considered ginger a superior medicine, adding it to combination remedies for its tonifying and spiritually uplifting properties. People throughout the world have learned to value its warming effect and ability to stimulate digestion, settle upset stomachs, and relieve aches and pains. Ginger is an effective treatment for nausea and motion sickness. It strengthens the mucosal lining of the upper gastrointestinal tract that protects against the formation of ulcers, and it has a wide range of actions against intestinal parasites.[1]

Ginger *(Zingiber officinale Roscoe)* is technically a rhizome, or underground stem, rather than a root. Its characteristic aroma is due to a volatile oil, and its pungency is attributed to ginger oleoresin, a mixture of volatile oil and resin. Components of oleo-resin, known as gingerols, have been found to possess a variety of sedative properties when given to laboratory animals.[2]

In a double-blind, randomized, placebo-controlled trial by Danish researchers, 80 Naval cadets unaccustomed to sailing in heavy seas were given 1 g of ginger root or a placebo every hour for four hours. The ginger root reduced the tendency toward vomiting and cold sweating as opposed to the placebo. Contrary to other anti–motion-sickness medications, no side effects were reported.[3]

David Taylor reported that 80 percent of the world's population relies on traditional medicinal systems and not on Western medicine, and that many of these traditional uses have herbal medicines as key ingredients. Ginger has been shown to be effective against motion sickness and morning sickness and is used in China to treat dysentery and inflammation of the testes.[4]

Danish researchers evaluated 30 women with hyperemesis gravidarium (excessive vomiting during pregnancy) by giving them 250 mg of ginger or lactose four times daily during the first four days of treatment. There was a two-day interruption (washout) period, and then the alternative medication was given for four days. Researchers found that 70.4 percent of the women preferred the ginger therapy, which provided significantly greater relief of their symptoms. The ginger was more effective than placebo in diminishing and/or limiting the symptoms of hyperemesis gravidarium.[5]

A study discussed in *Travel Medicine* involved 1,500 volunteers on a whale safari in a randomized, double-blind trial comparing seven antimotion drugs, including ginger. Although all the medications were effective, the incidence of seasickness symptoms after being given ginger was approximately 12 percent, compared with an estimated rate of 80 percent for those given a placebo.[6]

Ginger's ability to relieve gastrointestinal upset can be helpful in reducing the symptoms of irritable bowel syndrome, according to Robert M. Giller, M.D. Some patients have achieved relief with ginger capsules while others have not, but he believes it is certainly worth a try.[7]

Anisakis, acquired mainly through eating sushi or raw fish, is a significant important parasitic infection in Japan that is showing up increasingly in the United States. Although the extent of the problem is not known, there is no effective drug treatment to eliminate the parasites, which typically become embedded in the stomach or bowel wall. A study in laboratory glassware showed that an extract of ginger and two of its constituents caused more than 90 percent of the larvae to lose spontaneous movement within four hours and to be destroyed completely within 16 hours. Pyrantel pamoate, an antinematodal drug, was not effective, even in relatively high concentrations. This explains why ginger is traditionally eaten with sushi in Japan.[8]

A Danish researcher has stated that ginger consumption may provide relief from rheumatoid arthritis by reducing pain and improving movement of joints in arthritic patients. Ginger may be effective by reducing the amounts of prostaglandins and leukotrienes.[9]

Melchor Barros, M.D., a physician in Chicago, maintains that a slice or a piece of ginger works exceptionally well for throat irritation and itchiness. He recommends ginger as a throat lozenge.[10]

Nausea and vomiting are common side effects following major surgery. M. E. Bone et al. reported that ginger helps relieve postoperative nausea and vomiting following gynecological surgery. The double-blind study involved 60 women between the ages of 16 and 65. The researchers found that the administration of drugs to prevent vomiting following surgery was significantly greater in the placebo group than in the women receiving ginger.[11]

A typical capsule contains 250 mg of standardized ginger rhizome. For motion sickness, the recommended dosage is two capsules one half hour prior to the trip for adults and children over the age of six, then two capsules every four hours. The capsules are not recommended for children under the age of six. To avoid stomach discomfort, the recommended dose is one capsule one half hour before the expected onset of discomfort, then one capsule every four hours as needed.

References

1. Weil, Andrew, *8 Weeks to Optimum Health* (New York: Alfred A. Knopf, 1997), 117ff.

2. Tyler, Varro E., and Steven Foster, *Tyler's Honest Herbal* (New York: Haworth Herbal Press, 1999), 147ff.

3. Grontved, Acksel, et al., "Ginger Root Against Sea Sickness: A Controlled Trial on the Open Sea," *Acta Otolaryngology Stockholm* 105: 45–49, 1988.

4. Taylor, David, "Crossroads," *Environmental Health Perspectives* 104(9): 924–28, Sept. 1996.

5. Fisher-Rasmussen, Wiggo, "Ginger Treatment of Hyperemesis Gravidarium," *European Journal of Obstetrics and Gynecology and Reproductive Biology* 38: 19–24, 1990.

6. Schmid, R., et al., "Whale Safari," *Travel Medicine* 1(4): 203, 1994.

7. Giller, Robert M., and Kathy Matthews, *Natural Prescriptions* (New York: Ballantine Books, 1994), 223.

8. Schulick, Paul, *Ginger: Common Spice and Wonder Drug* (Brattleboro, Vt: Herbal Free Press Ltd., 1996), 48–49.

9. Srivastava, K. C., "Effect of Onion and Ginger Composition on Platelet Thromboxane Production in Humans," *Prostaglandins, Leukotrienes, and Essential Fatty Acids* 35: 183–85, 1989.

10. Barros, Melchor, "Soothing Sore Throats Gingerly," *Cortland Forum* 86: 16, 67, April 1995.

11. Bone, M. E., "Ginger Root—A New Antiemetic," *Anesthesia* 45: 669–71, 1990.

38

Ginkgo Biloba

A native of southwestern China, *Ginkgo biloba* is a member of the Ginkgoales family, which dates from the Permian period of the Paleozoic era, between 225 and 280 million years ago. In addition to the use of its bilobed, fan-shaped leaves for medicinal purposes, ginkgo is a familiar ornamental tree in parks and along city streets. These trees are males, since the female trees produce nuts, which fall to the ground and smell like rancid butter. The nuts are a delicacy in the Far East.

The *Ginkgo biloba* extract, standardized to contain 24 percent ginkgoflavonglycosides, has shown remarkably beneficial effects in improving many symptoms associated with aging, especially those linked to reduced blood flow to the brain—dizziness, ringing in the ears (tinnitus), headache, short-term memory loss, and depression.[1]

The extract has also been shown to be useful in treating dementia, impotence, multiple sclerosis, neuralgia, intermittent claudication, premenstrual syndrome, macular degeneration, diabetic retinopathy, and other conditions.

To meet the rising demand for ginkgo leaves, a German company has established plantations on the Atlantic coast of France and in South Carolina. On both sites, 25 million trees produce about 4,000 tons of dried leaves annually. Over 25 million trees are cultivated in China for the same purpose. Ginkgo is also cultivated in Japan and South Korea and is used worldwide as an ornamental tree. Ginkgo is resistant to urban pollution and grows naturally in the mountainous forests in China. Contrary to some reports, ginkgo is not an endangered species.[2]

In a review of the role of herbal medicine, David Taylor reported that 80 percent of the world's population relies on traditional medicine and not on Western medicine. Concerning *Ginkgo biloba,* he said that it has been shown to increase brain tolerance to oxygen deficiency, increase blood flow, improve memory and mental alertness, stimulate circulation, and reduce cardiovascular risk. It may also inhibit deteriorating vision in the elderly.[3]

In a study published in the *Journal of the American Medical Association,* Pierre L. LeBars, M.D., Ph.D., and colleagues at the New York Institute for Medical Research, Tarrytown, and other facilities, reported that 37 percent of the patients diagnosed with dementia showed some improvement after 52 weeks of getting *Ginkgo biloba* extract when compared to placebo. The 202 patients were randomly assigned to the treatment group, taking 120 mg/day of the extract, or a placebo, for one year. In addition, after the 52-week study, 27 percent of the patients taking ginkgo achieved a four-point improvement on the Alzheimer's Disease Assessment Scale, a standard test. A similar improvement was recorded for 14 percent in the control group.[4]

The ginkgo extract contains multiple compounds thought to act synergistically on diverse processes involved in the homeostasis of inflammation and oxidative stress. This provides membrane protection and neurotransmission modulation, which may be the basis of the extract's effects on the central nervous system.

Ginkgo biloba extract (EGb 761) is among the most popular over-the-counter medications in Europe and is available in health food stores in the United States. The European medical community has recognized the extract as an effective treatment for cerebral insufficiency. In some studies, the benefits to the central nervous system were similar to those of other psychoactive compounds classified as cognitive activators. Since the extract has shown therapeutic effects in the treatment of dementia, it has earned the approval of the German health authorities for the treatment of dementia. Therapeutic doses have ranged from 40 to 240 mg/day.[5]

At the Free University of Berlin, Germany, a double-blind study evaluated 216 Alzheimer's patients who received daily a dose of 240 mg of *Ginkgo biloba* extract or a placebo. The research team confirmed that the clinical benefit was evident in the 156 patients who completed the study with the extract.[6]

An extensive review in *The Lancet* reported that 12 symptoms related to cerebral insufficiency are said to be relieved by ginkgo, including difficulties with concentration and memory, absent-mindedness, confusion, lack of energy, tiredness, decreased physical performance, depressed mood, anxiety, dizziness, tinnitus, and headache.[7] The authors reported that important constituents in ginkgo are flavonoids and terpenoids, and the herb prevents free radicals and lipid peroxidation. Typical dosages are 120 to 200 mg/day. For intermittent claudication, there have been 15 controlled trials, 8 of which have been in

Germany and 5 in France. While two studies are of acceptable quality, all have shown positive benefit. No serious side effects have been reported. In a few cases, patients experienced mild gastrointestinal complaints, headache, and allergic skin reactions. Ginkgo extract can be given to patients with mild to moderate symptoms of cerebral insufficiency, with doses ranging from 120 to 160 mg/day in three divided doses. Treatment should continue for four to six weeks before positive results are noticed.

Researchers at Johann Wolfgang Goethe University in Frankfurt, in a double-blind study, evaluated Alzheimer's-type dementia patients who were given either a placebo or 240 mg/day of *Ginkgo biloba* extract (EGb 761) for three months. There was improvement in the treatment group using standard testing procedures, but there was a deterioration in the placebo group.[8]

In an animal model, it was reported that treatment with ginkgo extract at doses of 50 to 100 mg/kg protected the animals against a memory deficit found in the control group one month following cranial irradiation. Administration of 100 mg/kg of the extract significantly facilitated the learning ability of a second test group started one month after total cranial irradiation. The researchers suggested that the antistress effects of the extract accounted for the better performance of the treated animals.[9]

Since *Ginkgo biloba* has free radical–scavenging properties, its antioxidant action inhibits or reduces the morphological impairments to the retina of the eye that are observed after lipid peroxide release, according to French researchers. Therefore, ginkgo may be beneficial in the prevention and treatment of retinopathies in degenerative diseases of the eye related to oxidative stress.[10]

Ginkgo biloba extract is an efficient and multifunctional antioxidant that protects against oxidative stress. For example, the extract appears to have an antioxidant-scavenging effect against hydroxyl radicals and nitric oxide. In animals, the extract can prevent damage of the retina in rats that were made diabetic from an injection of alloxan, a drug that causes low blood sugar.[11]

In a placebo-controlled, double-blind study, 33 patients with chronic peripheral arterial occlusive disease participated in a physical training program three times weekly for 24 weeks. During the trial they were given either a placebo or 160 mg/day of ginkgo extract. The incidence of pain-free walking was higher in the extract group than in the placebo group.[12]

Armenian workers exposed to radiation while working at Chernobyl between 1986 and 1987 were given 40 mg of ginkgo extract three times daily for two months. The therapy reduced the clastogenic activity, which originally was 10 times higher than the reference range, to near normal levels. The treatment continued for up to one year. In about one-third of the workers, however, the clastogenic factor test became positive once again, suggesting that the process that produces these factors is not stopped indefinitely. Clastogen (e.g., certain chemicals, X rays, ultraviolet light, etc.) causes breaks in chromosomes.[13]

Ginkgo biloba extracts may be effective in treating erectile dysfunction due to restricted blood flow. In an experimental study, 60 patients with erection problems who had not responded to injections of papaverine (a vasodilator) of up to 50 mg were treated with 60 mg/day of ginkgo extract for 12 to 18 months. After four weeks of treatment, penile arterial blood flow was evaluated by duplex sonography every four weeks. The first signs of increased blood flow were observed after six to eight weeks. Following six weeks of therapy, 50 percent of the men had regained potency; 20 percent responded to a new trial of papaverine; and 25 percent showed improved arterial flow but did not respond to papaverine. There was no change in the remaining 5 percent.[14]

In a French study involving 70 patients with inner ear dysfunction, 47 percent given ginkgo extract became symptom free, compared to 18 percent of the controls. Following three months of therapy, the effectiveness of the extract on the intensity, frequency, and duration of the disorder was statistically significant. The usual dosage of the extract is 40 mg three times a day.[15]

Researchers in Mexico have reported that ginkgo is useful in treating brain-injured patients, since the herb shows little toxicity in animals and man. The active ingredients in the extract are terpenes (ginkgolides, bilobalicides, and flavonol-heterosides). The study supporting this theory came from two animal studies in which there were injuries to the motor centers of the brain.[16]

A French research team evaluated 15 patients undergoing aortic valve replacement. These volunteers were given 320 mg/day of ginkgo or a placebo for five days. The extract significantly reduced the more delayed leakage of myoglobin, an iron-containing protein in muscles similar to hemoglobin. The data suggest the usefulness of the extract in reducing oxidative stress in cardiovascular surgery, and suggest a role of the highly bioavailable terpene constituent in the extract.[17]

A case report discussed a patient who had had symptoms of unipolar depression for more than 30 years, beginning at age 17. During a 10-month period, the patient was given about 135 mg of ginkgo, in which 33 mg was taken in the morning and 17 mg thereafter every two hours. The patient was also given valerian, hops, zinc, and vitamin B_6. After 10 months of therapy, the patient felt remarkably better. *Ginkgo biloba* may inhibit biogenic amines, helping to maintain brain neurotransmitters.[18]

References

1. "Ginkgo Biloba Extract," *Natural Medicine Journal* 1(8): 7, Oct. 1998.
2. Schmid, Wilhelm, "Ginkgo Thrives," *Nature* 386: 765, April 24, 1997.

3. Taylor, David, "Herbal Medicine at the Crossroads," *Environmental Health Perspectives* 104(9): 924–28, Sept. 1996.

4. LeBars, Pierre L., et al., "A Placebo-Controlled, Double-Blind, Randomized Trial of an Extract of *Ginkgo Biloba* for Dementia," *Journal of the American Medical Association* 278(16): 1327–32, Oct. 22/29, 1997.

5. Itil, Turan, and David Martorano, "Natural Substances in Psychiatry (*Ginkgo Biloba* in Dementia)," *Psychopharmacology Bulletin* 31(1): 147–58, 1995.

6. Kanowski, S., et al., "Proof of Efficacy of the *Ginkgo Biloba* Special Extract EGb 761 in Outpatients Suffering from Mild to Moderate Primary Degenerative Dementia of the Alzheimer-Type or Multi-Infarct Dementia," *Pharmacopsychiat* 29: 47–56, 1996.

7. Kleijnen, Jos, and Paul Knipschild, "*Ginkgo Biloba*," *The Lancet* 340: 1136–39, Nov. 7, 1992.

8. Maurer, K., et al., "Clinical Efficacy of *Ginkgo Biloba* Special Extract EGb 761 in Dementia of the Alzheimer Type," *Journal of Psychiatric Research* 31(6): 645–55, 1997.

9. Lamproglou, I., et al., "Cognitive Dysfunction Induced by Cranial Irradiation: Effect of *Ginkgo Biloba* Extract (EGb 761) in 4-Month-Old Male Rats," *Advances in Ginkgo Biloba Extract Research* 6: 73–87, 1997.

10. Droy-Lefaix, Marie-Therese, et al., "Antioxidant Effect of a *Ginkgo Biloba* Extract EGb 761 on the Retina," *International Journal of Tissue Reactions* 17(3): 93–100, 1995.

11. Marocci, Lucia, et al., "Antioxidant Action of *Ginkgo Biloba* Extract EGb 761," *Methods in Enzymology* 234: 462–75, 1994.

12. Bulling, B., "The Treatment of Peripheral Arterial Occlusive Disease with Walking (Blood-Vessel) Training and *Ginkgo Biloba* Extract (EGb 761)," *Advances in Ginkgo Biloba Extract Research* 3: 143–50, 1994.

13. Emerit, I., et al., "*Ginkgo Biloba* Extract (EGb 761) and Adaptation to Radiation," *Advances in Ginkgo Biloba Extract Research* 6: 21–29, 1997.

14. Sikora, R., et al., "*Ginkgo Biloba* Extract in the Therapy of Erectile Dysfunction," *Journal of Urology* 141: 188A, 1989.

15. Haguenauer, J. P., et al., "Treatment of Equilibrium Disorders with *Ginkgo Biloba* Extract: A Multi-Center Double-Blind Drug vs. Placebo Study," *Presse Medica* 15(31): 1569–72, 1986.

16. Brailowski, S., et al., "Effects of *Ginkgo Biloba* Extract in Two Models of Cortical Hemiplegia in Rats," *Restorative Neurology and Neuroscience* 3: 267–74, 1991.

17. Pietri, Sylvia, et al., "*Ginkgo Biloba* Extract (EGb 761) Pretreatment Limits Free Radical–Induced Oxidative Stress in Patients Undergoing Coronary Bypass Surgery," *Cardiovascular Drugs and Therapy* 11: 121–31, 1997.

18. Sealey, R., "Surviving Unipolar Depression—the Effectiveness of *Ginkgo Biloba*," *Journal of Orthomolecular Medicine* 11(3): 168–72, 1996.

39

Ginseng

The legendary Chinese emperor Shen Nung, who reportedly lived as long ago as the third century B.C., documented several hundred plant-derived medicines that continue to be used in the Orient. In the 16th century A.D., herbalist Li Shih-chen compiled the Chinese materia medica known as the Great Pharmacopeia. One of the respected herbs in this compendium is ginseng, which contains compounds thought to stimulate the nervous system, enhance circulation, and increase the secretion of hormones. Saponins, found in various species of ginseng, are potent glucosides that act on the nervous system as either a depressant or a stimulant, depending on the dosage.[1] There are a number of varieties of ginseng, including Asian ginseng *(Panax ginseng)*, American ginseng *(Panax quiquefolius)*, and Siberian ginseng *(Eleutherococcus senticosus)*. References can

also be found for Chinese ginseng, Korean ginseng, and others.

Both Chinese ginseng and North American ginseng have similar restorative qualities, although Chinese ginseng is more of a stimulant and sexual energizer, and American ginseng may be more active as an adaptogen, according to Andrew Weil, M.D. Among Chinese and Koreans, ginseng is highly regarded as a tonic for the elderly, since it can improve appetite and digestion, tone skin and muscles, and restore depleted sexual energy.[2]

"Ginseng is generally safe, but the Oriental variety can raise blood pressure in some individuals, as well as cause irritability," Weil added. "People who experience those side effects should lower the dose or switch to American ginseng (which is preferred by many Orientals). I recommend ginseng frequently to people who have low vitality or have been weakened by chronic illness or old age."

Asian ginseng and Siberian ginseng are said to improve athletic performance, although it takes up to a month before benefits kick in. Animal studies have repeatedly confirmed that the herb stimulates the immune system. Ginseng is used by Russian cosmonauts and Asian Olympic athletes as an adaptogen or energy-enhancing tonic, since it increases resistance to all types of stress. It is also highly regarded for reducing fatigue and improving alertness, coordination, memory, and stress-coping abilities.[3]

In a double-blind study, nurses who took Asian ginseng when they switched from a day shift to a night shift demonstrated higher scores in physical and mental performance and had better moods than those on a placebo, according to Harold H. Bloomfield, M.D. Studies indicate that ginseng can lower blood cholesterol and has an anticlotting factor that might decrease the risk of a heart attack. But ginseng is not recommended for those with manic-depressive illness, heart palpitations, asthma, or emphysema. It is also not recommended for pregnant women. The usual dosage is 100 mg of ginseng extract standardized to 13 percent ginsenosides twice daily, he said.[4]

Compared to Asian ginseng, American ginseng is said to be "cooler" or less stimulating, and is thought to be more appropriate for counteracting the stress experienced by overworked, burned-out, adren-

ally depleted young adults, Bloomfield continued. The dosage for American ginseng is the same as for Asian ginseng.

Siberian ginseng, which is not specifically a ginseng, has a wide spectrum of benefits, including promoting adaptation to climatic extremes of heat, cold, and altitude; increasing workload; improving visual and aural acuity; and protecting against radiation and depression, Bloomfield said. Siberian ginseng benefits stressed adrenal and pituitary glands, and it is especially useful for people suffering from mild anxiety and insomnia. The recommended dosage is 180 to 360 mg of the extract, in divided doses, for two to three months, followed by a two-week break.

In a lab glassware experiment at Okayama University Medical School in Japan, ginseng completely inhibited hydroxyl radical formation. This antioxidant effect may explain why ginseng is responsible for so many pharmacologic actions in clinical practice.[5] A hydroxyl radical is a dangerous free radical that will attack almost any molecule in the body and cause the breakdown of membrane lipids and proteins.

Other researchers found that *Panax ginseng* is a pulmonary vasodilator that protects the lungs in animals against free radical injury.[6]

Danish researchers injected laboratory animals with ginseng, followed two weeks later with a challenge with *Pseudomonas aeruginosa*, a bacterium that mimics the predominant pathogen in cystic fibrosis. The ginseng-treated animals showed significantly improved bacterial clearance in the lungs, and there were fewer mast cells in the lungs. Mast cells are large cells that occur in connective tissue. Ginseng may be a promising remedy for the treatment of *P. aeruginosa* lung infections in cystic fibrosis patients.[7] *P. aeruginosa* is a bacterium also commonly found in wound infections, infected burn lesions, and urinary tract infections.

Recent studies suggest that ginseng serves as an antioxidant and organ-protective agent associated with enhanced nitric acid synthesis in the endothelium of the lungs, heart, and kidney.[8] Nitric oxide, a potentially toxic compound composed of oxygen and nitrogen, is found in cigarette smoke and pollution and may cause a genetic mutation that could lead to cancer.

Ginseng root *(Panax ginseng)* contains at least 1.5 percent ginsenosides, according to the *Complete German Commission E Monographs*. As a tonic, it is used for invigoration and fortification during fatigue and disability, as well as for declining capacity for work and concentration. It is also used during convalescence. Side effects and interactions with other drugs are unknown.[9]

A ginsenoside from *Panax ginseng* has shown significant inhibitory effects against platelet activating factor (PAF), which is involved in many inflammatory and allergic processes. Until now, no saponins have exhibited this activity.[10]

At the University of Milan, researchers tested 227 patients to see if ginseng would prevent a cold or flu. Volunteers were given a daily dose of 100 mg of ginseng or a placebo for 12 weeks. The researchers found 15 cases of cold or flu in the ginseng group, compared with 42 in the placebo. After eight weeks of therapy, antibodies to infections rose to an average of 171 units in the placebo group, compared to 272 units in the treatment group. Natural killer cell activity after 8 and 12 weeks was almost twice as high in the ginseng group, compared to the control group. Out of 227 volunteers, only nine side effects were reported: one in the placebo group and eight in the ginseng volunteers, which consisted of insomnia, nausea, gastric pain, and anxiety. Natural killer cells are the first line of defense against infections and cancer.[11]

References

1. Mason, Jerry, "Drugs: Some Do Grow on Trees," *Medical and Health Annual* (Chicago: Encyclopaedia Britannica, 1993), 141–42.

2. Weil, Andrew, *Spontaneous Healing* (New York: Alfred A. Knopf, 1995), 179–80.

3. Duke, James A., *The Green Pharmacy* (Emmaus, Pa.: Rodale Press, 1997), 132–33.

4. Bloomfield, Harold H., *Healing Anxiety with Herbs* (New York: HarperCollins, 1998), 103ff.

5. Zhang, Daxian, et al., "Ginseng Extract Scavenges Hydroxyl Radical and Protects Unsaturated Fatty Aids from Decomposition Caused by Iron-Mediated Lipid Peroxidation," *Free Radical Biology in Medicine* 20(1): 145–50, 1996.

6. Rimar, S., et al., "Pulmonary Protective and Vasodilator Effects of a Standardized *Panax ginseng* Preparation Following Artificial Gastric Digestion," *Pulmonary Pharmacology* 9: 205–09, 1996.

7. Song, Zhijun, et al., "Ginseng Treatment Reduces Bacterial Load and Lung Pathology in Chronic *Pseudomonas Aeruginosa* Pneumonia in Rats," *Antimicrobial Agents and Chemotherapy* 41(5): 961–64, May 1997.

8. Gillis, C. Norman. "Panax Ginseng Pharmacology: A Nitric Oxide Link?" *Biochemical Pharmacology* 54: 1–8, 1997.

9. Blumenthal, Mark, ed., *The Complete German Commission E Monographs* (Boston: Integrative Medicine Communications and American Botanical Council [Austin, Texas], 1998, 138–39.

10. Jung, K. J., et al., "Platelet Activating Factor Antagonist Activity of Ginseno-sides," *Biological Pharmacology Bulletin* 21: 79–80, 1998.

11. Scaglione, F., et al., "Efficacy and Safety of the Standardized Ginseng Extract G-115 for Potentiating Vaccination Against Common Cold and/or Influenza Syndrome," *Drugs in Experimental and Clinical Research* 22(2): 65–72, 1996.

40

Glucosamine Sulfate

Osteoarthritis affects more than 15 million Americans annually. Its frequency increases with age and occurs universally in those over the age of 75. By 2030, those afflicted who are over the age of 65 are expected to constitute at least 17 percent of the population and account for about 40 percent of the total drug expenditures in the United States. Since glucosamine is a primary constituent in cartilage, it has been shown to be effective in strengthening cartilage. In one study, 1.5 g/day of oral glucosamine compared to oral ibuprofen at 1.2 g/day showed that while glucosamine was slower to achieve therapeutic effect, it was superior to the drug at the end of the eight-week trial.[1]

Michael T. Murray, N.D., wrote that glucosamine, a naturally found substance in joint structures, appears to be nature's best remedy for osteoarthritis. Glucosamine's action on joints is responsible for stimulating the manufacture of substances necessary for joint repair. It also exerts a protective effect against joint destruction, and when taken as glucosamine sulfate as a supplement, it is selectively taken up by joint tissues to exert a powerful therapeutic effect on osteoarthritis.[2]

"While NSAIDs offer purely symptomatic relief and may actually promote the disease process," Murray added, "glucosamine sulfate addresses the cause of osteoarthritis. By getting to the root of the problem, glucosamine sulfate not only alleviates the symptoms, including pain; it also helps the body to repair damaged joints."

Researchers at the Southern Regional Area Health Education Center in Fayetteville, North Carolina, did a Medline search from January 1975 through March 1997. They found that glucosamine has produced consistent benefit (about 50 percent overall improvement in symptom scores) in patients with osteoarthritis and, in some cases, may be equal or superior to ibuprofen in controlling symptoms. Glucosamine sulfate may provide pain relief, reduce tenderness, and improve mobility in patients with the disease. Studies have tended to involve small numbers of volunteers, and long-term trials concerning safety, efficacy, and optimal doses are warranted. The most frequently used dosage of glucosamine sulfate in the trials was 500 mg three times daily.[3]

Successful treatment of osteoarthritis must control pain and slow down or reverse the progression of the disease. Biochemical and pharmacological data, along with human and animal studies, have demonstrated that glucosamine sulfate can satisfy both criteria. The supplement's primary role in halting or reversing joint degeneration seems to be its ability to serve as an essential substrate for, and to stimulate the biosynthesis of, the glycosaminoglycans and the hyaluronic acid backbone required for the formation of proteoglycans found in the structural matrix of joints. The combination of glucosamine sulfate and chondroitin sulfate supplements in the treatment of degenerative joint disease has become a popular protocol in treating arthritic conditions of the joints.[4] Glycosaminoglycans are chains of modified sugars; proteoglycans form the structure of collagenous tissue.

Researchers at Case Western Reserve University School of Medicine and University Hospitals in Cleveland reviewed the literature concerning the roles of glucosamine sulfate and chondroitin sulfate. After evaluating 13 studies, it was concluded that clinical trials of the two substances showed substantial benefit in the treatment of osteoarthritis. Glucosamine was found superior to placebo in seven trials, and in two studies comparing glucosamine to ibuprofen, glucosamine was superior in one and equivalent in the other. Dosages generally used are 1,500 mg/day of glucosamine sulfate and 1,200 mg/day of chondroitin sulfate. Consumers are urged to check the dosages listed on the labels.[5]

Glucosamine sulfate stimulates cartilage regeneration, protects against joint destruction, and alleviates the symptoms of osteoarthritis. However, it is not an analgesic and several weeks are required before noticeable relief can be obtained.[6]

A large-scale Portuguese study involving 252 doctors evaluated how effective glucosamine was in treating 1,208 patients with osteoarthritis. The patients were given three daily doses, totaling 1.5 g of glucosamine, for 36 to 64 days, with an average of 50 days. Pain improved throughout the study, and 95 percent reported a "sufficient" or "good" clinical response. Glucosamine continued to work 6 to 12 weeks after the study ended, with 86 percent of the patients reporting no side effects. Of the small number who reported side effects, such as gastrointestinal discomfort, the discomfort generally disappeared within one to three weeks.[7]

In 1994, German researchers conducted a double-blind study involving 252 patients with osteoarthritis of the knee. During weekly clinical visits, the volunteers received either 1.5 g/day of glucosamine sulfate for four weeks or a placebo. The researchers said that glucosamine sulfate was significantly more effective than placebo in improving pain and movement in patients with osteoarthritis of the knee. In another 1994 study, 329 patients were evaluated with either 1.5 g/day of glucosamine sulfate or 20 mg/day of the drug piroxicam (Feldene). It was confirmed that glucosamine sulfate outperformed the drug.[8]

Supplemental glucosamine aids in the synthesis of connective tissue. This is especially beneficial for athletes, since repair and growth of connective tissue is an ongoing process. When glucosamine is taken orally by athletes, it gives injured connective tissue time to rebuild its collagenous matrix.[9]

The production of hyaluronic acid by fibroblasts in the early stages of wound healing is said to be of critical importance. Hyaluronic acid is a cementing substance in subcutaneous tissue. Glucosamine given by mouth during the first few days after surgery or trauma enhances hyaluronic acid production and promotes faster wound healing.[10]

Researchers at the Naval Special Warfare Group Two in Norfolk, Virginia, evaluated 34 Navy personnel from the diving and special warfare community who complained of chronic pain in the knees and lower back. During the 16-week trial, the volunteers were given either 1,500 mg/day of glucosamine, 1,200 mg/day of chondroitin, and 228 mg/day of manganese ascorbate; or a placebo. The combination therapy relieved symptoms of osteoarthritis in the knee. Further research is needed to determine the therapy's effectiveness for spinal degenerative joint disease.[11]

The symptoms of osteoarthritis are common complaints in patients with temporomandibular disorders (TMD). For a number of years in veterinary medicine, glucosamine and chondroitin sulfates have been used to treat osteoarthritis, and these supplements may be useful in treating humans with TMD if the problem is related to osteoarthritis.[12] TMD is a spasm of the chewing muscles, which brings on pain and other symptoms in the head, jaw, and face. The problem begins when the temporomandibular (jaw) joints and their muscles and ligaments do not mesh properly. The problem is also exacerbated by clenching or grinding teeth or an incorrect bite. With or without the accompanying pain, joint noises are annoying to both the patient and people sitting near them at mealtime.

Glucosamine sulfate and chondroitin sulfate supplements are available individually in health food stores or other markets, and they are also found in combination with other ingredients. This seems to be a breakthrough therapy for osteoarthritis, but little research has been done as to whether the two supplements can benefit other forms of arthritis, such as rheumatoid arthritis.

References

1. Heyneman, C. A., and R. S. Rhodes, "Glucosamine for Osteoarthritis: Cure or Conundrum?" *Annals of Pharmacotherapy* 32: 602–03, May 1998.

2. Murray, Michael T., *Natural Alternatives to Over-the-Counter and Prescription Drugs* (New York: William Morrow and Co., 1994), 74–75.

3. deCamara, C. C., and G. V. Dowless, "Glucosamine Sulfate for Osteoarthritis," *Annals of Pharmacotherapy* 32: 580–87, May 1998.

4. Kelly, G. S., "The Role of Glucosamine Sulfate and Chondroitin Sulfates in the Treatment of Degenerative Joint Disease," *Alternative Medicine Review* 3: 27–39, Feb. 1998.

5. Deal, C. L., and R. W. Moskowitz, "Nutraceuticals as Therapeutic Agents in Osteoarthritis: The Role of Glucosamine, Chondroitin Sulfate, and Collagen Hydrolysate," *Rheumatic Disease Clinics of North America* 25: 379–95, May 1999.

6. Pizzorno, Joseph E., Jr., "Natural Medicine Approach to Treating Osteoarthritis," *Alternative and Complementary Therapies,* Jan./Feb. 1995, 93–95.

7. Theodosakis, Jason, Brenda Adderly, and Barry Fox, *The Arthritis Cure* (New York: St. Martin's Press, 1997), 39.

8. Loes, Michael, Gary Wikholm, Megan Shields, and David Steinman, *Arthritis: The Doctors' Cure* (New Canaan, Conn.: Keats Publishing, 1998), 84ff.

9. Gastelu, Daniel, and Fred Hatfield, *Dynamic Nutrition for Maximum Performance* (Garden City Park, N.Y.: Avery Publishing Group, 1997), 105.

10. McCarty, M. F., "Glucosamine for Wound Healing," *Medical Hypotheses* 47: 273–75, 1996.

11. Leffler, C. T., et al., "Glucosamine, Chondroitin, and Manganese Ascorbate for Degenerative Joint Disease of the Knee or Lower Back: A Randomized, Double-Blind, Placebo-Controlled Pilot Study," *Military Medicine* 164: 85–91, Feb. 1999.

12. Shankland, W. E. II, "The Effects of Glucosamine and Chondroitin Sulfate on Osteoarthritis of the TMJ: A Preliminary Report of 50 Patients," *Cranio.* 16: 230–35, Oct. 1998.

41

Glutamine

L-glutamine, considered nonessential, is one of the 20 amino acids that serve as building blocks for proteins. However, it can be considered essential in a variety of health care problems. While glutamine is the most prevalent amino acid in plasma, it is in short supply during severe illnesses. Glutamine is manufactured in the body by glutamic acid, another amino acid, and the brain and muscle synthesize it to rid the body of ammonia, a toxic metabolic by-product. Supplements of glutamine are available over the counter, and it is often added to sports drinks.

A research team at Brigham and Women's Hospital in Boston evaluated 43 patients admitted to the Bone Marrow Transplant Unit. The patients received the standard tubal feeding or an isonitrogenous parenteral nutrition solution containing glutamine, which was given one day after the bone marrow transplant. The glutamine-laced feeding improved nitrogen balance, length of the hospital stay was shorter, and incidence of microbial hospital infections was significantly lower. Hospital charges were $21,095 less per patient, and room and board charges were significantly reduced in the glutamine-supplemented group at $51,484 versus $61,591 in the standard-feeding group. Further, the cost savings at this hospital for 22 patients who received glutamine-supplemented feedings were estimated to be $10,687 per patient, or $235,114 total. Glutamine therapy could realize notable financial benefits and savings for the hospital and additional revenue.[1]

The overall metabolism of protein is reflected in the body's nitrogen balance. Nitrogen, an almost inert gas, enters the body from various dietary protein sources, and the by-products of nitrogen metabolism are excreted in the urine, feces, and dermal loss. It is the total of nitrogen in versus nitrogen out, or nitrogen balance, that demonstrates tissue growth, degradation, and maintenance.

At the University of Hohenheim in Stuttgart, Germany, researchers found significant evidence that supplemental glutamine dipeptide positively influences nitrogen excretion, immune status, gut integrity, morbidity, rehabilitation, and recovery. Therefore, glutamine can be considered an indispensable amino acid during stress. In one study in which the patients were in an intensive care unit, supplementation with glutamine brought a 15 percent reduction of total hospital care, which was $6,373 per patient when expressed as cost per survivor. This amounted to 50 percent less than seen with conventional intravenous feeding. The researchers concluded that a positive effect on the immune system and the gastrointestinal tract can be achieved with glutamine supplements between 10 and 13 g/day.[2]

Researchers at Metro Health Medical Center, Cleveland, Ohio, reported that for patients with cirrhosis of the liver, glutamine supplementation may improve glutamine uptake and oxidation in the intestine, while preserving the gut mucosal barrier and reducing the absorption of endotoxin, a poisonous substance found in bacteria in the gut. For these patients, glutamine may be an essential amino acid for obtaining positive nitrogen balance and preventing malnutrition.[3]

Although some consider glutamine a nonessential amino acid, it may be essential during inflammatory conditions such as infection and injury. In patients undergoing cytotoxic therapy for cancer, glutamine has been shown to improve nitrogen balance, decrease infections, and reduce hospitalizations. In premature infants, glutamine given intravenously has led to a shorter time on a ventilator and decreased total tube feedings.[4]

Glutamine supplements bring decreased morbidity in very low-birth-weight infants whose feedings include the amino acid. In a randomized study, infants were given enteral glutamine supplementation in three different amounts ranging from 500 to 1,250 g/day. Hospital-acquired sepsis was 30 percent in the control group, compared to only 11 percent in the glutamine group. Sepsis is the spread of bacteria or other products, a frequent problem in hospitals.[5]

Glutamine supplements protect lymphocytes and reduce gut permeability in patients with advanced esophageal cancer during chemotherapy treatments. A study in Japan involved 12 patients with esophageal cancer who received either 30 g/day of glutamine at the beginning of radiochemotherapy and for a subsequent 28 days, or a control treatment. The supplement prevented a reduction in lymphocyte count, among other things. Lymphocytes are a type of white blood cell and an important constituent of the immune system.[6]

Researchers at the University of São Paulo, Brazil, reported that burn patients experience extensive nitrogen loss, malnutrition, markedly increased metabolic rate, and immunologic deficiency. These patients have frequent infections, poor wound healing, increased hospital stays, and increased death rates. This calls for nutritional support high in protein and high-energy diets given shortly after injury. Supplementing with glutamine, arginine (another amino acid), and omega-3 fatty acids at levels two to seven times those in the normal diet of a healthy person can be beneficial in normalizing the pathophysiological alterations in burn patients. The Shriners' diet for burn patients, as an example, is high in protein, low in fat, linoleic-acid restricted, and enriched with omega-3 fatty acids, arginine, cysteine, histidine, vitamin A, and vitamin C. This diet brings fewer infections and shorter stays in the hospital.[7]

During catabolic states, glutamine metabolism is considerably altered, and its tissue and plasma pools are depleted. Catabolism is the breaking down of complex chemical compounds into simpler ones. In laboratory animals fed glutamine, there was a reduction in the number of *E. coli* in peritoneal fluid, as well as a reduction of bacterial cultures in the liver.[8]

Researchers in Italy have found that glutamine supplementation in acute leukemia patients—before, during, and after chemotherapy—is feasible and possibly associated with better tolerance to chemotherapeutic treatments. In one study involving 22 patients between the ages of 24 and 62, it was found that the severity of diarrhea and its duration (a side effect of the therapy) were significantly reduced in those getting glutamine supplements, and none reported severe diarrhea. The usual dosage was 6 g of L-glutamine dissolved in water three times daily during meals, taken three days prior to chemotherapy treatments.[9]

In certain situations, amino acids can be beneficial in the treatment of low blood sugar, wrote Ralph Golan, M.D. As an example, if chromium, biotin, and the B complex have not been effective in reducing sugar cravings, glutamine may be of help. He recommends 500 to 1,000 mg two or three times daily. Glutamine can be taken 1½ hours before or after any protein foods or on an empty stomach. Entry into the brain can be enhanced if amino acids are taken with a little carbohydrate, such as crackers or diluted fruit juice.[10]

In uncontrolled human and animal studies, glutamine at 1 g/day has been shown to reduce voluntary alcohol consumption, according to Michael Murray, N.D., and Joseph Pizzorno, N.D. This research is over 40 years old, however. The authors suggested that this therapy is promising, since glutamine is safe and relatively inexpensive.[11]

Although anecdotal, the late Roger J. Williams, Ph.D., reported that J. B. Trunell gave an alcoholic patient glutamine, which is tasteless, on the sly. The results were dramatic. The patient abruptly stopped drinking and got a job. Two years later, the patient did not crave alcohol. Glutamine, which is present in proteins, is often destroyed and converted into glutamic acid when proteins are broken down, but glutamic acid is not effective in treating alcoholics, Trunell said. Williams, who discovered pantothenic acid, the B vitamin, urged researchers to follow up on this as a possible treatment for alcoholics. At the time of his discussion with Trunell, glutamine was too expensive to use in trials, but the cost has gone down dramatically since.[12]

For athletes, glutamine is important for recovery and healing. It produces a strong anticatabolic effect, which seems to neutralize the cortisol that accompanies strenuous exercise and permits more efficient anabolism. Cortisol is a steroid hormone that is highly catabolic. Catabolism is the breakdown of constituents in the diet into simpler substances and the consequent release of energy. This is the process by which the body supplies itself with needed energy. The buildup of substances is referred to as anabolism.[13]

When a muscle is in a protein catabolic state, glutamine supplies diminish. There is a 40 percent reduction of the amino acid after surgical trauma, and an 80 to 90 percent reduction with a critical illness. When 20 g/day of glutamine are added to feeding tubes after surgery, this reduces nitrogen losses and slows the drop in muscle glutamine and protein synthesis.[14]

A research team in England noted that there is an increased risk of infection in athletes who undergo prolonged, strenuous exercise. For example, there is a decrease in plasma glutamine after these exercises. To test their theory, they gave 200 runners and rowers a drink containing 5 g L-glutamine in water, or a placebo, immediately after and two hours after strenuous exercise. The researchers found that 81 percent reported no infections with glutamine therapy, compared to 49 percent of controls. Taking glutamine after prolonged exercise may make it available for key cells of the immune system during a critical time of infection.[15]

Depending on your health situation, glutamine can be an important amino acid. It benefits people of all ages and, according to the research given here, it's a substance that deserves additional study.

References

1. MacBurney, Maureen, et al., "A Cost-Evaluation of Glutamine-Supplemented Parenteral Nutrition in Adult Bone Marrow Transplant Patients," *Journal of the American Dietetic Association* 94(11): 1263–66, Nov. 1994.

2. Furst, Peter, et al., "Glutamine Dipeptides in Clinical Nutrition," *Nutrition* 13(7/8): 731–37, 1997.

3. Teran, J. Carlos, et al., "Glutamine—A Conditionally Essential Amino Acid in Cirrhosis," *American Journal of Clinical Nutrition* 62: 897–900, 1995.

4. Wilmore, D. W., and J. K. Shabert, "Role of Glutamine in Immunologic Responses," *Nutrition* 14(7/8): 618–26, 1998.

5. Neu, Josef, et al., "Enteral Glutamine Supplementation for Very Low Birth

Weight Infants Decreases Morbidity," *Journal of Pediatrics* 131: 691–99, 1997.

6. Yoshida, Shogo, et al., "Effects of Glutamine Supplements and Radio-chemotherapy on Systemic Immune and Gut Barrier Function in Patients with Advanced Esophageal Cancer," *Annals of Surgery* 227(4): 485–91, April 1998.

7. DeSouza, D. A., and L. J. Greene, "Pharmacological Nutrition After Burn Injury," *Journal of Nutrition* 128: 797–803, 1998.

8. Smith, Robert J., "Glutamine-Supplemented Nutrition," *Journal of Parenteral and Enteral Nutrition* 21(4): 183–84, 1997.

9. Muscaritoli, M., et al., "Oral Glutamine in the Prevention of Chemotherapy-Induced Gastrointestinal Toxicity," *European Journal of Cancer* 33(2): 319–20, 1997.

10. Golan, Ralph, *Optimal Wellness* (New York: Ballantine Books, 1995), 192.

11. Murray, Michael, and Joseph Pizzorno, *Encyclopedia of Natural Medicine,* rev. 2nd ed. (Rocklin, Calif.: Prima Publishing, 1998), 217.

12. Williams, Roger J., *Nutrition Against Disease* (New York: Pitman Publishing Co., 1971), 172ff.

13. Gastelu, Daniel, and Fred Hatfield, *Dynamic Nutrition for Maximum Performance* (Garden City Park, N.Y.: Avery Publishing Group, 1997), 39.

14. Wernerman, Jan, and Folke Hammerqvist, "Clinical Experience with Glutamine Supplementation," *Nutrition* 10(2): 176–77, 1994.

15. Castell, L. M., et al., "Does Glutamine Have a Role in Reducing Infections in Athletes?" *European Journal of Applied Physiology* 73: 488–90, 1996.

42

Glutathione

A primary antioxidant, glutathione works with an enzyme, glutathione peroxidase, to inactivate hydrogen peroxide and oxidized fats, preventing them from liberating potentially damaging reacting agents. Containing three amino acids—the sulfur amino acid cysteine, glycine, and glutamic acid—glutathione quenches destructive free radicals. It also assists the synthesis of leukotrienes, which are very potent inflammatory agents.[1]

Glutathione is the body's recycling star. It can recycle degraded (oxidized) vitamin C back into fresh ascorbic acid, and it can do the same for spent (oxidized) vitamin E. Our bodies also contain large amounts of glutathione peroxidase, the selenium-containing, selenium-dependent enzyme that deactivates free radicals, especially the dangerous lipid-peroxide ones such as rancid cholesterol that can form in

arteries. In mopping up dangerous chemicals inside our bodies, glutathione attaches itself to toxic substances like epoxides; halides (chlorine, bromine, fluorine, etc.); and heavy metals such as lead, cadmium, and mercury, and dispatches them in the urine.[2]

Glutathione can protect the liver against damage from alcohol and hepatitis, and can possibly prevent liver cancer. Italian researchers found that glutathione levels are very low in tumors and in tumor-free tissue of patients with liver cancer. Eye surgeons often bathe the inside of the eye chambers with high concentrations of glutathione instead of a saline solution. There seems to be no toxicity with glutathione, even in high doses. One researcher monitored patients with liver damage who were taking 1 g/day of glutathione and found no problems.

There is increasing evidence that free radical damage may be an important cause of some of the adverse effects of disease and advancing age. Much of the clinical evidence to support such a hypothesis is related to the protective effect observed in those with diets high in antioxidants and those given antioxidant supplements. To test this theory, researchers at Queen Elizabeth Hospital and the University of Birmingham in England evaluated glutathione levels in the young and the elderly, both those in good health and those who were sick. As might be expected, glutathione levels were found to be higher in the young, healthy adults when compared with the healthy elderly. Elderly outpatients had lower levels than healthy adults. The researchers concluded that aging is associated with a decrease in plasma antioxidants and an increase in oxidative damage, even in those who are apparently healthy. Disease, especially severe illnesses requiring hospitalization, is associated with greater changes in antioxidants and evidence of oxidative damage. Oxidative stress may have an important role in the cause of disease, and antioxidants may play a potential therapeutic role.[3]

At the University of Michigan in Ann Arbor, researchers evaluated blood glutathione levels of 33 volunteers over the age of 60. Higher levels of the antioxidant were associated with fewer numbers of illnesses, higher levels of self-rated health, lower cholesterol, lower body mass index, and lower blood pressure. Those diagnosed with arthritis, diabetes, and heart disease had the lowest levels of glutathione. Glutathione, plus age, and a measure of suppressed anger, accounted for 39 percent of the variance of an index of morbidity. The study seems to be the first showing an association between higher glutathione levels and higher levels of physical health in a community-based sample.[4]

At the University of Rome, researchers studied 20 infertile men who were given either 600 mg/day of glutathione or a placebo. Glutathione produced a statistically significant positive effect on sperm motility, kinetic parameters, and structure of sperm. Glutathione should be considered ideal therapy for infertile men. It may work by inhibiting lipid peroxidation of the sperm membrane.[5]

Mitochondrial glutathione plays a distinctive role in protecting against free radical damage associated with aging. In fact, oxidative damage to mitochondrial DNA is related to oxidation of mitochondrial glutathione. Mitochondria are the principal energy source of cells. Therefore, antioxidant supplementation may be a rational way of partially protecting against age-related impairment.[6]

In laboratory glassware, glutathione has helped to halt oxygen-induced damage to retinal tissue. Good food sources of the antioxidant are green, yellow, and red vegetables; however, canned and frozen vegetables lose much of their glutathione during processing. Georg Weber, M.D., Ph.D., of Harvard Medical School has stated that some children with severe seizures and repeated infections have low blood levels of glutathione peroxidase. Giving these children 50 to 150 mg/day of selenium significantly reduces the seizures, since glutathione peroxidase is a selenium-dependent antioxidant enzyme.[7]

At University Hospital in Amsterdam, samples of inflamed mucosa were taken from nine patients with chronic sinusitis during endoscopic sinus surgery, and compared with mucosa of 10 healthy controls. A significant reduction in glutathione and uric acid levels was noted in mucosal samples of the chronic sinusitis patients, compared to controls. The reduction of glutathione and uric acid in patients with chronic sinusitis may lead to a reduced antioxidant defense and increase their susceptibility to certain pathogens.[8]

Researchers at the Netherlands Kancer Institute in Amsterdam said that 600 mg/day of N-acetylcysteine is safe and can be recommended for clinical chemo-prevention against lung cancer due to its ability to enhance glutathione levels and modulate the detoxification of DNA repair.[9]

A study in Germany examined the peroxidative damage from cyclosporin, an antitubercular drug. The damaging effects of the drug can be prevented or reduced by giving glutathione, vitamin E N-acetyl-cysteine, or extracts of *Ginkgo biloba*.[10]

Researchers at the Medical College of Pennsylvania evaluated 32 adult patients with cystic fibrosis and compared red blood cell (RBC) glutathione concentrations with 8 healthy matched controls. While the RBC glutathione concentrations in the two groups were not significantly different, it was noted that there was more variability in RBC glutathione concentration in those with cystic fibrosis. RBC glutathione was also inversely and significantly correlated for testing the patient's lung function. The study suggests that there is variability in ery-throcyte antioxidants in patients with cystic fibrosis, and RBC glutathione may be a beneficial marker for evaluating the severity of the disease and a rationale for prescribing antioxidant supplementation.[11]

It has been a puzzle for many years as to why some patients with HIV infection live for many years while others become ill and die. Leonore Herzenberg, Ph.D., and colleagues at Stanford University School of Medicine in California, believe that glutathione levels in CD4 cells affect survival.[12] Scientists have known for some time that levels of glutathione are low in CD4 cells of people with HIV. Herzenberg suggests that glutathione levels are predictive of survival. In studying 204 HIV-infected patients, she said that in patients with fewer than 200 CD4 cells and low glutathione levels, the mortality rate was 60 to 80 percent in three years. In those with similarly low CD4 cell counts but with normal glutathione levels, the mortality rate within three years was about 20 percent.

Herzenberg said that acetylcysteine, which is used to treat acetaminophen overdose, can replenish glutathione levels. She and Leonard Herzenberg, Ph.D., also at Stanford, and John James, publisher of *AIDS Treatment News,* have asked the FDA to consider requiring that glutathione-depleting substances such as acetaminophen carry a label stating the potential hazard to those with HIV.

In comparing 24 HIV-infected children with 24 healthy controls, researchers in Puerto Rico reported that the HIV-infected children were deficient in plasma glutathione levels. Low concentrations of glutathione are directly correlated with CD4 cell counts and inversely correlated with viral loads in HIV-infected children. Therefore, the researchers said, glutathione may be involved in the progression of HIV.[13]

Researchers in Italy evaluated 10 patients with chronic hepatitis C, of which 55 were HIV positive and 50 were HIV negative, for glutathione levels. Liver, blood, and lymphocyte glutathione levels were considerably reduced in the hepatitis patients with HIV, compared to the healthy controls. In all patients with hepatitis C, glutathione tissue levels were deficient in those addicted to drugs. This depletion may be a factor in the resistance to interferon therapy, and in the resistance of HIV-positive patients to antiviral drugs, suggesting the possible need for glutathione supplements.[14]

Since glutathione levels decrease as we age, it is obvious why this antioxidant is important to good health. A good antioxidant formula should contain cysteine, glutathione, selenium, vitamin E, vitamin C, vitamin A or beta-carotene, zinc, manganese, bioflavonoids, and methyl donors such as N-dimethylglycine. The antioxidants are especially important because they probably protect us from aging, cardiovascular disease, arthritis, cancer, Alzheimer's disease, diabetes, lung problems, and many other conditions.[15] For dosages concerning glutathione, ask your health care professional.

References

1. Ronzio, Robert A., *The Encyclopedia of Nutrition and Good Health* (New York: Facts on File, 1997), 214.
2. Kronhausen, Eberhard, et al., *Formula for Life: The Anti-Oxidant Free-Radical Detoxification Program* (New York: William Morrow and Co., 1989), 118ff.
3. Nuttall, S. L., et al., "Glutathione: In Sickness and in Health," *The Lancet* 351: 645–46, Feb. 28, 1998.
4. Julius, Mara, "Glutathione and Morbidity in a Community-Based Sample of Elderly," *Journal of Clinical Epidemiology* 47(9): 1021–26, 1994.
5. Lenzi, A. "Placebo Controlled, Double-Blind, Cross-Over Trial of Glutathione Therapy in Male Infertility," *Human Reproduction* 8(10): 997–1001, 1993.
6. Sastre, Juan, et al., "Glutathione, Oxidative Stress, and Aging," *Age* 19: 129–39, 1996.
7. Feinstein, Alice, ed., *Healing with Vitamins* (Emmaus, Pa.: Rodale Press, 1996), 242, 371.

8. Westerveld, Gerrit-Jan, et al., "Anti-oxidant Levels in the Nasal Mucosa of Patients with Chronic Sinusitis and Healthy Controls," *Archives of Otolaryngology Head and Neck Surgery* 123: 201–04, 1997.

9. Zandwijk, Nice van, "N-Acetylcysteine (NAC) and Glutathione (GSH): Antioxidant and Chemopreventive Properties, with Special Reference to Lung Cancer," *Journal of Cellular Biochemistry* S22: 24–32, 1995.

10. Barth, S., et al., "Influences of *Ginkgo Biloba* on Cyclosporin-A Induced Lipid Peroxidation in Human Liver Microsomes in Comparison to Vitamin E, Glutathione, and N-Acetylcysteine," *Biochemical Pharmacology* 41: 1521–26, 1991.

11. Mangione, Salvatore, et al., "Erythrocyte Glutathione in Cystic Fibrosis: A Possible Marker of Pulmonary Function," *Chest* 105(5): 1470–73, May 1994.

12. Voelker, Rebecca, "Glutathione and Survival," *Journal of the American Medical Association* 277(12): 951, March 26, 1997.

13. Rodriguez, Jose F., et al., "Plasma Glutathione Concentrations in Children Infected with Human Immunodeficiency Virus," *Pediatric Infectious Disease Journal* 17(3): 236–41, 1998.

14. Barbaro, Giuseppe, et al., "Hepatic Glutathione Deficiency in Chronic Hepatitis C: Quantitative Evaluation in Patients Who Are HIV Positive and HIV Negative and Correlations with Plasmatic and Lymphocytic Concentrations and with the Activity of the Liver Disease," *American Journal of Gastroenterology* 91(12): 2569–73, 1996.

15. Atkins, Robert C., *Dr. Atkins' Health Revolution* (Boston: Houghton Mifflin Co., 1988), 332.

43

Golden Root

Used for hundreds of years in China, Russia, and the Far East, *Rhodiola rosea* (golden root) is fairly new to the United States. Clinical tests have shown that it can ward off fatigue and increase mental and physical energy and performance, as well as treat a variety of sexual disorders in men, such as weak erections, premature ejaculation, sexual impotency, and also sleep disturbances. One three-month clinical trial revealed significant improvement in sexual functions, including the normalizing of prostate gland fluids, energy levels, and the relieving of insomnia.[1]

Rhodiola consists of more than 40 species of alpine plants that normally grow 3,000 to 5,500 miles above sea level in the mountainous regions of the Far East. Russian scientists have identified a number of constituents in the plants, including

beta-sitosterol, gallic acid, daucosterol, and others.[2]

When highland villagers in China climb from a 2,500-mile altitude up to 4,475 miles, they are subject to considerable stress on their hearts and lungs. *Rhodiola kirilowii,* another variety of the plant, can relieve many of these stresses.[3]

Using laboratory animals, Russian scientists reported that *Rhodiola rosea* extracts provided protection to the animals' hearts and lungs during various stress tests, thereby preventing damage to the middle muscular layer of the heart (myocardium).[4] Researchers in Russia also tested ginseng, chinopanax tincture, eleutherococcus, *Rhodiola rosea,* and leuzea on experimental animals with diabetes. They found that both golden root and ginseng increased the blood levels of insulin and decreased the level of glucagon, a protein hormone produced by the islets of Langerhans, which promotes an increase in the sugar content of the blood by accelerating the rate of glycogen breakdown in the liver.[5]

In a small study involving 12 bladder cancer patients, Russian researchers reported that oral doses of *Rhodiola rosea* extract improved the tissue lining of the urinary tract and T cell immunity, among other things. Relapses were common but statistical differences were said to be insignificant.[6]

Since the liver can regenerate itself, researchers at the Academy of Medical Sciences, Tomsk, Russia, investigated whether *Rhodiola rosea* extracts would inhibit the growth of tumors in rats with Pliss lymphosarcoma who had had a partial hepatectomy, or removal of a portion of the liver. The treatment inhibited the growth of tumors by 37, 39, and 59 percent, respectively. Metastases, or the movement of a tumor to other parts of the body, decreased by 42, 50, and 75 percent, respectively.[7]

Other research has found that *Rhodiola rosea* extracts inhibit the growth of Erlich's tumor and Pliss lymphosarcoma. The extracts aid in the production of immune factors by the liver, thus inhibiting the activity of tumor cells in both laboratory glassware and in the body.[8]

A research team in Russia wanted to know if extracts of *Rhodiola rosea, Panax ginseng,* and ganoderma mushroom could prevent tumor formation in tissues predisposed to hereditary tumors. They found that

the least activity was shown by extracts from ganoderma, while those from *Rhodiola rosea* were the most effective. Their study can serve as the basis for further investigations by using the extracts on inbred animals and in a clinical setting for the prevention of and natural therapy against tumors.[9]

Rhodiola rosea (golden root) is available over the counter in various formulations. The suggested dosage is one or two tablets or capsules prior to physical or mental workouts, or follow the directions on the label.

References

1. "Another Viagra?" *Daily News,* May 19, 1998, 6.
2. "Epihalochine: Isolation, Structure, and Anti-Hypoxic Activity," *Chemico-Pharmaceutical Journal* (Russia) 25(1): 55–57, 1991.
3. Zhang, Z., et al., "The Effect of Rhodiola Kirilowii (Regel.) Maximum on Preventing Mountain Reactions: A Comparison of Cardiopulmonary Function in Villagers at Different Altitude Areas," *China Journal of Chinese Materia Medica* 14(11): 47–50, 1989.
4. Maslova, L. V., et al., "Accumulation of Technetium-Pyrophosphate and Level of Cyclic Nucleotides in the Myocardium During Its Adaptation to Stress Damage," *Pathophysiology and Experimental Therapy* 3: 53–55, 1989.
5. Molokovski, D. S., et al., "Effect of Adaptogenic Phytopharmaceuticals in

Experimental Aloxan Diabetes," *Problems of Endocrinology* (Russia) 35: 82–87, 1989.

6. Bocharova, O. A., et al., "The Effect of *Rhodiola rosea* Extract on the Incidence of Recurrences of a Superficial Bladder Cancer," *Urol Nefro* (Moscow) 2: 46–47, 1995.

7. Udintsev, S. N., and V. P. Shakhov, "The Role of Humoral Factors of Regenerating Liver in the Development of Experimental Tumors and the Effect of *Rhodiola rosea* Extract on This Process," *Neoplasma* 38: 323–31, 1991.

8. Udintsev, S. N., and V. P. Shakhov, "The Inhibitory Effect of Partial Hepatectomy on the Growth Rate of Erlich's Tumor and Pliss Lymphosarcoma," *Problems of Oncology* (Russia) 35(9): 1072–75, 1989.

9. Bocharova, O.A., et al., "Testing Plant-Based Drugs for Prevention and Nontoxic Therapy of Cancer Disease on Experimental Models," *Biological Abstracts* 98(5), 1994.

44

Goldenseal

Goldenseal was used by Native Americans for a variety of applications. The Cherokees used it to treat sore eyes, mouth ulcers, tuberculosis, and edema or swelling. When mixed with bear fat, it became an insect repellent. Settlers in the West began appropriating the herb as an antiseptic and wound-healing medication, and it was later used in a commercial tonic for gastric ailments.[1]

Today, the supply of goldenseal is scarce, due to both overzealous harvesting and drought. It continues to be highly regarded for cleansing the liver and blood, and as a remedy for colds and flu and for alcoholics. When consumed in a tea, goldenseal is recommended for mouth sores, including cracked, bleeding lips and canker sores. A commercial eyedrop that includes berberine, a constituent in the herb, has been suggested for reducing eye irritation, presumably because it constricts the blood vessels in the eyes. While the herb is said to be safe in reasonable amounts, it may induce uterine contractions and is not recommended for pregnant women. Herbal preparations are made from the root and rhizome. In addition to berberine, goldenseal contains a number of other alkaloids, including hydrastine, canadine, and hydrastinine.

According to Andrew Weil, M.D., goldenseal is the most useful component in the herbal medicine chest. He recommends goldenseal powder, which can be sprinkled directly onto a wound, since it is a good disinfectant and also promotes scar formation. As a rinse for irritated or inflamed mucous membranes, Weil suggests that you mix one-quarter teaspoon of salt and one-half teaspoon, or the contents of one goldenseal capsule, in a cup of warm water. This mixture can be used as a gargle for sore throat or as a mouth rinse for canker sores, sore tongue, tonsillitis, or gingivitis. Since the herb does not always completely dissolve, he recommends using sterile water and straining out any floating particles.[2]

"Taken internally," Weil said, "goldenseal tones the digestive system and has a reputation as a blood purifier. I sometimes recommend it to people who are debilitated, have weak digestive systems, or who are susceptible to recurrent infection. But I find its internal effects are less impressive than the external applications."

Healing herbs such as goldenseal, and alternative therapies represent a $40 billion market annually, with consumers picking up most of the tab. That explains why hospitals and entrepreneurs are not waiting for insurers to expand their coverage before venturing on their own into alternative medicine.[3]

Berberine and other goldenseal alkaloids are well documented in scientific literature for their antibiotic activity, reported Michael T. Murray, N.D. For example, berberine is an effective antibiotic against a range of harmful organisms, such as *Staphylococcal* sp., *Streptococcus* sp., *Chlamydia* sp., *Corynebacterium diphtheria, Salmonella typhi, Vibrio cholerae, Diplococcus pneumonia,* and *Candida albicans.*[4] "Goldenseal has also shown remarkable immunostimulatory activity," Murray added. "Foremost is its ability to increase the blood supply to the spleen and the release of immune-potentiating compounds."

Murray went on to say that berberine has also been shown to be a potent activator of macrophages, the cells responsible for destroying bacteria, viruses, fungi, and tumor cells. Improved macrophage activity is one of the reasons why goldenseal is effective in reducing fever. As a dried root tea, he recommends 1 to 2 g. For a tincture, use 1 to 1½ teaspoons. As a powdered solid extract, the recommendation is 250 to 500 mg.

A good treatment for bronchitis and pneumonia is a combination of goldenseal and bromelain, according to Julian Whitaker, M.D. Bromelain is one of a group of peptide hydrolases often administered orally in the treatment of inflammation and edema of soft tissues. Whitaker added that the combination supports the historical use of goldenseal for infections of the mucous membranes; that is, the linings of the oral cavity, throat, sinuses, bronchi, lungs, and genitourinary and gastrointestinal tracts. For a standardized extract of 5 percent hydrastine, the recommended dosage for bronchitis or pneumonia is 400 to 800 mg, three times daily.[5]

Also known as hydrastis, goldenseal has been used by Native Americans as both a clothing dye and a medicinal herb, stated Sheldon Saul Hendler, M.D., Ph.D. The herb has been applied topically to treat acne, eczema, hemorrhoids, and cold sores; served as a bitter tonic; and used as a douche for uterine bleeding. Caution should be taken if the herb is used as a douche.[6]

Very high doses of goldenseal are said to cause nausea, vomiting, a decrease in white blood count, and feelings of pins and needles in the hands and feet, Hendler said. Some of goldenseal's derivatives may eventually prove quite useful.

Several years ago, goldenseal tea gained considerable publicity under the claim that it prevented the detection of morphine in urine samples following heroin use. This idea became popular among some heroin addicts who were patients in methadone or other drug rehabilitation programs. However, scientific studies have shown that goldenseal neither prevents morphine detection in urine specimens nor flushes that compound out of the body.[7] The suggestion that goldenseal could mask the presence of illicit drugs or their metabolites in urine was purloined from a novel written in 1900 by John Uri Lloyd of the Lloyd Brothers Pharmacy in Cincinnati, Ohio. Because of Lloyd's stature in the pharmaceutical industry, a number of letters were written to pharmacy journals discussing the potential role of goldenseal. These references spotlighted the herb's myth and its connection with illicit drugs.[8]

References

1. Guinness, Alma E., ed., *Family Guide to Natural Medicine* (Pleasantville, N.Y.: The Reader's Digest Association, 1993), 310–11.
2. Weil, Andrew, *Natural Health, Natural Medicine* (Boston: Houghton Mifflin, 1990), 239–40.
3. Blecher, M. B., and K. Douglass, "Gold in Goldenseal," *Hospital Health Network* 71: 50–52, Oct. 20, 1997.
4. Murray, Michael T., *Natural Alternatives to Over-the-Counter and Prescription Drugs* (New York: William Morrow and Co., 1994), 151–52.
5. Whitaker, Julian, *Dr. Whitaker's Guide to Natural Healing* (Rocklin, Calif.: Prima Publishing, 1995), 174–75.
6. Hendler, Sheldon Saul, *The Doctors' Vitamin and Mineral Encyclopedia* (New York: Simon & Schuster, 1990), 307.
7. Foster, Steven, and Varro E. Tyler, *Tyler's Honest Herbal* (New York: Haworth Herbal Press, 1999), 195ff.
8. Eskinazi, Daniel, ed., *Botanical Medicine* (Larchmont, N.Y.: Mary Ann Liebert, 1999), 20.

45

Grape Seed Extract

In the entry on red wine later in this book, I refer to the so-called French Paradox: The French eat slightly more fat than Americans, yet they suffer fewer heart attacks. While the French do eat fruits, their higher intake of saturated fats and cholesterol surpasses that of other countries that report a low incidence of heart attacks.[1]

"The French have a fondness for butter, cream, sauces, patés, an enormous variety of cheeses, and rich, buttery baked goods such as croissants," explained Antonio M. Gotto Jr., M.D., of Baylor College of Medicine in Houston. "Even more puzzling, the death rate from heart disease in southwestern France—where foie gras—the enlarged livers of force-fed ducks and geese—is commonly eaten and the intake of saturated fat is said to be the highest in the industrialized world—is even lower than in other parts of France."

Gotto's research suggests that the French are protected by the constituents in the large amounts of red wine they consume, which averages almost 99 bottles per person annually, compared with nine bottles per person in the United States. They are also protected by the grape skins and grape seed extracts that are part of the winemaking process.

One of the most beneficial groups of plant flavonoids is the proanthocyanidins (also called procyanidins), which provide a variety of health benefits, according to Michael Murray, N.D., and Joseph Pizzorno, N.D. Collectively, mixtures of proanthocyanidin molecules are called procyanidolic oligomers, or PCO. PCO extracts are being used in the treatment of venous and capillary disorders, such as venous insufficiency, varicose veins, capillary fragility, diabetic retinopathy, and macular degeneration.[2]

In animal studies, the authors continued, PCO extracts have been shown to prevent damage to the lining of an artery, lower blood cholesterol levels, and shrink cholesterol deposits in an artery. PCO extracts in a supplement form, 50 mg/day, should be thought of as a necessary food in the prevention and treatment of heart disease and stroke.

Researchers at Creighton University in Omaha, Nebraska, conducted a test to determine the chemoprotective properties of grape seed extract, vitamin C, vitamin E, superoxide dismutase, catalase, and mannitol against biochemically generated superoxide anion and hydroxyl radical. At a concentration of 100 mg/l, the extract exhibited 78 to 81 percent inhibition of superoxide anion and hydroxyl radical. Under similar conditions, vitamin C inhibited the two oxygen free radicals by about 12 to 19 percent, while vitamin E inhibited the two radicals by 36 to 44 percent. The combination of superoxide dismutase (an enzyme that reduces potentially harmful oxygen free radicals) and catalase (an enzyme involved in the decomposition of hydrogen peroxide) inhibited superoxide anion by about 83 percent, while mannitol (a slightly sweet crystaline alcohol) registered an 87 percent inhibition of hydroxyl radical. The study demonstrated that grape seed extract is a more potent scavenger of oxygen free radicals than either vitamin C or vitamin E.[3]

Laboratory studies at the University of Connecticut School of Medicine at Storrs show that grape seed extract, in this case Activin, reduces tissue damage caused by cardiac ischemia/reperfusion injury. The study also revealed that pretreatment with the extract improves aortic blood flow and reduces creatine kinase levels, which are markers for coronary tissue damage. The extract's protective effects are traced to its ability to scavenge harmful free radicals in the body.[4]

At a conference on antioxidants held at Tufts University in Boston in 1998, it was reported that constituents in grape seeds constitute a unique class of antioxidants, since they have been proven in clinical trials to be beneficial in fighting specific cardiovascular diseases.[5]

Researchers at the University of Birmingham in the United Kingdom pointed out that coronary artery disease remains the major cause of mortality and morbidity in the Western world. The oxidation of LDL cholesterol by free radicals is protected by antioxidants, and, in times of antioxidant deficiency, is more apt to be oxidized. Since patients with high cholesterol levels are at a higher cardiovascular risk, they require more antioxidant protection.[6]

The English researchers evaluated 20 young volunteers who were given two capsules containing 300 mg of grape seed extracts or a placebo for five days. Blood samples were drawn at the beginning and end of the study and assayed for antioxidant activity as well as vitamin C and vitamin E levels. After a halt in the study for about two weeks, the trial was repeated with the alternate therapy. The extract had no effect on blood levels of the vitamins, but it increased total antioxidant activity in the blood.

Using cholesterol-fed rabbits, a research team in Japan found that feeding a proanthocyanidin-rich extract from grape seeds significantly reduced severe atherosclerosis in the animals' aortas. The study suggests that proanthocyanidins might trap reactive oxygen species in plasma and intestinal fluid of the arterial wall, thereby inhibiting oxidation of LDL cholesterol as well as inhibiting atherosclerotic activity.[7]

Catechins and their oligomers, known as proanthocyanidins, are natural products that have shown some biological properties as captors of free radicals, and for their use in preventing certain vascular diseases. Mature grape seeds contain a considerable amount of these compounds, up to 28 g/kg, which are only partially extracted during red and rosé winemaking. Therefore, grape seeds, which are by-products of winemaking, can be considered an easily available source of catechins and proanthocyanidins for pharmaceutical and cosmetic applications.[8]

A variety of grape seed supplements are available over the counter. The suggested dosage ranges from 50 to 300 mg/day, with a maintenance dose in the range of 50 to 100 mg/day.

References

1. Gotto, Antonio M., Jr., et al., "A Look at Eating Habits and Heart Disease Around the World," *Medical and Health Annual* (Chicago: Encyclopaedia Britannica, 1993), 49–50.

2. Murray, Michael, and Joseph Pizzorno, *Encyclopedia of Natural Medicine,* rev. 2nd ed. (Rocklin, Calif.: Prima Publishing, 1998), 94–95.

3. Bagchi, D., et al., "Oxygen Free Radical Scavenging Abilities of Vitamin C and E, and a Grape Seed Proanthocyanidin Extract in Vitro," *Research Communications in Molecular Pathology and Pharmacology* 95(2): 179–89, Feb. 1997.

4. "Grape Seed Extract Protects Heart," *Nutritional Outlook,* May 1999, 56.

5. Tyler, Varro E., "Herb News," *Prevention,* Nov. 1999, 105ff.

6. Nuttall, S. L., et al., "An Evaluation of the Antioxidant Activity of a Standardized Grape Seed Extract, Leucoselect," *Journal of Clinical Pharmacy and Therapy* 23: 385–89, Oct. 1998.

7. Yamakoshi, J., et al., "Proanthocyanidin-Rich Extract from Grape Seeds Attenuates the Development of Aortic Atherosclerosis in Cholesterol-Fed Rabbits," *Atherosclerosis* 142: 139–49, Jan. 1999.

8. Alonso, Emilia, et al., "Suitability of Water/Ethanol Mixtures for the Extraction of Catechins and Proanthocyanidins from *Vitis vinifera* Seeds Contained in a Winery By-Product," *Seed Science and Technology* 19: 545–52, 1991.

46

Green Tea

Tea, a beverage that has been consumed for thousands of years, was originally introduced around 2735 B.C., when leaves from a tea plant happened to fall into boiling water at a reception hosted by the Chinese emperor Shen Nung. Tea is renowned for its specific polyphenols and an enzyme, polyphenol oxidase, which is activated when the leaves of the plant are bruised during chopping and rolling at harvest time. When the leaves are dried, the result is green tea.[1]

The most important compound in green tea is epigallocatechin-3 gallate (EGCG), which accounts for about 50 to 60 percent of the catechins, or antioxidant polyphenols, in green tea. Tea *(Camellia sinensis)* also contains caffeine, about 40 to 50 percent of that found in coffee.

Epidemiological studies show that people who consume five cups or more of green tea daily are at lower risk for various types of cancer. This is because the polyphenols in the tea have antibacterial and antiviral properties. Green tea protects against stomach cancer by inactivating the bacterium *Helicobacter pylori*. It also protects against esophageal cancer by destroying cancer-causing nitrosamines. Those who drink four or more cups of tea daily have the equivalent benefit of eating two of the recommended intake of five to nine fruits and vegetables daily.

Green tea, made by steaming or pan-frying tea leaves and then drying them, accounts for almost 20 percent of world production and is especially popular in China and Japan. When used for medicinal purposes, 5 to 10 ml of green tea are steeped in a cup of boiling water for 15 minutes. A cup of black or green tea contains 10 to 80 mg of caffeine, depending on its production, storage, and preparation.[2]

Green tea provides more catechins than black tea, since some of these compounds are destroyed during "sweating," a natural fermentation process that darkens the leaves and changes their aroma and flavor to make black tea. Oolong tea falls in between, having a color, flavor, and catechin content between green and black tea. In addition to their significant anticancer and antibacterial properties, catechins lower cholesterol levels in the blood and improve lipid metabolism.[3]

At a 1998 meeting of the American Association for Cancer Research, 10 papers were presented extolling the value of green tea. While green tea offers protection against cancers of the breast, skin, stomach, lung, colon, and prostate, black tea, derived from the same plant, also seems beneficial. Zhi-Yuan Wang, Ph.D., of Columbia University in New York, stated that both green and black tea antioxidants (polyphenols) may offer protection against sunburn and possibly even skin cancer.[4]

Green tea's cancer-fighting properties may be due to its component, EGCG, which prevents the growth of new blood vessels. Using laboratory animals, researchers in Sweden found that mice given green tea in their water had between 35 and 70 percent less blood vessel growth than the animals drinking only water.[5]

A study at the Shanghai Cancer Institute in China and the National Cancer Institute in Bethesda, Maryland, found that drinking green tea was associated with a 60 percent reduction in esophageal cancer among nonsmoking men and women.

The normal amount of green tea consumed by the Japanese and other green tea–drinking cultures is about three cups daily, or about 3 g of soluble components, providing roughly 240 to 320 mg of polyphenols. To achieve some degree of protection, a person would have to consume an equivalent of the green tea or green tea polyphenols that are consumed in population studies. For a green tea extract standardized for 80 percent polyphenols and 55 percent EGCG, this means a daily dose of 300 to 400 mg.[6]

In a laboratory study in Tokyo, researchers suggested that green tea may inhibit bladder tumor growth. Other teas used in the experiment did not provide sufficient protection.[7]

Green tea polyphenols possess strong chemopreventive properties against a variety of animal tumors as well in some epidemiological trials. At least two epidemiological studies have shown that people who consume green tea regularly may have a decreased risk of developing prostate cancer.[8]

Researchers at the Medical College of Ohio and the University of Toledo in Ohio have found a component in green tea that may prevent the development of cancer in humans. Green tea also contains epigallocatechin (EGC) and epicathechin-3 gallate (ECG). Human cancers need specific enzymes to invade cells and form metastases (the spreading of cancer cells to various parts of the body). One of these enzymes, urokinase, is inhibited by the EGCG in green tea, which reduces the size of the tumor and possibly even causes complete remission of cancer.[9]

At a 1999 meeting of Digestive Disease Week, researchers at the University of California at San Diego reported that EGCG in green tea stopped the growth of human colorectal cancer cells and destroyed them in laboratory glassware. Therefore, green tea should be considered a possible preventive agent against cancer.[10]

D. James and Dorothy Morré of Purdue University at West Lafayette, Indiana, have studied the reaction between EGCG and an enzyme, quinol oxidase (NOX), which controls cell growth, and their relation to cancer. NOX is an overactive enzyme that regulates how fast cells enlarge after they divide.[11] James and Morré found that EGCG in black and green tea inhibit NOX activity, but since green tea has an EGCG content higher than that of black tea, the effects of green tea were 10 times more powerful. NOX cells zapped by EGCG can divide, but they do not grow after dividing and thus die.

French researchers have reported that in a laboratory setting, the free radical–scavenging ability of green tea showed antiradical activity comparable to rutin, a bioflavonoid, and vitamin E. EGCG produced the major antiradical activity in green tea.[12]

Since green tea contains potent antioxidant compounds, epidemiological data

have reported that the tea provides greater antioxidant protection than vitamin C and vitamin E against cardiovascular disease. In one Japanese study, men aged 40 and older who drank nine cups of green tea daily had increases in HDL cholesterol and decreases in LDL cholesterol.[13]

Because of its high content of flavonoids and polyphenols, green tea has been shown to inhibit xanthine oxidase, an enzyme responsible for producing uric acid. Decreasing uric acid content is one way of preventing gout attacks. In fact, green tea flavonoids inhibited xanthine oxidase levels similar to those achieved by the drug allopurinol.[14]

Green tea may provide protection against the onset and severity of arthritis, according to researchers at Case Western Reserve University, Cleveland, Ohio. An antioxidant-rich polyphenolic constituent isolated from green tea has been shown to possess anti-inflammatory and anticarcinogenic properties in experimental animals. In three different experiments, mice given green tea in their water exhibited significantly reduced incidence of arthritis (33 to 50 percent), compared to animals who drank only water (84 to 100 percent).[15]

A study at Saitama Cancer Center Research Institute in Japan studied 1,371 men aged 40 and over concerning their green tea intake and its relationship to cardiovascular disease and disorders of the liver. Increased consumption of green tea brought a decrease in blood levels of total cholesterol and triglycerides and a better

HDL:LDL cholesterol ratio. The men who drank more than 10 cups of green tea had lower amounts of hepatological markers in their blood, aspartate aminotransferase, alanine transferase, and ferritin. Green tea may be protective against cardiovascular disease and disorders of the liver as well as the development of cancer.[16]

Also at Saitama, researchers evaluated 8,552 Japanese people over the age of 40 during a nine-year follow-up. There were 384 cancer cases during that time and the researchers found that green tea provided protection against cancer, especially among women who drank more than 10 cups daily. The average annual incidence of cancer was significantly lower among women who drank large amounts of green tea. The relative risk of developing cancer was lower among females and males with the highest consumption, but the preventive effect was not statistically relevant for males.[17]

Green tea supplements are available over the counter in a variety of forms. In addition, there are various blends for making your own green tea at home.

References

1. Weisburger, John H., "Beneficial Effects of Tea in Chronic Disease Prevention," paper presented at the Third International Symposium on Green Tea, Seoul, Korea, Sept. 1, 1995.

2. Kaegi, Elizabeth, "Unconventional Therapies for Cancer: Green Tea," *Canadian Medical Association Journal* 158(8): 1033–35, April 21, 1998.

3. Weil, Andrew, *Eight Weeks to Optimum Health* (New York: Alfred A. Knopf, 1997), 71.

4. "Studies Tout Cancer-Fighting Properties of Green and Black Tea," *Medical Tribune*, May 8, 1998, 13.

5. Leigh, Suzanne, "Substance Found in Green Tea Prevents Blood Vessel Growth," *Medical Tribune*, May 6, 1999, 2.

6. "Green Tea," *American Journal of Natural Medicine* 4(5): 18–19, June 1997.

7. Sato, D., "Inhibition of Urinary Bladder Tumors Induced by N-butyl-N-(4-hydroxybutyl)-Nitrosamine in Rats by Green Tea," *International Journal of Urology* 6: 93–99, Feb. 1999.

8. Gupta, S., et al., "Prostate Cancer Chemoprevention by Green Tea: In Vitro and In Vivo Inhibition of Testosterone-Mediated Induction of Ornithine Decarboxylase," *Cancer Research* 59: 2115–20, May 1, 1999.

9. Jankun, Jerzy, et al., "Why Drinking Green Tea Could Prevent Cancer," *Nature* 387(5): 561, June 1997.

10. Frei, Shoshana, "Component of Green Tea Halts Cancer Cell In Vitro," *Medical Tribune*, June 10, 1999, 12.

11. Melton, Marissa, "The Power of Tea," *U.S. News and World Report*, Dec. 21, 1998, 58.

12. Fourneau, C., et al., "Radical Scavenging Evaluation of Green Tea Extracts,"

Phytotherapy Research 10: 529–30, 1996.

13. Yand, T. T. C., et al., "Hypocholesterolemic Effects of Chinese Tea," *Pharmacological Research* 35: 505–12, 1997.

14. Aucamp, J., "Inhibition of Xanthine Oxidase by Catechins from Tea *(Camellia sinensis)*," *Anticancer Research* 17: 4381–86, 1997.

15. Haqqi, T. M., et al., "Prevention of Collagen-Induced Arthritis in Mice by a Polyphenolic Fraction from Green Tea," *Proceedings of the National Academy of Sciences, USA* 96: 4524–29, April 13, 1999.

16. Imai, K., and K. Nakachi, "Cross Sectional Study of Effects of Drinking Green Tea on Cardiovascular-Liver Diseases," *British Medical Journal* 310: 693–96, 1995.

17. Imai, K., "Cancer-Preventive Effects of Drinking Green Tea Among a Japanese Population," *Preventive Medicine* 26: 769–75, 1997.

47

5-HTP

On November 17, 1989, the FDA recalled all dietary supplements containing a daily dose of 100 mg of manufactured L-tryptophan, the essential amino acid. Until that point, the supplement had been used by tens of thousands of consumers without problems, ostensibly for insomnia. The recall was made after more than 1,000 cases of eosinophilia-myalgia syndrome (EMS), and a number of deaths, were traced to a single batch of L-tryptophan. The offending batch was made by Showa Denko Company in Japan, which had used a new, genetically engineered strain of the bacterium *Bacillus amyloliquifaciens,* a 50 percent reduction in the amount of activated charcoal used in one of the purification steps, and other procedures that had not been used before.[1]

Since then, consumers have turned to 5-hydroxytryptophan (5-HTP), available in Europe since the 1970s. It has been researched for more than 30 years and is now available over the counter. Derived from an African herb, 5-HTP is reportedly manufactured differently from the original L-tryptophan. Tryptophan is found in such foods as turkey, chicken, yogurt, cheese, and bananas.

5-HTP is a brain chemical that is the intermediate step between tryptopohan and serotonin. Low levels of serotonin, an important brain chemical, are associated with depression, obesity, carbohydrate cravings, bulimia, insomnia, sleep apnea, migraine headaches, premenstrual syndrome, fibromyalgia, and other health conditions, according to Michael T. Murray, N.D.[2]

Studies have shown that 5-HTP is equal or better than standard antidepressant drugs, such as Prozac, Paxil, and

Zoloft. In a study involving weight loss, women taking 5-HTP lost an average of 4.39 pounds in six weeks and an average of 11.63 pounds after 12 weeks. 5-HTP has also been shown to be a better treatment for insomnia than melatonin. Double-blind studies have reported that 5-HTP can relieve pain associated with fibromyalgia, Murray added.

For depression, weight loss, headaches, and fibromyalgia, Murray recommends 50 mg of 5-HTP three times daily. If there is no response after two weeks, increase the dosage to 100 mg three times a day. For insomnia, the general dosage is 100 to 300 mg 30 to 45 minutes before retiring. Begin with the lower amount for at least three days before taking more.

5-HTP may be used to help obese patients lose weight. Researchers at the University of Rome in Italy evaluated 20 obese patients who were randomly given either 900 mg/day of 5-HTP or a placebo. The study involved two consecutive six-week trials in which no systematic diet was followed the first week. A recommended diet was eaten the second week. The patients lost weight during both weeks, and there was a consistent finding of reduced carbohydrate intake and early satiety. The supplement was well tolerated, and the researchers suggested that 5-HTP may be used safely to treat obesity.[3]

The same researchers reported that by inhibiting carbohydrate intake, 5-HTP may be safely utilized to improve the health of non-insulin-dependent diabetes mellitus patients. Twenty-five overweight diabetics were given either 750 mg/day of 5-HTP or a placebo for two consecutive weeks. Brain tryptophan availability in the diabetics was significantly reduced when compared to healthy controls. The patients taking 5-HTP significantly decreased their daily energy intake by reducing carbohydrate and fat intake and reducing body weight.[4]

French researchers evaluated 19 patients with Friedreich's ataxia. The patients were given either 100 or 300 mg/day of 5-HTP or, in those weighing 60 kg, the dose was either 900 mg/day or a placebo. Friedreich's ataxia is an inherited disorder in which degeneration of nerve fibers in the spinal cord causes loss of coordinated movement and balance.[5] In the treatment group, there was a significant decrease in kinetic scores, indicating improved coordination. The data suggest that 5-HTP is useful in treating patients with this medical condition.

On September 24, 1998, the FDA reported that the Mayo Clinic had found some impurities in 5-HTP products. One of the impurities was identified as "peak X," and the FDA urged manufacturers of 5-HTP to ensure that their products are safe.[6]

Appearing on the TV newsmagazine program *Dateline* on April 7, 1999, Michael T. Murray, said that 5-HTP is perfectly safe, based on many clinical trials. He suggested that anyone taking megadoses of 5-HTP should have their blood checked every three months for any signs of peak X.[7]

Based on the available evidence, 5-HTP seems to be an ideal supplement for tackling a plethora of health problems. Ask your health care provider for guidelines for your specific problem.

References

1. Roufs, James B., "Review of L-Tryptophan and Eosinophilia-Myalgia Syndrome," *Journal of the American Dietetic Association* 92(7): 844–50, July 1992.

2. Murray, Michael T., "Boost Your Mood and Feel Great," *Let's Live,* Sept. 1998, 40–43.

3. Cangiano, Carlo, et al., "Eating Behavior and Adherence to Dietary Prescriptions in Obese Adult Subjects Treated with 5-Hydroxytryptophan," *Journal of the American College of Nutrition* 56: 863–67, 1992.

4. Cangiano, Carlos, et al., "Effects of Oral 5-Hydroxytryptophan on Energy Intake and Micronutrient Selection in Non-Insulin Dependent Diabetic Patients," *International Journal of Obesity* 22: 648–54, 1998.

5. Trouillas, Paul, et al., "Levoratory Form of 5-Hydroxytropthan in Friedreich's Ataxia: Results of a Double Blind Drug Placebo Cooperative Study," *Archives of Neurology* 52: 456–60, 1995.

6. FDA/Department of Health and Human Services press release, Sept. 24, 1998.

7. *Dateline,* April 7, 1999.

48

Horse Chestnut

Horse chestnut *(Aesculus hippocas-tanum)*, also known as *Hippo-castanum vulgare,* is an entirely different tree from sweet chestnut *(Castanea vesca)*. The prefix *horse* is believed to derive from the plant's use in treating coughs in horses and other animals. It may also be derived from the Welsh *gwres,* meaning hot or pungent. While the tree is chiefly grown for ornamental purposes, its bark, fruit, and seeds are used for a variety of medicinal purposes, including fevers, ulcers, rheumatism, neuralgia, and hemorrhoids.[1] More recently, it has been used to treat varicose veins.

Botanists have isolated horse chestnut's most active compound, aescin, and experiments with laboratory animals have found it useful in treating varicose veins and hemorrhoids. Aescin is thought to strengthen capillary cells and to reduce fluid leakage.[2]

A dry extract manufactured from horse chestnut seeds is being used in the treatment of varicose veins, as reported in *The Complete German Commission E Monographs.* There are no known contraindications, special cautions, or interactions with other drugs. Daily dosage is calculated at 100 mg aescin (escin), corresponding to 250 to 312.5 mg extract twice daily in delayed release form.[3]

"Using placebo as reference, a significant reduction of transcapillary leakage has been demonstrated in pharmacological studies involving human subjects, and a significant improvement in the symptoms of chronic venous insufficiency—tiredness, heaviness and tension, itching, pain, and swelling in the legs—in various randomized double-blind studies and/or cross-over studies," the commission reported.

Researchers in England studied 240 patients, of which 194 suffered from chronic venous insufficiency. The volunteers were divided into groups. One was given compression therapy, and another received 50 mg of horse chestnut seed extract twice daily. A third group acted as controls. Following 12 weeks of therapy, the lower leg volume of the more severely affected limbs decreased an average of 46.7 ml in the compression therapy group, and 43.8 ml with the horse chestnut seed extract. Horse chestnut seed extract provides an alternative treatment to compression therapy for edema or swelling in the legs.[4]

At the University of Exeter in the United Kingdom, researchers combed the literature for the efficacy of horse chestnut seed extract in treating chronic venous insufficiency and varicose veins. The extract was found to be superior in all placebo-controlled trials, decreasing lower leg volume and reducing leg circumference at the calf and ankle. Symptoms of leg pain, itching, and feelings of fatigue and tenseness were reduced. Five comparative studies found horse chestnut seed extract equally effective when pitted against a medication for swollen extremities, and one study suggested that the extract and compression therapy were also equally effective. Adverse side effects were considered mild and infrequent in those getting the extract. The available data imply that horse chestnut seed extract is superior to placebo and is as effective as the various medications in alleviating signs and symptoms of chronic venous insufficiency, and that the extract represents a treatment option worth considering.[5]

Native to Asia and southeastern Europe, horse chestnuts were used by the Turks to treat their horses' respiratory problems. By the 18th century, horse chestnuts had been introduced to North America. Native Americans crushed the fruits to ease the pain and inflammation of hemorrhoids.[6]

According to *The Family Guide to Natural Medicine,* "Today, horse chestnuts are used in the treatment of a number of circulatory problems, including varicose veins, blood clots, and hemorrhoids." An extract sold commercially is popular in Europe for arthritis and other complaints, and there is some scientific evidence that horse chestnuts may indeed have anti-inflammatory properties. Horse chestnut extract is also available as a salve, which may be applied to ease sore muscles and leg cramps. These remedies are widely available in Germany and are just beginning to be marketed in the United States.

In a double-blind, randomized trial, German researchers evaluated 137 postmenopausal women who complained of chronic venous insufficiency. Following one week of placebo administration, the patients were given either 1,000 mg/day of oxerutins, or 600 mg/day of horse chestnut extract for four weeks, followed by 500 mg/day of horse chestnut extract for 12 weeks. The women were then evaluated for an additional six weeks. Both compounds were judged therapeutic in reducing fluid leakage in the legs.[7]

A dietary supplement for leg health is now available over the counter. Containing horse chestnut seed extract, the capsules are designed to promote leg vein health and circulation in the legs, and to protect against swelling in the lower extremities. Other supplements are also available.

References

1. Grieve, Maude, *A Modern Herbal* (New York: Dover Publications, 1971), 192–93.

2. Duke, James A., *The Green Pharmacy* (Emmaus, Pa.: Rodale Press, 1997), 445–46.

3. Blumenthal, Mark, ed., *The Complete German Commission E Monographs* (Boston: Integrative Medicine Communications and American Botanical Council [Austin, Texas], 1998), 148–49.

4. Diehm, C., et al., "Horse Chestnut Seed Extract an Option for Treating Edema," *The Lancet* 347: 292–94, 1996.

5. Pittler, M. H., and E. Ernst, "Horse-Chestnut Seed Extract for Chronic Venous Insufficiency. A Criteria-Based Systemic Review," *Archives of Dermatology* 134: 1356–60, Nov. 1998.

6. Guinness, Alma E., ed., *Family Guide to Natural Medicine* (Pleasantville, N.Y.: The Reader's Digest Association, 1993), 312.

7. Rehn, D., et al., "Comparative Clinical Efficacy and Tolerability of Oxerutins and Horse Chestnut Extract in Patients with Chronic Venous Insufficiency," *Arzneimittelforschung* 46: 483–87, May 1996.

49

Huperzine A

With the graying of America, many older people will succumb to Alzheimer's disease (AD), a degenerative disorder that attacks the brain and leads to dementia. Alzheimer's affects an estimated four million people in the United States. If current demographic trends continue, researchers believe that the number of people affected by the disease will double every 20 years.[1]

Huperzine A (HupA), an alkaloid compound found in club moss (*Huperzia serrata*), was discovered in the herbal medicine Qian Ceng Ta. It has been used in China for centuries to treat fever and inflammation, and some researchers now think it could be even more effective than the two FDA-approved drugs in treating Alzheimer's, according to Andrew A. Skolnick. While HupA does not exhibit any antifever or anti-inflammatory proper-

ties, it does seem to be a potent inhibitor of acetylcholinesterase (AChE). In addition to being more selective and possibly less toxic than the two AChE inhibitors currently approved for treating AD—tacrine hydrochloride and donepezil—HupA has several other pharmacological properties of clinical interest.[2]

HupA is a potent blocker to acetylcholinesterase, an enzyme that helps break down acetylcholine, a neurotransmitter necessary for memory and function. AChE normally plays an essential housekeeping role by breaking down excess acetylcholine; however, biopsy and postmortem examinations have shown a substantial loss of certain neurons in the brains of Alzheimer's patients. Whatever acetylcholine is produced in the brains of AD patients is quickly broken down by AChE and the shortage of the neurotransmitter apparently contributes to the patients' memory loss and other cognitive defects, Skolnick reported.

HupA seems to bind more tightly and specifically to acetylcholinesterase than other AChE inhibitors, according to Joel Sussman, Ph.D., of the Weizmann Institute and Protein Data Bank at Brookhaven National Laboratory in Upton, New York. It is as though this natural substance was ingeniously designed to fit into the exact spot in acetylcholinesterase where it will do the most good. Added Alan Kozikowski, Ph.D., of Georgetown University's Institute of Cognitive and Computational Sciences, who first synthesized HupA in 1991, compared to tacrine and donepezil, HupA has a longer half-life and the AChE-HupA complex has a slower rate of dissociation, which may make it a more effective therapeutic agent.

In *Acta Pharmacologica Sinica*, Xi-Can Tang of the Shanghai Institute of Materia Medica in China reported that HupA is a potent and selective inhibitor of AChE, with rapid absorption and penetration into the brains of laboratory animals. Further, HupA exhibited a broad range of memory-enhancing activities in the animal models. The study suggests that HupA is a promising candidate for clinical trials as a symptomatic treatment for AD.[3] A study by Si-Sun Xu and colleagues at Zhejiang Medical University in Shanghai showed that HupA is a promising supplement for symptomatic treatment of AD.[4]

Alan A. Mazurek, M.D., of Mercy Medical Center in Rockville Centre, New York, has conducted an open label study with Huperzine A on his patients with dementia and memory loss. Most of the volunteers continued to take their prescribed medications during the study. Twenty-two patients were given 50 mcg of HupA b.i.d. (twice a day); two patients got 100 mcg b.i.d.; and five patients were increased to 100 mcg b.i.d.[5] "In approximately 29 patients, more than half have shown an improvement or an arrest of progression of their dementia, which represents a significant result," Mazurek said. "More studies are needed to determine the exact dosage and further usefulness of Huperzine A, but it clearly is a major advancement in the treatment of dementia and memory loss."

HupA has been found to be a potent inhibitor of cholinesterase, which penetrates into the brain and produces increases of acetylcholine, norepinephrine, and dopamine in rat brains. It may be a more suitable drug for treatment of AD than physostigmine, a reversible inhibitor of cholinesterases that prevents the destruction of acetylcholine.[6]

Since HupA can inhibit the transport of choline in the brain, this permits more to be available for synthesis of acetylcholine, the neurotransmitter necessary for maintaining normal eye function. Related to the B complex of vitamins, choline is a precursor of acetylcholine. HupA may be a better therapeutic drug than other AChE inhibitors—such as physostigmine, neostigmine, or tacrine—for the treatment of glaucoma.[7]

A limited number of studies have shown that HupA significantly improves muscle weakness associated with myasthenia gravis, a neuromuscular disorder characterized by weakness and marked fatigability of skeletal muscle. In a 1986 study involving 128 myasthenia gravis patients treated with HupA, 99 percent demonstrated controlled or improved clinical symptoms of the disease. Except for nausea in a few patients, side effects were minimal when compared with those produced by prostigmin.

Huperzine A has been recommended as a prescription drug in China since the 1990s, and it is said to have been used by more than 100,000 people with no serious side effects. In a double-blind trial in China, HupA, at a dose of 200 mcg twice daily, produced measurable improvements in memory, cognitive function, and behavioral factors in 58 percent of Alzheimer's patients. In the placebo group, only 36 percent showed an improvement.[8]

As a preventive or treatment for Alzheimer's disease, HupA is a welcome addition to the roster of natural supplements.

References

1. Khachaturian, Zaven S., and Teresa Radebaugh, "Alzheimer's Disease," *Medical and Health Annual* (Chicago: Encylopaedia Britannica, 1995), 222ff.

2. Skolnick, Andrew A., "Old Chinese Herbal Medicine Used for Fever Yields Possible New Alzheimer's Disease Therapy," *Journal of the American Medical Association* 277(10): 776, March 12, 1997.

3. Tang, Xi-Can, "Huperzine A (Shuangyiping): A Promising Drug for Alzheimer's Disease," *Acta Pharmacologica Sinica* 17(6): 481–84, Nov. 1996.

4. Xu, Si-Sun, et al., "Efficacy of Tablet Huperzine A on Memory, Cognition, and Behavior in Alzheimer's Disease," *Acta Pharmacologica Sinica* 16(5): 291–95, Sept. 1995.

5. Mazurek, Alan A., "An Open-Label Trial of Huperzine A in the Treatment of Alzheimer's Disease," unpublished, 1997.

6. Zhu, X. D., and E. Giacobini, "Second Generation Cholinesterase Inhibitors: Effect of (L)-Huperzine-A on Cortical Biogenic Amines," *Journal of Neuroscience Research* 41: 828–35, 1995.

7. Bagchi, Debasis, and Jean Barilla, *Huperzine A: Boost Your Brain Power* (New Canaan, Conn.: Keats Publishing, 1998), 34–35.

8. "Huperzine A: A New Treatment for Alzheimer's Disease from China," *Natural Medicine Journal*, March 1999, 22.

50

IP6

The National Cancer Society reported that in 1998, the latest year tabulated, an estimated 564,000 Americans were expected to succumb to cancer. That amounts to more than 1,500 deaths each day. Cancer is the second leading cause of death in the United States, ranking second only to heart disease.

As scientists frantically search for possible cures for the many types of cancer, a naturally occurring constituent whose chemical composition consists of inositol, with six phosphate groups, is showing great promise as a cancer fighter. The new substance, IP6, also known as inositol hexaphosphate, is found naturally in whole-grain cereals such as rice, oats, wheat, and corn, as well as legumes such as beans. Inositol is associated with the B complex of vitamins, and since its chemical structure is similar to glucose, it is referred to as a "sugar."

A 15-year laboratory study by AbulKalam M. Shamsuddin, M.D., Ph.D., of the University of Maryland School of Medicine at Baltimore, along with colleagues at the National Cancer Institute, found that IP6 inhibits cell growth and shrinks existing tumors by almost 50-fold. Treated cells showed signs of returning to normal. IP6 works as an antioxidant to suppress the body's production of free radicals and inhibits lipid peroxidation that damages cells and promotes cancer. IP6 has also been shown to inhibit kidney-stone formation, lower lipid levels in the blood, prevent fatty liver, protect the heart muscles during a heart attack, and prevent hardening of the arteries. The study was designed to determine whether or not IP6 can inhibit the growth of rhabdomyosarcoma, the most common soft-tissue sarcoma in children.[1]

Several epidemiological studies have shown a strong correlation between nutrient composition of the diet and cancer of the colon. Bandaru S. Reddy, Ph.D., and colleagues at Alabama A&M University at Normal, and the American Health Foundation, Valhalla, New York, decided to test this theory using IP6 and green tea. In tests on laboratory animals, green tea had a marginal effect on colon cancer, and IP6 significantly reduced the incidence of precancerous lesions of the colon.[2]

A study at the University of Maryland School of Medicine in Baltimore investigated whether a high-fiber bran diet containing high IP6 is as effective as pure IP6 in preventing chemically induced rat mammary carcinogenesis.[3]

Rats were divided into five groups. Three groups were given diets consisting of 5, 10, and 20 percent fiber, while a fourth group received a diet containing a carcinogen. The fifth group was administered 0.4 percent IP6 in drinking water, an amount equivalent to IP6 in 20 percent bran. The trial lasted 29 weeks. Tumor incidence was reduced by 16.7, 14.6, and 11.4 percent in the animals fed the 5, 10, and 20 percent bran diets, respectively. However, the animals given 0.4 percent pure IP6 in drinking water—the same amount as in the highest 20 percent bran group—had a 33.5 percent reduction in tumor incidence and 48.8 percent fewer tumors. In practical terms, ingesting IP6 may be a more pragmatic approach for cancer prophylaxis than gorging on enormous quantities of fiber.

Prostate cancer is one of the most prominent cancers in males in industrialized countries. In 1994, the American Cancer Society predicted that 200,000 men would contract the disease and that 38,000 would die from it. Once the cancer spreads to the regional lymph nodes, the prognosis is generally poor. With this in mind, Shamsuddin and Guang-Yu Yang, of the University of Maryland School of Medicine, investigated the effects of IP6 on growth inhibition and differentiation of human prostate cancer cells in laboratory glassware. They found that IP6 does indeed inhibit the growth of cancer cells in vitro. Since IP6 is an antioxidant and a natural dietary ingredient in cereals and legumes, it is a strong candidate for adjuvant chemotherapy and prevention of prostate cancer. As most prostate cancers remain clinically silent and are common in the elderly, these are important reasons for targeting this population for preventive measures so as to stop the development of cancer, or to reverse it if it has already been found. Studies of the modulation of tumor markers by chemopreventive agents such as IP6 may help in planning strategies for combating the disease.[4]

Considered with the anticancer action against breast cancer, this study on prostate cancer shows the potential of IP6. Since breast and prostate cancers are hormone dependent, treatment modalities would suggest a hormone approach. But IP6 is just as effective in both types of cancer, the researchers said.

A study at the Hormel Institute, University of Minnesota at Austin, confirmed the anticancer activity of IP6 in skin cancer cells. Also spotlighted was the molecular mechanism responsible for the cancer-fighting action of IP6. This mechanism may be the blocking of cell transformation and activator protein (AP-1), which is said to play a significant role in the development of tumors.[5]

In the *American Journal of Clinical Nutrition,* Shamsuddin wrote, "Ohkawa, et al., demonstrated that administration of 20 grams of rice bran to humans for up to three years resulted in a strikingly decreased incidence of kidney stones without significantly affecting the serum mineral concentrations. Recent papers from my laboratory showed a consistent and reproducible anticancer action of IP6 in at least two models of experimental colon cancer. Support for this anticancer action is beginning to come from others. . . . I for one would therefore have no hesitation in taking an extra gram or two of IP6 daily to prevent cancer of the colon (or breast, if I were female)."[6,7]

In another experiment, Shamsuddin and his colleagues injected human liver cancer cells into mice. In 71 percent of the animals that did not receive IP6 before being exposed to the cancer, a solid tumor growth appeared. But no tumors were found in the mice receiving the same number of liver cancer cells that had been pretreated in glassware with IP6 for 48 hours before being injected. Exposing the cancerous tumor cells to IP6 had stopped them from out-of-control growth and from forming a tumor. For the mice with detectable tumors, when the tumors reached 8 to 10 mm in diameter—which, in a human, would be about the size of a basketball—an IP6 injection was made into the growth daily for 12 days. The researchers reported that the tumor weight in the IP6-treated animals was 3.4-fold less than that in the control mice who didn't receive an IP6 treatment.[8]

"The most intriguing finding in this experiment," Shamsuddin continued, "was that a single treatment of cancer cells with IP6 resulted in complete loss of the ability of these cells to form tumors. On the other hand, the untreated cells formed tumors in the mice. Even more exciting was the effect on preexisting liver cancers. When they were treated directly with IP6, they regressed. This experiment showed that IP6 can be used to treat highly malignant liver cancers as well." The liver cancer study was reported at the 1998 annual meeting of the American Association of Cancer Research and reprinted in the November/December 1998 issue of *Anti-Cancer Research.*[9]

Since most of the research on IP6 has been done in the laboratory, doctors familiar with the potential for treating patients with cancer are eager to publicize their results. Admittedly anecdotal, the results are often startling. A 34-year-old patient was diagnosed with glioma-astrocytoma, a fast-growing brain tumor. Instead of chemotherapy, the patient opted to take 10 doses of radiation, but the cancer remained. In September 1998, the patient began taking 6 to 15 tablets of IP6 and inositol daily, along with grape seed extract, methylsulfonylmethane (MSM), and folic acid. By early 1999, no traces of the brain tumor could be found.[10]

A leukemia patient in Fort Benning, Georgia, began taking 16 capsules of IP6 and inositol per day at the beginning of her fifth month of chemotherapy. Since the weekly chemotherapy treatments were not helping, she stopped them after eight months but continued to take IP6 and inositol and Essiac tea. Her leukemia is now in remission and her spinal tumor has decreased in size.

In Blue Bell, Pennsylvania, a prostate cancer patient reported that his cancer was in remission after only five weeks of taking six tablets of IP6 and inositol daily, along with other dietary supplements. His PSA (prostate-specific antigen) levels have gone down 95 percent.

A patient in Seymour, Tennessee, who suffered from lung cancer that had spread to the spine and rib cage, underwent 31 treatments of radiation and chemotherapy, along with Alexia, a derivative of aloe vera that builds the immune system. In June 1998, he began taking six tablets of IP6 and inositol per day. Four months later, the cancer had pulled away from the spine and the lung cancer was in remission.

"The lack of remuneration is the reason behind the one deficiency in the scientific portfolio of IP6—the lack of clinical trials in humans," said Michael T. Murray, N.D. "With the prospect of large, well-designed clinical studies unlikely, it was only 'natural' for IP6 to present itself as a nutritional supplement; one I predict will soon become very popular."[11]

Murray hopes the lack of human research will be rectified with time. In the meantime, he plans to recommend IP6 supplementation to his patients with cancer and those who are at high risk for developing cancer. "As I have said in previous editorials, I believe that we need to move away from requiring a substance to have absolute proof before we feel confident in recommending it to patients. Instead, I believe that we need to proceed when we have reasonable certainty. The two primary criteria should be safety and possible benefits. The cost of the therapy should also be included. What we know about IP6 at present is that it is a relatively inexpensive natural substance that poses no documented health risk, yet holds the promise of being a real answer to one of the most deadly diseases on the planet—cancer. There is no downside, and based on the work of Dr. Shamsuddin and others the potential upside is enormous."

For those who are susceptible to cancer, kidney stones, fatty liver, hardening of the arteries, and so forth—or have those disorders now—ask your doctor to review the many published studies on IP6.

References

1. Vucenik, Ivana, et al., "Novel Anticancer Function of Inositol Hexaphosphate: Inhibition of Human Rhabdomyosarcoma in Vitro and in Vivo," *Anticancer Research* 18: 1377–84, 1998.

2. Challa, Anjana, et al., "Interactive Suppression of Aberrant Crypt Foci Induced by Azoxymethane in Rat Colon by Phytic Acid and Green Tea," *Carcinogenesis* 18(10): 2023–26, 1997.

3. Vucenik, Ivana, et al., "Comparison of Pure Inositol Hexaphosphate and High-Bran Diet in the Prevention of DMBA-Induced Rat Mammary Carcinogenesis," *Nutrition and Cancer* 28(1): 7–13, 1997.

4. Shamsuddin, AbulKalam M., and Guang-Yu Yang, "Inositol Hexaphosphate Inhibits Growth and Induces Differentiation of PC-3 Human Prostate Cancer Cells," *Carcinogenesis* 16(8): 1975–79, 1995.

5. Huang, Chuanshu, et al., "Inositol Hexaphosphate Inhibits Cell Transformation and Activator Protein I Activation by Targeting Phosphatidylinositol-3 Kinase," *Cancer Research* 57: 2873–78, July 15, 1971.

6. Shamsuddin, AbulKalam M., "Phytate and Colon-Cancer Risk," *American Journal of Clinical Nutrition* 55: 478–85, 1992.

7. Ohkawa, T., et al., "Rice Bran Treatment for Patients with Hypercalciuric Stones Experimental and Clinical Studies," *Journal of Urology* 132: 1140–45, 1984.

8. Shamsuddin, AbulKalam M., *IP6: Nature's Revolutionary Cancer-Fighter* (New York: Kensington Books, 1998), 90ff.

9. "IP6 May Reduce Tumors," *Nutritional Outlook,* May 1999, 56.

10. "Stories of IP6/Inositol: The Effects of a Natural Cancer Fighter on Cancer Patients Across the United States," AdInfinitum press release, March 1999.

11. Murray, Michael T., "Clinical Commentary on IP6," *Natural Medicine Journal,* June 1998, 16–17.

51

Ipriflavone

Osteoporosis is a debilitating disease that affects more than 1.5 million older men and women annually. In response, consumers are continuously searching for ways to strengthen their bones and help avoid broken hips, arms, and wrists. Osteoporosis develops when bone resorption exceeds bone formation, resulting in a loss of bone mass and density. Fortunately, there may be a solution as near as your local health food store: ipriflavone.

Ipriflavone was synthesized in the 1960s. It is devoid of estrogenic activity in humans and animals, although it increases estrogenic activity in the uterus. Clinical studies have shown that ipriflavone inhibits bone resorption and enhances bone formation. The substance has been used at doses of 600 mg/day in double-blind, placebo-controlled studies in postmenopausal and senile osteo-porosis, and it has shown a reduction in bone turnover, resulting in a significant bone-spurring effect at the lumbar and radial levels. No significant side effects have been reported. Ipriflavone may inhibit bone resorption through its effect on osteoclasts and its inhibition of recruitment and/or differentiation of preosteoclasts. Osteoclasts are large cells associated with bone resorption. Ipriflavone seems to be a new nonhormonal approach for prevention and treatment of postmenopausal and senile osteoporosis.[1]

An Italian study found two substances that help to treat osteoporosis. One is designed to decrease bone resorption and the other is supposed to enhance bone formation. In the 1970s, it was found that ipriflavone, a derivative of the naturally occurring class of isoflavones, enhanced the amount of calcium retained in bones when given orally to animals. In a Japanese trial, a daily dose of 600 mg was found to be an optimal therapeutic regimen for the treatment of osteoporosis. Other trials have used dosages of 1,200 mg/day. The consensus is that ipriflavone seems to be safe and a rational alternative to estrogen replacement therapy in preventing bone loss in acute ovarian-deficient states and in the postmenopausal period in estrogen-deficient osteoporosis.[2]

Actually, ipriflavone with low doses of estrogen has been suggested as an excellent therapy. Vitamin D and its metabolites may also have a positive effect on bone status. Researchers have reported that vitamin D is an indirect stimulator of bone resorption both in humans and in laboratory glassware. In addition, vitamin D stimulates calcium absorption in the gastrointestinal tract, promotes mineralization, and increases calcium absorption while inhibiting bone resorption.

In a study in Siena, Italy, 56 women with low vertebral density, who were postmenopausal for less than five years, were randomly selected to receive either 200 mg of ipriflavone three times daily or a placebo. They were also given 1,000 mg of calcium daily. Vertebral bone density declined after two years in women taking only calcium but did not change in those receiving ipriflavone. Ipriflavone prevents the rapid bone loss following early menopause. When given alone, it does not produce estrogenic effects, but it is known to inhibit bone resorption.[3]

Ipriflavone, similar to soy isoflavonoids, is approved for the treatment and prevention of osteoporosis in Japan, Hungary, and Italy, according to Michael T. Murray, N.D., and Joseph E. Pizzorno, N.D. In one study, 200 mg of ipriflavone three times daily increased bone density by 2 percent and 5.8 percent after 6 and 12 months, respectively. The study involved 100 women with osteoporosis. In a one-year study, women with osteoporosis were given 600 mg/day of ipriflavone. This produced a 6 percent increase in bone mineral density after 12 months, compared with 0.3 percent in the controls.[4]

At Semmelweis Medical University in Budapest, researchers reported that ipriflavone has been used as a medical treatment for otosclerosis, or the growth of spongy bone in the inner ear, which may cause deafness. Quercetin, the bioflavonoid, also seems promising for the control of otosclerotic bone-remodeling disturbances.[5]

If you are concerned about preventing or treating osteoporosis, ask your physician for guidelines concerning ipriflavone.

References

1. Reginster, Jean-Yves L., "Ipriflavone: Pharmacological Properties and Usefulness to Postmenopausal Osteoporosis," *Bone and Mineral* 23: 223–32, 1993.
2. Brandi, Maria Luisa, "New Treatment Strategies: Ipriflavone, Strontium,

Vitamin D Metabolites, and Analogs," *American Journal of Medicine* 95(Suppl. 5A): 69S–74S, Nov. 30, 1993.

3. Gennari, C., et al., "Effect of Ipriflavone—a Synthetic Derivative of Natural Isoflavones—on Bone Mass Loss in the Early Years After Menopause," *Menopause: The Journal of the North American Menopause Society* 5(1): 9–15, 1998.

4. Murray, Michael T., and Joseph E. Pizzorno, *Encyclopedia of Natural Medicine,* rev. 2nd ed. (Rocklin, Calif.: Prima Publishing, 1998), 720.

5. Sziklai, Istvan, and Otto Ribari, "Flavonoids After Bone-Remodeling in Auditory Ossicle Organ Cultures," *ACTA Otolaryngology Stockholm* 115: 296–99, 1995.

52

Iron

Based on data gathered from 24,894 people aged one year or older by the National Center for Health Statistics and other agencies, iron deficiency is rather common in the United States. The problem is most acute in adolescent girls, women of childbearing age, and toddlers. That translates into 7.8 million adolescent girls and women of childbearing age, an estimated 3.3 million of whom have iron deficiency anemia. Estimates for toddlers show about 700,000 with iron deficiency, approximately 240,000 of whom have iron deficiency anemia.[1] Iron deficiency is related to anemia, fatigue, curved nails, behavioral problems, depression, learning problems, dizziness, inattention in school, heavy menstruation, swollen ankles, and other health problems.

Although iron is one of the most plentiful minerals in the earth's crust, iron deficiency is one of the most common nutritional prob-

lems in both developing and developed nations, according to Elaine R. Monsen of the University of Washington at Seattle. Iron is a critical component of one of the world's most costly liquids: blood. The physiologic demand for iron is markedly lower in males than in growing children and in women during their reproductive years, and yet iron intake is considerably higher in men than in children or premenopausal women. And the amount of iron consumed is many times greater than the amount absorbed. Iron is not readily excreted through the usual routes of urine, bile, and sweat. Rather, the primary exit is through the shedding of cells from the skin or gastrointestinal tract, or through blood loss, as in menstrual blood or chronic or acute hemorrhage.[2]

"The ultimate irony of iron may be apparent only when we finally understand this abundant yet not abundantly absorbed and less abundantly excreted metal that is essential for life," Monsen continued. "Too much is lethal; too little is incompatible with life. This delicate balance is achieved by close control of iron absorption and, at the same time, exquisite regulation of iron excretion."

Iron deficiency is found in between 20 and 40 percent of pregnant women. Therefore, the American College of Obstetrics and Gynecology recommends that women be given a daily dose of 30 mg of iron during the second and third trimesters of pregnancy. In one study, 22 patients who did not improve with oral iron supplements were given intravenous iron shots, which improved their iron stores. Side effects of intravenous iron included flushing, headaches, joint pains, and lymph node complications, but there were no effects on the pregnancies.[3]

At the Conservatoire National des Arts et Metiers in Paris, and other facilities, researchers studied the effect of iron supplements on the iron status of new mothers and on biochemical iron status and clinical and anthropometric measures of their infants. Used as background was a study by Scholl et al.,[4] which found an association between iron deficiency anemia and pregnancy outcome, but not between iron deficiency without anemia. The researchers reported that women with iron deficiency anemia had three times the risk of giving birth to an infant with low birth weight. No significant difference in birth weight according to maternal iron-supplementation status was found, but differences existed in length of the baby at birth and in Apgar scores, which were higher in newborns whose mothers had received iron supplements.[5] Named after American anesthesiologist Virginia Apgar (1909–74), the Apgar score uses numerical values (0, 1, or 2) to measure an infant's progress in five categories: heart rate, breathing, muscle tone, response stimulation, and skin color. A total score of 8 to 10 indicates the infant is doing well.

Infants with iron deficiency anemia may suffer long-lasting consequences for behavioral development. Laboratory work with rats has shown that iron deficiency during gestation or early postnatal life directly affects the brain, while early neurophysiologic data in humans infer a direct effect on the central nervous system.[6]

Four pediatricians in the New York City area, in evaluating 504 children between the ages of 1 and 3, found that more than one-third (35 percent) had iron insufficiency; 7 percent were iron deficient without anemia; and 10 percent had iron deficiency anemia. Iron deficiency is related to mental and psychomotor impairment during the first two years of life.[7]

In a study of 78 girls with mildly low iron levels but no anemia, those who were given four iron supplements a day for eight weeks showed improvements on tests measuring their memory and their ability to recall new vocabulary words, compared to the teens who were given a placebo. Even in the absence of anemia, iron supplements improve some aspects of cognitive functioning in iron-deficient adolescent girls, according to Ann B. Bruner, M.D., and colleagues at Johns Hopkins School of Medicine in Baltimore. Adolescent girls are often lacking in the mineral because they do not eat foods high in iron, such as prunes, raisins, red meat, liver, and whole-wheat products.[8]

A growth spurt and menstrual status had adverse effects on iron stores in adolescent girls who had low intakes of the mineral, but long-term supplementation with calcium did not affect iron stores. It has long been suspected that a high-calcium diet might inhibit iron stores in the body, but researchers have found that supplements of calcium citrate maleate at an amount approaching the RDA (1,500 mg/day for adolescent girls) did not have a detrimental effect on the iron reserves of these girls.[9]

The avoidance of red meat increases the risk of iron and zinc deficiencies, and low concentrations of serum ferritin (iron-containing protein) mean the possibility of low zinc stores, reported researchers at the University of Texas at Galveston. Their study involved 38 healthy, nonpregnant premenopausal women between the ages of 19 and 40.[10]

People with excessive amounts of iron—often middle-aged men—are at risk of developing heart disease. However, periodic blood donations seem to correct the problem, as well as monitoring iron-rich foods in the diet. Researchers at the University of Kuopio in Finland conducted a study that found that depleting iron results in an increased resistance to lipid peroxidation. This lends support to the role of iron overload and the etiology of coronary heart disease. If the antioxidative effect of donating blood is confirmed, then periodic donations may be a safe and inexpensive therapy in the prevention and treatment of free radical–initiated diseases, especially in those with hemochromatosis, a metabolic disorder in which large amounts of iron are stored in the body.[11] When damaged fats and cholesterol form toxic compounds such as lipid peroxides and oxidized cholesterol, they damage artery walls and contribute to the progression of hardening of the arteries and coronary heart disease.

At least 30 years ago, a connection was found between iron status and restless leg syndrome. Researchers at Johns Hopkins Sleep Center in Baltimore went through four years of patient records and found 18 women and 9 men ages 29 to 80 who had been evaluated for ferritin levels about the same time they were diagnosed with restless leg syndrome. Those with the lower ferritin levels correlated with the greater severity of restless leg syndrome and decreased sleep efficiency. Raising blood ferritin levels to above 50 mcg/L may help to improve the problem.[12]

Up to 27 percent of healthy children engage in breath-holding spells that are understandably frightening to their parents. However, 88 percent of the children given iron supplements showed a significant reduction in these spells. In the children given a placebo, only 6 percent had fewer episodes. Iron deficiency may impact on oxygen uptake to the lungs, which reduces available oxygen to the tissues.[13]

From available data, three groups of people seem to be at greatest risk of developing altered body iron status when they exercise: (1) female athletes who may not be getting sufficient iron from their diets; (2) distance runners who may also be neglecting their intake of iron-rich foods; and (3) vegetarian athletes who also may be ignoring iron-rich foods. Iron losses in humans are about 1 mg/day and must be replaced by an equivalent amount of iron derived from the diet. The typical Western diet provides an average of 6 mg of heme and nonheme iron per 1,000 kcals of energy intake daily. Heme iron, which is more readily absorbed, is from animal sources; nonheme iron is from vegetable sources and iron-fortified foods.[14]

In a study at National Taiwan University, Taipei, 55 Chinese Buddhist vegetarians and 59 nonvegetarian medical students were evaluated. Iron deficiency was found to be more prevalent among the vegetarians. The researchers said that a vegetarian diet rich in soybeans and restricted in animal foods is limited in bioavailable iron and is not adequate for maintaining iron balance in men and women.[15]

At McGill University in Montréal, Canada, researchers found that Ethiopian children who ate food cooked in iron pots were less likely to have iron-deficient blood, compared to their friends who ate similar food cooked in aluminum pots. Following a one-year study, iron deficiency anemia rates fell from 57 to 13 percent in the children eating from iron cookware, but only 55 to 39 percent in the control group. If larger studies showed similar results, this could lead to advances in child, adolescent, and maternal health at a rather low cost, commented Bernard Brabin of the Liverpool, England, School of Tropical Medicine.[16]

Based on animal studies, it has been suggested that iron supplements should not be given daily, but rather weekly or twice weekly, since the intestinal mucosal cells are not able to absorb therapeutic doses of iron given daily because of blockage of the absorption by the iron retained in the mucosal walls. After reviewing the literature on the subject, Leif Hallberg of the University of Gothenburg, Sweden, found no scientific basis for changing the well-established regimen of daily supplementation of iron deficient populations to a weekly regimen. This is especially important for pregnant women, he said, since a weekly regimen can seriously harm both the mother and the fetus. He added that the so-called mucosal block is nonexistent.[17]

Food sources of iron include meat, poultry, fish, iron-fortified cereals, and some vegetables and fruits, such as raisins and prunes. Suggested daily intake ranges from 10 to 12 mg for boys; 10 mg for men over age 19; 15 mg for girls and women to age 50; 10 mg for women over age 50; 30 mg for pregnant women; and 15 mg for breast-feeding women.

Like other minerals, iron has a somewhat contradictory nature, meaning that you can get too little as well as too much. For a lingering health problem that may involve iron, confer with your holistic doctor.

References

1. Locker, Anne C., et al., "Prevalence of Iron Deficiency in the United States," *Journal of the American Medical Association* 277(12): 973–76, March 26, 1997.

2. Monsen, Elaine R., "The Ironies of Iron," *American Journal of Clinical Nutrition* 69: 831–32, 1999.

3. Jancin, Bruce, "IV Iron Works Where Oral Supplementation Fails," *Family Practice News* 26(13): 29, July 1, 1996.

4. Scholl, T. O., et al., "Anemia vs. Iron Deficiency: Increased Risk of Preterm Delivery in a Prospective Study," *American Journal of Clinical Nutrition* 55: 985–88, 1992.

5. Preziosi, Paul, et al., "Effect of Iron Supplementation on the Iron Status of Pregnant Women: Consequences for Newborns," *American Journal of Clinical Nutrition* 66: 1178–82, 1997.

6. Holst, Mary-Clare, "Developmental and Behavioral Effects of Iron Deficiency Anemia in Infants," *Nutrition Today* 33(1): 27–36, Jan./Feb. 1998.

7. Eden, Alvin N., and Mohammad A. Mir, "Iron Deficiency in 1- to 3-Year-Old Children: A Pediatric Failure?" *Archives of Pediatric and Adolescent Medicine* 151: 986–88, Oct. 1997.

8. Mann, Denise, "Iron-Deficient Girls May Suffer Memory Problems," *Medical Tribune* 37(19): 18, Nov. 7, 1996.

9. Hich-Ernst, Jasminka Z., et al., "Iron Status, Menarche, and Calcium Supplementation in Adolescent Girls," *American Journal of Clinical Nutrition* 66: 880–87, 1998.

10. Yokoi, Katsuhiko, et al., "Iron and Zinc Nutriture of Premenopausal Women: Association of Diet with Serum Ferritin and Plasma Zinc Disappearance," *Journal of Laboratory and Clinical Medicine* 124: 852–61, 1994.

11. Salomen, J. T., et al., "Lowering of Body Iron Stores by Blood Letting and Oxidation Resistance of Serum Lipoproteins: A Randomized Cross-Over in Male Smokers," *Journal of Internal Medicine* 237: 161–68, 1995.

12. Murray, Michael, "Iron for Restless Legs Syndrome," *Natural Medicine Journal* 2(5): 21, Summer 1999. Also, R. R. Sun et al., "Iron and the Restless Legs Syndrome," *Sleep* 21: 371–77, 1998.

13. Daoud, A. S., et al., "Effectiveness of Iron Therapy on Breath-Holding Spells," *Journal of Pediatrics* 130: 547–50, 1997.

14. Beard, John L., "Iron Nutrition and Exercise," Workshop on the Role of Dietary Supplements for Physically Active People, National Institutes of Health, Bethesda, Maryland, June 3–4, 1996.

15. Shaw, Ning-Sing, et al., "A Vegetarian Diet Rich in Soybean Products

Compromises Iron Status in Young Students," *Journal of Nutrition* 125: 212–19, 1995.

16. Seppa, Nathan, "Iron Pots Help Fend Off Anemia," *Science News* 155(11): 175, March 13, 1999.

17. Hallberg, Leif, "Combating Iron Deficiency: Daily Administration of Iron Is Far Superior to Weekly Administration," *American Journal of Clinical Nutrition* 68: 213–17, 1998.

53

Isoflavone

Isoflavone is a nonnutrient plant substance found in rather high concentrations in soy products and many other plants. Two examples of isoflavones are genistein and daidzein. Their general shape is similar to the steroid hormone estrogen, the female sex hormone. It is believed that isoflavones block estrogen from binding to various sites, a needed step in hormone-dependent cancers such as those of the breast, ovary, and endometrium. They may also stimulate the production of an estrogen-binding protein in blood, or they may block liver enzymes that activate compounds that may become carcinogenic. Vegetarians who consume tofu and other soy products are thought to have a lower risk of cancer.[1]

An overview of phytoestrogens in *Australian Family Practice* reported that the main classes of phytoestrogens include isoflavones, found in soybeans, lentils, and beans, and in soybean products such as soy meal and flour, tofu, and soy milk. Tofu has a greater concentration of isoflavones than soy milk. In the gastrointestinal tract, lignans and isoflavone precursors are metabolized to form heterocyclic phenols that are similar to estrogens. The most estrogenically active isoflavones are genistein and daidzein. Soy consumption may be useful in preventing and/or treating menopausal symptoms, hot flashes, osteoporosis, cardiovascular disease, and cancer. An increase of 30 to 50 mg of isoflavones is possible when consuming one serving of a soy food or two servings of soy milk (200 mg each), or four slices of soy-enriched bread. This would match consumption comparable to intakes in Asian communities.[2]

Between 1980 and 1990, the intake of soy products by Americans increased about

40 percent; this may be below the amount necessary for a reduction in cancer risk, since the average intake by Americans is only 3 g/day. Consumption of 3.7 ounces of tempeh provides an average of 0.5 mg of isoflavones per kg of body weight per day. A study at the Fred Hutchinson Cancer Research Center in Seattle studied 17 healthy men 20 to 40 years of age who consumed either 112 g of tempeh or 125 g of unfermented soy during control feedings. Urinary excretion of isoflavonoids was higher and excretion of lignans was lower when the volunteers consumed the soy diets instead of their regular diets.[3]

Isoflavones are found in soybeans and soybean products in concentrations ranging up to 300 mg/100 g. In analyzing food questionnaires from 102 Caucasian, Native Hawaiian, Chinese, Japanese, and Filipino women, in conjunction with overnight urinary samples, it was found that Japanese women excreted more daidzein, genistein, and glycitein than Caucasian women. Caucasian women excreted a little more coumestrol. Since diet history has a strong correlation with isoflavone excretion, the questionnaire is often used in evaluating dietary risk factors for breast cancer.[4]

Excretion of isoflavonoids in the urine of Japanese women was found much higher than in American and Finnish women. That is because Japanese women consume such soy products as tofu, miso, aburage, atuage, koridofu, soybeans, and boiled beans. The high intake may partly explain why hot flashes and other menopausal complaints are reduced in Japanese women. Although isoflavonoids have a weak estrogenic effect, high amounts could have biological effects, especially in postmenopausal women with low levels of estrogen.[5]

Six premenopausal women 21 to 29 years of age with regular ovulatory cycles were given 60 g/day of soy protein, which contained 45 mg of isoflavonoids, for one month. There was a significant increase in the time from menstruation to ovulation (follicular phase) and/or delayed menstruation. Midcycle surges of luteinizing hormone and follicle-stimulating hormone were significantly suppressed during the dietary intervention and were similar to tamoxifen, an antiestrogen used for those at high risk of breast cancer. The delayed menstruation is apparently why Japanese women have fewer menopausal complaints. There was also a 9.6 percent reduction in cholesterol in the isoflavone-rich diet.[6]

Miso, a Japanese soybean paste, has been reported to prevent gastric and mammary cancer and chronic nephritis, which is chronic inflammation of the kidney. Researchers, using laboratory mice, found that miso acted as an antioxidant by scavenging free radicals. Miso contains such antioxidants as vitamin E, isoflavones, and saponins, as well as other antioxidants that are not destroyed by heating miso soup preparations.[7] Researchers at Guy's Hospital in London ascertained the antioxidant action of various phytoestrogenic isoflavones and found that genistein has the greatest scavenging ability.[8]

Isoflavones appear to lower LDL cholesterol and help protect against coronary heart disease, according to a research team at the University of Sydney in Australia. Flavonoids reduce the formation of free radicals and help protect or regenerate other antioxidants. The mineral boron may have a beneficial effect in coronary heart disease by causing increases in the concentration of plant estrogen.[9]

At Tufts University in Boston, researchers studied a meta-analysis (a compilation of studies) of 38 human trials. When soy is substituted for animal protein in the diet, it was found that the levels of cholesterol, LDL cholesterol, and triglycerides are lowered without affecting HDL cholesterol. The average soy intake was 47 g/day. Thirty grams of soy can be obtained by drinking two cups of soy milk or consuming 112 g of tofu. Soy seems to be more beneficial for those who have high cholesterol levels.[10] Genistein and daidzein may reduce the risk of cancer by enhancing the activity of natural killer cells, which play key roles in the destruction of cancer cells and infectious microbes.[11]

If soy products are not to your liking, you are not alone. Soy is definitely an acquired taste. But you can still benefit by taking over-the-counter supplements. Look for a supplement that contains genistein and daidzein, and try to avoid soy products that are from genetically modified soybeans. You can find genistein supplements and other soy products, such as tofu, tempeh, and meat substitutes, at your local health food store.

References

1. Ronzio, Robert A., *The Encyclopedia of Nutrition and Good Health* (New York: Facts on File, 1997), 253.

2. Murkies, Alice, "Phytoestrogens—What Is the Current Knowledge?" *Australian Family Physician* 27(Suppl. 1): S47–S51, 1998.

3. Hutchins, Andrea M., et al., "Urinary Isoflavonoid, Phytoestrogens, and Lignan Excretion After Consumption of Fermented and Unfermented Soy Products," *Journal of the American Dietetic Association* 95(5): 545–51, May 1995.

4. Maskarinec, G., et al., "Dietary Soy Intake and Urinary Isoflavone Excretion Among Women from a Multiethnic Population," *Cancer Epidemiology, Biomarkers, and Prevention* 7: 613–19, 1998.

5. Aldercreutz, Herman, and Esa Hamalainen, "Dietary Phyto-Estrogens and the Menopause in Japan," *The Lancet* 339: 1233, May 16, 1992.

6. Cassidy, Aedin, et al., "Biological Effects of a Diet of Soy Protein Rich in Isoflavones on the Menstrual Cycle of Premenopausal Women," *American Journal of Clinical Nutrition* 60: 333–40, 1994.

7. Santiago, Librado A., et al., "Japanese Soybean Paste Miso Scavenges Free

Radicals and Inhibits Lipid Peroxidation," *Journal of Nutrition Science and Vitaminol* 38: 297–304, 1992.

8. Ruiz-Larrea, M. Bergona, et al., "Antioxidant Activity of Phytoestrogenic Isoflavones," *Free Radical Research* 26: 63–70, 1997.

9. Samman, Samir, et al., "Minor Dietary Factors in Relation to Coronary Heart Disease—Flavonoids, Isoflavones, and Boron," *Journal of Chemical Biochemistry and Nutrition* 20: 173–80, 1996.

10. Russell, Robert M., "Soy Protein and Nutrition," *Journal of the American Medical Association* 277(23): 1876–78, June 18, 1997.

11. Zhang, Y., et al., "Daidzein and Genistein Glucuronides In Vitro Are Weakly Estrogenic and Activate Human Natural Killer Cells at Nutritionally Relevant Concentrations," *Journal of Nutrition* 129: 399–405, 1999.

54

Kava

The attributes of kava (sometimes called kava-kava) were recorded in 1777 by George Foster, a naturalist aboard Captain James Cook's ship as it visited various islands in the South Pacific. Kava *(Piper methylsticum),* derived from the root of a Polynesian pepper tree, was cultivated throughout the islands as a tranquilizer, ceremonial beverage, and feel-good drink.

The herbal remedy was given a boost in respectability on February 26, 1998, when the *Wall Street Journal* referred to it as a "superstar." The newspaper quoted Virginia chiropractor Arthur Fierro as saying that he uses kava to treat patients suffering from anxiety or depression. Ferro is convinced the results are just as effective as those with medications such as Prozac and Valium.[1]

In evaluating 101 patients suffering from anxiety of nonpsychotic origin, researchers in Germany found that an extract of kava was superior to placebo. The trial lasted for 25 weeks, and there was a noticeable improvement in the treatment group from week eight on. The volunteers received either a capsule containing 90 to 100 mg of extract, a capsule containing 70 mg of kavalactones (the active ingredients in kava), or a placebo, three times daily. Few side effects were noted in the kava patients. Kava extract is an alternative to tricyclic antidepressants and benzodiazepines recommended for anxiety disorders, since it does not have the tolerance problems associated with the drugs.[2]

A study by Nirbhay N. Singh, Ph.D., and colleagues at the Medical College of Virginia at Richmond reported that kava extract also was superior to placebo in treatment of anxiety. A group of 20 was given two capsules of kava twice daily, while a control group of 31 received two look-alike capsules twice daily. Each dose contained 120 mg of kavalactones.[3] "Our data show that anxiety can be significantly reduced with a moderate dose of kava without any side effects," Singh said. "Our findings confirm the belief that kava products may offer an alternative to benzodiazepines in the reduction of anxiety states of adults. Clinical studies suggest that the pharmacological activity of kava is comparable to the benzodiazepines, but it is not addictive and it does not lead to untoward side effects such as addiction."

In a July 15, 1998, review of several popular herbs, *Family Practice News* reported that kava seems to be one of the most potent anxiolytic (anxiety relieving) agents. It also has muscle-relaxant, anticonvulsant, and analgesic (pain reducing) properties.[4]

Writing in *The Green Pharmacy,* James A. Duke, Ph.D., quoted pharmacognosist (natural product pharmacist) Albert Leung, Ph.D., and herbalist Steven Foster as saying that kava contains two pain-relieving chemicals—dihydrokavain and dihydromethysticin—that are as effective as aspirin. Since the herb is known to relax the uterus, it is used to treat menstrual cramps.[5]

Drinking large amounts of nonstandardized kava liquid preparations can lead to a dry, scaly skin rash known as kava dermopathy. Problems with balance have also been reported. The risk of this rash or equilibrium problems develops only at kavalactone dosages in excess of several grams (2,000 mg or more) daily. The herb is also not recommended for pregnant or lactating women.[6]

In *Healing Anxiety with Herbs,* psychiatrist Harold H. Bloomfield, M.D., stated health boards in England, Germany, Switzerland, and other European nations have approved kava for the treatment of anxiety and insomnia. Although kava can relieve a wide range of anxiety symptoms, researchers are not certain how it works. It may work to soothe an overactive amygdala, the brain's alarm center, thereby relieving anxiety and elevating mood.[7]

Bloomfield referred to a 1996 double-blind study in which two groups of 29 patients with anxiety syndromes were given 100 mg of kava extract standardized to 70 percent kavalactones three times a day for four weeks. Anxiety symptoms in the treatment group were significantly reduced, and no adverse reactions were reported. Kava supplements should not be taken longer than 25 weeks and should not be combined with benzodiazepine tranquilizers without medical supervision. The herb is not recommended for those suffering from Parkinson's disease.

"Kava reduces anxiety without causing the lethargy, diminished concentration, and fuzziness so often associated with synthetic tranquilizers," Bloomfield continued. "Though caution is always indicated, people who are taking appropriate doses of kava can generally drive an automobile or focus on work without experiencing any sedation. With the growing availability of high-quality kava products, this natural tranquilizer could soon become a first-rate treatment for mild to moderate anxiety."

Kava supplements are available in capsules, extracts, and teas. Liquid extracts and capsules come in various strengths, usually from 100 to 250 mg, with the percentage of kavalactones ranging from 30 to 70 percent.

If you are suffering from mild depression or insomnia, kava just might bring you relief.

References

1. Petersen, Andrea, "The Making of an Herbal Superstar," *Wall Street Journal,* Feb. 26, 1998, B1.

2. Volz, H. P., and M. Kieser, "Kava-Kava Extract WS 1490 vs. Placebo in Anxiety Disorders—A Randomized Placebo-Controlled 25-Week Outpatient Trial," *Pharmacopsychiatry* 30: 1–5, 1997.

3. Singh, Nirbhay N., et al., "Kavatrol Reduces Daily Stress and Anxiety in Adults," unpublished, 1997.

4. Sherman, C., "Herbal Anxiolytics Have Novel Mechanisms," *Family Practice News,* July 15, 1998, 30.

5. Duke, James A., *The Green Pharmacy* (Emmaus, Pa.: Rodale Press, 1997), 327–28, 349.

6. Brown, Donald J., *Herbal Prescriptions for Better Health* (Rocklin, Calif.: Prima Publishing, 1996), 145ff.

7. Bloomfield, Harold H., *Healing Anxiety with Herbs* (New York: HarperCollins Publishers, 1998), 12ff.

55

7-Keto DHEA

Produced by the adrenal glands, testes, and ovaries, dehydroepiandrosterone (DHEA) is a hormone that is synthesized from cholesterol. DHEA is also converted into metabolites such as testosterone and estrogens. Today there is a new kid on the block—7-Keto DHEA—an analog of DHEA, which cannot be converted into active androgenic or estrogenic hormones. This supplement is gaining wider acceptance among consumers who are concerned about taking supplementary hormones.

Developed at the University of Wisconsin at Madison by Henry A. Lardy, Ph.D., 7-Keto DHEA has been shown in laboratory studies to be more potent than DHEA in boosting the immune system, enhancing memory, raising energy, reducing weight, increasing lean muscle mass, and fighting the ravages of aging.

A study at the Chicago Center for Clinical Research examined the effects of 7-Keto DHEA on several endocrine and safety parameters in 23 healthy men ranging in age from 18 to 49. The study lasted for eight weeks, and the dose was increased each week to a maximum of 100 mg twice daily during the final four weeks. At the end of the trial, dihydrotestosterone, estradiol, cortisol, and insulin levels were virtually the same among the volunteers as when the study began. All hormone levels were within normal limits. The study suggests that 7-Keto DHEA is well tolerated at doses up to 200 mg/day, and it does not produce clinically important sex hormone changes in healthy men.[1]

Since DHEA is a memory enhancer, researchers at the University of Wisconsin at Madison compared DHEA and 7-Keto DHEA. Using aging, two-year-old laboratory mice, Henry Lardy, Ph.D., and colleagues trained the animals to negotiate the Morris water maze procedure before beginning the experiment. The mice were then given 20 mg/kg of DHEA, the same amount of 7-Keto DHEA, or a placebo, and then positioned in the maze to see how well they could remember the exercise and how long it would take them to finish it. In this experiment, 7-Keto DHEA won out handily. The control animals finished the exercise in 34 seconds; DHEA-treated mice took 22 seconds; and the 7-Keto DHEA animals needed only 7.6 seconds.[2]

In a second experiment, Lardy gave the control mice scopolamine, a sedative, to dull their memory. The mice protected with 7-Keto DHEA were able to negotiate the water maze in 6.5 seconds, compared to 11.5 seconds for those on DHEA therapy, and 22 seconds for the mice getting the scopolamine-administered diet. These encouraging results indicate that 7-Keto DHEA may be a useful supplement for treating memory loss and Alzheimer's disease.

According to Henry Lardy, 7-Keto DHEA shows promise as a weight-loss supplement. In the 1995 *Annals of the New York Academy of Sciences* Lardy indicates that 7-Keto DHEA may promote fat loss by enhancing thermogenic activity; that is, raising body heat to burn calories. In effect, the supplement activates thermogenic enzymes in the livers of laboratory animals, causing them to lose weight without altering their food intake.[3] 7-Keto DHEA is thought to reduce cortisol, the body's primary stress hormone, which helps to curb a person's appetite.

Since DHEA is converted into testosterone, there has been some concern as to whether it might affect human prostate cancer cells. But 7-Keto DHEA, a natural metabolite of DHEA, does not affect these cells. This was determined in another study conducted by Lardy and colleagues at the University of Rochester Medical Center. 7-Keto DHEA was found to have no effect on human prostate cancer cells, although another derivative of DHEA, called delta-5 androstenediol (Adiol), can raise the amount of testosterone in the body to unhealthy levels. This could pose a risk for prostate cancer. While Adiol was found to activate androgen receptor target genes in prostate cancer cells, thereby encouraging prostate cancer growth, 7-Keto DHEA did not demonstrate this effect.[4]

Using laboratory glassware, researchers at the University of Minnesota and the University of Wisconsin have found that 7-Keto DHEA augments interleukin-2 production by human lymphocytes. Interleukin is a protein secreted by T cells to fight infections. This suggests that 7-Keto DHEA should be considered as therapy for HIV-infected individuals, and a clinical trial investigating the safety of the supplement is now in progress.[5]

While we await the results of various human trials now under way, there may be many benefits in taking 7-Keto DHEA supplements now. The fact that it does not apparently produce excessive levels of testosterone and estrogen is of interest to those who wish to avoid taking hormone supplements. The usual dosage ranges from 50 to 200 mg/day.

References

1. Davidson, M. H., et al., "Safety and Endocrine Effects of 3-Acetyl-7-Oxo DHEA (7-Keto DHEA)," paper presented at Experimental Biology 98, April 19–22, 1998, San Francisco.

2. Shi, J., and H. Lardy, "3-beta-Hydroxyandrost-5-Ene-7, 17-Diome (7-Keto DHEA) Improves Memory in Mice," ibid.

3. Lardy, H., et al., "Ersosteroids: Induction of Thermogenic Enzymes in Liver of Rats Treated with Steroids Derived from Dehydroepiandrosterone," *Proceedings of the National Academy of Sciences* 92: 6617–19, 1995.

4. Ibid.

5. Nelson, Robert, et al., "Dehydro-epiandrosterone and 7-Keto DHEA Augment Interleukin 2 Production by Human Lymphocytes In Vitro," paper presented at Fifth Conference on Retroviruses and Opportunistic Infection, Feb. 1–5, 1998, Chicago.

56

Lactobacillus Acidophilus

If you have recurring problems with candidiasis, cystitis, thrush, diarrhea, flatulence, hiatal hernia, Crohn's disease, traveler's diarrhea, constipation, and other seemingly unrelated health problems such as asthma, rhinitis (nasal catarrh), and ear infections in children, there may be a logical connection between these conditions. Antibiotics, which are often necessary to control infections, inactivate *Lactobacillus acidophilus,* a beneficial bacterium, in the intestines and vagina, resulting in yeast infections and a sluggish digestive system. Other drugs, pesticides, processed foods, contaminated water, and numerous environmental toxins also compromise the gastrointestinal tract and damage the intestinal microflora. *Lactobacillus acidophilus* is an important deterrent because it is nonpathogenic, nontoxic, and a natural inhabitant in the intestinal tract.

Soon after birth, the digestive tract is colonized by a variety of microorganisms, among the first being the lactobacilli, which originate in the maternal vagina during the birth of the child. During the mother's puberty, Doderlein's bacillus, considered identical to *Lactobacillus acidophilus,* establishes itself as a predominant vaginal microorganism. In addition, it provides inoculum to the infant during birth.[1] In a breast-feeding infant, a stable microflora establishes itself in the intestinal tract within a few days. Tests on newborns' fecal content show that the microflora are mostly *Lactobacillus bifidus* (bifidobacteria). For a bottle-fed infant, the fecal microflora is similar to that of adults. While the stomach contains only a few indigenous organisms, the small intestine is home to numerous bacterial flora, with *Lactobacillus acidophilus* being the most prominent. This bacteria survives the passage through the powerful gastric juices in the stomach, and moves on to the intestines, where it grows.

In women, the normal vaginal flora includes *Lactobacillus acidophilus, Lactobacillus bifidus, Lactobacillus fermenti,* and *Lactobacillus plantarum.* Abnormal flora sometimes found in the vagina include *Candida albicans, Trichomonas vaginalis,* and *Hemophilus vaginalis.* Because of antibiotics, hormonal imbalances, inadequate enemas, contacts with contaminated individuals, and a defective immune system, these abnormal flora continue to grow, ostensibly because they have replaced the beneficial flora that have been killed off. Vaginitis can be treated with the appropriate lactobacilli and streptococci, because they inhibit the existing infection, restore the normal lactic acid flora, and lower the pH of vaginal secretions to a normal level.

Lactobacilli or their cousins, bifidobacteria, demonstrate anticancer activity by inhibiting the growth or activity of cancer-producing bacteria, and some strains produce chemicals that inhibit tumor growth. Declining levels of bifidobacteria in the elderly allow the toxin-producing *Clostridium* species to accumulate. *Clostridium* has been implicated in cancer of the large bowel. Taking bifidobacteria in a dose of three billion organisms per day lowers the level of clostridia in the bowel and also reduces the concentration of chemicals thought to promote cancer.[2]

At Geneva University Hospital in Switzerland, researchers found *Candida albicans* infections in the stools, vaginas, skin, and mouths of 60 patients with asthma. Two other yeasts, *Epidermophyton* and *Trichophyton,* were also present. Studies using *Lactobacillus* and other agents may be useful in activating these agents, since researchers are convinced that 8 to 10 percent of patients with asthma and rhinitis are sensitive to these yeasts.[3]

Although the mechanism remains elusive, researchers at Oklahoma State University at Stillwater have found that certain strains of *Lactobacillus acidophilus* act directly on cholesterol in the gastrointestinal tract and may therefore be beneficial in reducing cholesterol levels in the blood.[4]

According to researchers in Australia, probiotic organisms such as *Lactobacillus acidophilus* can inhibit *Helicobacter pylori,* a harmful bacteria that may cause peptic ulcers.[5]

In a double-blind trial at the University of California at Davis, 18 patients with irritable bowel syndrome and a mean age of 44.1 years were given capsules containing *Lactobacillus acidophilus* for six weeks, followed by a two-week washout, or rest period. They then continued with the acidophilus supplement for an additional six weeks. The acidophilus product brought a significantly therapeutic benefit to 50 percent of the patients.[6]

Supplemental use of *Lactobacillus acidophilus* is crucial in the treatment of diarrhea of any kind, but especially in the case of antibiotic-associated diarrhea, reported Michael Murray, N.D., and Joseph Pizzorno,

N.D. The dosage of one to two billion viable acidophilus organisms daily is usually sufficient for most people. A larger dose—except when taking an antibiotic—may cause mild gastrointestinal problems, while smaller amounts may not be sufficient to colonize the gastrointestinal tract, they said.[7]

The use of antibiotics results in a severe form of diarrhea called oseudomembranous enterocolitis, Murray and Pizzorno added. This is caused by an overgrowth of a bacterium *(Clostridium difficele)*, which results from the death of the bacteria that normally keep this bacterium under control. "Although it is commonly believed that acidophilus supplements are not effective if taken during antibiotic therapy, research actually supports the use of *L. acidophilus* during antibiotic administration," the authors continued. "Reduction of friendly bacteria and/or infection with antibiotic-resistant bacteria may be prevented by administering *L. acidophilus* products during antibiotic therapy. A dosage of at least 15 to 20 billion organisms is required. We would still recommend taking *L. acidophilus* supplements at a different time than the antibiotic. In fact, take it as far away from the antibiotic as possible."

Those with lactose intolerance, an inability to digest milk products, may find relief with *L. acidophilus*, which contains lactic acid bacteria similar to those used for fermenting yogurt, according to Robert M. Giller, M.D. He suggests three capsules daily, along with other recommendations.[8]

A Finnish researcher has reported that radiation therapy in the lower pelvic region causes irritation of the gut mucosa, leading to diarrhea and intestinal fistulas. However, when the patients were given *L. acidophilus,* they experienced less diarrhea than the controls.[9]

Lactobacillus acidophilus has long been used in protecting against vaginal infections by maintaining an acid environment, as well as by producing metabolites such as hydrogen peroxide, which inhibits other vaginal microorganisms, according to studies in Israel. Using a yogurt containing *L. acidophilus,* researchers proved that acidophilus survives the digestive enzymes in the gastrointestinal tract and colonizes the rectum and vagina. Therefore, it is a recommended prophylaxis for vaginitis.[10] Hydrogen peroxide combines with catalase, an enzyme found in the mouth and skin, which releases oxygen that kills bacteria and cleanses infected areas.

In the Israeli trial, 46 patients with at least four documented cases of vaginitis were randomly assigned to one of two groups. Group 1 ate 150 ml/day of yogurt that contained *L. acidophilus* for two months, followed by two months without yogurt, and finally two months of eating 150 ml/day of pasteurized yogurt that did not contain *L. acidophilus*. Group 2 was given pasteurized yogurt for two months, then no yogurt for two months, and *L. acidophilus*-enriched yogurt for two months. While the women ate the yogurt containing *L. acidophilus,* there was an increase in the colonization of the rectum and vagina by the beneficial bacteria and consequently a reduction in bacterial vaginosis. There was no difference in candidal infections between the periods of ingesting yogurt that was just pasteurized, compared to that containing the lactobacillis, even though there was a reduction in the number of infections in both groups.

In 33 women with recurrent candida vaginitis at the Long Island Jewish Medical Center in New Hyde Park, New York, there was a threefold decrease in infections when the volunteers ate yogurt containing *L. acidophilus* for six months. The mean number of infections during that time was 2.54 in the placebo group and only 0.38 in the yogurt-treated group. The spread of the *Candida* infection decreased from a mean of 3.23 in the control group to 0.84 in the yogurt group during the six-month study.[11]

Commenting on the study in an editorial in the March 1, 1992 issue of *Annals of Internal Medicine*, David J. Drutz, M.D., said that there are two possibilities in which *L. acidophilus* may reduce vaginal colonization. First, *L. acidophilus* displaces *Candida* normally found in the gastrointestinal tract, thereby reducing the opportunity for autoinoculation of the vagina from the area surrounding the anus and the region from the vulva to the anus. Second, *L. acidophilus* may have colonized the vagina from the gastrointestinal tract, thereby inhibiting *Candida* colonization by its competing presence in the vagina. *L. acidophilus* dominates in the vagina, but it is not dominant in the gastrointestinal tract. Therefore, the best possibility for successful

colonization might be when antibiotic therapy has displaced the normal microflora.[12]

Researchers found that *L. acidophilus* and *L. plantarum* were the predominant organisms found in the vaginas of 47 of 53 healthy women, and in 30 of 192 women with bacterial infections of the vagina. It was found that 72 percent and 77 percent of the bacteria produced hydrogen peroxide in the two groups, respectively. The research team thought that hydrogen peroxide may be less bactericidal than previously thought in controlling vaginosis-related bacteria in the vagina.[13]

L. acidophilus supplements are available in capsules, tablets, powders, and liquids. Some formulas contain three kinds of friendly bacteria—*L. acidophilus, B. longum,* and *B. bifidum*—along with the digestive enzymes lipase, protease, and amylase. Other products contain *B. longum, L. acidophilus,* and fructooligosaccharides. You can find nondairy *L. acidophilus* formulas, as well as those that do not require refrigeration.

If you are using yogurt to prevent or treat candidiasis, it may not contain *L. acidophilus*. The beneficial bacteria are often destroyed by heat during the processing, leaving you with a tart-tasting snack and nothing more.

References

1. Murray, Frank, *Acidophilus and Your Health* (New Canaan, Conn.: Keats Publishing, 1998), 6ff.
2. Galland, Leo, *The Four Pillars of Healing* (New York: Random House, 1997), 198ff.

3. Gumowski, Pierre, et al., "Chronic Asthma and Rhinitis Due to *Candida albicans,* Epidermophyton, and Trichophyton," *Annals of Allergy* 59: 48–51, 1987.

4. Gilliland, S. E., et al., "Assimilation of Cholesterol by *Lactobacillus acidophilus,*" *Applied and Environmental Microbiology* 49(2): 377–81, Feb. 1985.

5. Midolo, D., et al., "In Vitro Inhibition of *Helicobacter pylori* NCTC 11637 by Organic Acids and Lactic Acid Bacteria," *Journal of Applied Bacteriology* 79: 475–79, 1995.

6. Halpern, Georges M., et al., "Treatment of Irritable Bowel Syndrome with Lacteol Fort: A Randomized, Double-Blind, Cross-Over Trial," *American Journal of Gastroenterology* 91(8): 1579–85, 1996.

7. Murray, Michael T., and Joseph E. Pizzorno, *Encyclopedia of Natural Medicine,* rev. 2nd ed. (Rocklin, Calif.: Prima Publishing, 1998), 435, 438.

8. Giller, Robert M., and Kathy Matthews, *Natural Prescriptions* (New York: Ballantine Books, 1994), 231ff.

9. Salminen, Eeva, Fifth International Meeting on Progress on Radio-Oncology, Turku, Finland, May 1995.

10. Shalev, Eliezer, et al., "Ingestion of Yogurt Containing *Lactobacillus acidophilus* Compared with Pasteurized Yogurt as Prophylaxis for Recurrent Candidal Vaginitis and Bacterial Vaginosis," *Archives of Family Medicine* 5: 593–96, Nov./Dec. 1996.

11. Hilton, Eileen, et al., "Ingestion of Yogurt Containing *Lactobacillus acidophilus* as Prophylaxis for Candidal Vaginitis," *Annals of Internal Medicine* 116(5): 353–57, March 1, 1992.

12. Drutz, David J., "Lactobacillus Prophylaxis for Candida Vaginitis," *Annals of Internal Medicine* 116(5): 419–20, March 1, 1992.

13. Fontaine, E. A., et al., "Lactobacilli from Women with or Without Bacterial Vaginosis and Observations on the Significance of Hydrogen Peroxide," *Microbial Ecology in Health and Disease* 9: 135–41, 1996.

57

Lecithin

Lecithin, whose name is derived from the Greek word for egg yolk, is also known as phosphatidylcholine, which has its own entry in this book. As a building block of cell membranes, lecithin helps build healthy cells. In bile, it acts like a soap to dissolve fats and soluble vitamins for digestion and absorption. One of lecithin's most important functions is to carry fat and cholesterol as part of the lipid transport particles of blood, namely LDL cholesterol, HDL cholesterol, and very low density lipoprotein cholesterol (VLDL).[1]

In animal models, lecithin and choline deficiency may result in a progression from liver dysfunction to fatty liver and possibly liver cancer. Abnormalities in lecithin and choline metabolism are thought to be involved in various neurodegenerative diseases such as Alzheimer's. A lack of choline and lecithin may cause neuronal membrane defects and amyloid deposition, which is associated with the progression of Alzheimer's. Amyloid is a waxy substance made up of protein and polysaccharides, and it is deposited in various organs and tissues under normal conditions. A choline-deficient diet can cause liver dysfunction, and diets with abnormal levels of methionine, an amino acid, and other nutrients involved in methyl group metabolism can mask a choline deficiency.[2]

Lecithin was as effective as choline in treating several patients with tardive dyskinesia, reported John H. Growdon, M.D., of the Tufts–New England Medical Center Hospital in Boston. Choline is a precursor of the neurotransmitter acetylcholine, while lecithin is a natural source of dietary choline. Tardive dyskinesia is a central nervous system disorder characterized by twitching of the face and tongue, as well as involuntary movements of the trunk and limbs.[3] In the study, choline suppressed involuntary movements in 9 of 20 patients with tardive dyskinesia, the researchers said. The team then gave lecithin granules to two patients with the disease who had previously improved with choline chloride, and one patient who had not taken it. The first two patients continued to take their regular medication but discontinued choline for about two weeks prior to taking the lecithin. The third patient did not take any kind of medication. All three patients experienced fewer twitches while taking lecithin, and blood levels of choline increased. The authors added that patients might prefer lecithin, since it does not have a bitter taste or the fishy odor associated with choline.

In a study involving five men with mild to moderate tardive dyskinesia, oral supplements of choline and lecithin improved abnormal movements in all the patients. Few side effects were attributed to the lecithin.[4] Although choline has not been officially declared a vitamin, it is associated with the B complex of vitamins.

John Dommisse, M.D., of Tucson, Arizona, has stated that lecithin is one of the nutrients that may reduce the symptoms of tardive dyskinesia. Other beneficial nutrients are vitamin E, vitamin B_3, vitamin B_6, and manganese. The disease may be related to the overuse of antipsychotic drugs.[5]

In a small study involving patients with Alzheimer's disease, lecithin, magnesium, vitamin C, B complex, and micronutrients enhanced memory and alleviated symptoms.[6]

On August 23, 1999, talk-show host Montel Williams announced that he had been diagnosed with multiple sclerosis (MS), a neurological disease for which there is no cure.[7] At his clinic in New York City, Robert C. Atkins, M.D., uses lecithin to treat MS patients. In his book *Dr. Atkins' Health Revolution,* he discussed a 35-year-old patient with MS who progressed nicely until he stopped using a key element in Atkins's therapy. Initial findings were that the patient had toxic levels of aluminum in his body, along with low blood sugar. The prolonged regimen included elimination of sugar from his diet to control hypoglycemia. In addition to lecithin, he was prescribed EAP, a calcium salt of the neurotransmitter colamine phosphate (10 ml given intravenously); potassium and magnesium orotates (pioneered by the late Hans Nieper, M.D.); evening primrose oil; octacosanol (rich in vitamin E); pantothenic acid, the B vitamin; and vitamins A and C.[8]

"Within one week the patient indicated he felt better," Atkins said. "By the end of the second week, he noted that his depression and mental tiredness were gone, his energy was returning, the tingling in his right hand was less, and his bladder pain was markedly reduced. By the end of the third week, the patient had no further dizziness or headaches and strength was returning to his right side. By the fourth week, he indicated that he felt like he had years earlier, with the exception of the foreshortening of his right leg and right hand, which had atrophied beyond natural correction."

In the four days the patient went without EAP, his headaches, weakness, and lethargy returned, Atkins said. "Somewhere along the line, the patient went off the regimen (for financial reasons) and he fell back to square one," Atkins continued. "There is no reason to assume he will not respond to calcium-EAP injections once again, if he decides to resume treatment. Since most of my patients do not live in Manhattan, the calcium-EAP injections must be given by their family doctors. It only takes two minutes." (Atkins's book was written in 1988. Of the first 60 doctors who were asked by the patients to give the injection, 51 refused.)

Roger J. Williams, Ph.D., of the University of Texas at Austin, said that the answer to solving cholesterol deposits was to consume more lecithin. Lecithin is a powerful emulsifying agent, and its presence in the blood tends to dissolve cholesterol deposits. When there is substantially more lecithin in the blood than cholesterol—a ratio of 1:2 to 1 is said to be favorable—the actual amount of cholesterol can be high without the blood plasma getting milky or showing a tendency to produce fatty deposits. Another researcher, L. M. Morrison, found that the cholesterol levels in the blood of 12 patients were lowered substantially when they consumed about an ounce of lecithin per day for three months.[9]

In 1951, J. Rinse, Ph.D., a consulting chemist who was 51 at the time, suffered an attack of angina pectoris and was told by his physician that he probably had only 10 years to live. He began researching his condition and developed "Dr. Rinse's Morning Feed," a mixture that includes 1 tablespoon of soybean lecithin, debittered brewer's yeast, raw wheat germ, and 1 teaspoon of bone meal, plus vitamin C, vitamin E, and other foods and nutrients. Rinse lived to be in his 90s. An anecdotal story, but dozens of people who used Rinse's "cereal" have claimed it has improved their health.[10]

Food sources of lecithin include red meat, eggs, liver, soybeans, peanut butter, apples, and oranges. As a maintenance dose, David Canty, Ph.D., recommends 1 or 2 tablespoons of granular lecithin daily, which supplies 1,725 to 3,450 mg of phosphatidylcholine and 250 to 500 mg of choline. These amounts represent between 30 and 60 percent of what people normally obtain from their diets.[11] For a serious health problem, ask your holistic doctor for dosage recommendations.

References

1. Ronzio, Robert A., *The Encyclopedia of Nutrition and Good Health* (New York: Facts on File, 1997), 267.
2. Canty, David J. "Lecithin and Choline in Human Health and Disease," *Nutrition Reviews* 52(10): 327–39, Oct. 1994.
3. Growdon, John H., et al., "Lecithin Can Suppress Tardive Dyskinesia,"

New England Journal of Medicine 298: 1029–30, May 1978.

4. Gelenberg, Alan J., et al., "Choline and Lecithin in the Treatment of Tardive Dyskinesia: Preliminary Results from a Pilot Study," *American Journal of Psychiatry* 136(6): 772, June 1979.

5. Dommisse, John, "Nutritional Treatment for Tardive Dyskinesia," *American Journal of Psychiatry* 148(2): 279, Feb. 1991.

6. Glick, J. Leslie, "Use of Magnesium in the Management of Dementias," *Medical Sciences Research* 18: 831–33, 1990.

7. Barron, James, "Sobering News for T.V. Host," *New York Times,* Aug. 24, 1999), B2.

8. Atkins, Robert C., *Dr. Atkins' Health Revolution* (Boston: Houghton Mifflin, 1988), 12–13, 272–74.

9. Murray, Frank, *Program Your Heart for Health* (New York: Larchmont Books, 1977), 221–222.

10. Ibid, 51ff.

11. Canty, David, "Lecithin and Choline Redeemed," *Nutrition Science News,* Oct. 1997.

58

Lemon Balm

The first recorded use of lemon balm *(Melissa officinalis)* as a therapeutic agent was around 300 B.C., in *Historia Plantarum*, compiled by Theophrasus of Ephesus, a pupil of Aristotle. Later, between A.D. 50 and 80, Plinus Secundus, a Roman, suggested the efficacy of melissa in his materia medica. The essential oils in the plant had long been used externally to treat insect bites and internally for abdominal colic and uterine spasms. In the 1960s, there was renewed interest in the herb, when dried extracts from its leaves inhibited smallpox, mumps, and Newcastle disease viruses.[1] The latter virus, isolated in 1927 in England, affects primarily birds and domestic fowl, and when it is transferred to humans, it causes an eye inflammation.

A rather common viral infection is herpes simplex, found in two forms. Herpes simplex virus Type 1 is associated with infections of the lips, mouth, and face (cold sores), while Type 2 is related to infections of the genitals and rashes that babies develop as they pass through the birth canal. There is considerable overlap between the two, however, since some lesions caused by Type 1 may be caused by Type 2 and vice versa. Both of the viruses are highly contagious, and infections are spread by direct contact with the sores or by the fluid they contain. A relative of the Herpes simplex virus is the varicella-zoster virus, which causes chicken pox (varicella) and herpes zoster (shingles).[2]

The initial trials to determine the efficacy of lemon balm in treating patients with Type 1 and Type 2 herpes infections were conducted at four dermatological clinics in Germany. The study involved 115 patients, 45 males and 70 females.

Each patient was instructed to apply lemon balm cream five times daily until the lesions healed. After eight days of therapy, 96 percent of the patients reported complete healing. Between four and six days, healing was noted in 60 to 87 percent of the volunteers.[3]

In another study, 116 outpatients with Type 1 and Type 2 infections applied the lemon balm cream or a placebo for between 5 and 10 days, depending on the healing of the lesions. After day 5, there were no symptoms in 24 patients using the cream, compared with 15 patients in the placebo group with no complaints. There were few side effects in the two groups. At the end of the study, the physicians reported that healing was "very good" in the melissa group, and some in the placebo group also reported no lesions. "The effect of melissa cream in the topical treatment of herpes simplex infections of the skin and transitional mucosa is statistically significant," the researchers said. "To be effective the treatment must be started in the very early stages of the infection."

Acyclovir is an effective drug treatment for genital herpes, but a lemon balm formulation is just as effective, according to A. Mohrig and R. G. Alken of Berlin, Germany. In the study using a melissa cream and a topical acyclovir 5 percent cream, the authors said, "Judging by this evaluation, it would seem that the lemon balm extract–based preparation has nothing to fear from the prospect of a direct comparison in a controlled study." To be effective, the cream should be applied up to about eight hours after onset of symptoms.[4]

A lemon balm cream similar to the one used to treat Type 1 and Type 2 herpes sores in Europe is available in health food stores and elsewhere in the United States. Another approach is to steep 2 or 3 teaspoons of finely cut lemon balm leaves in 150 ml of water. The tea can be applied with a cotton swab to the lesions several times daily.[5]

In *The Green Pharmacy*, James A. Duke, Ph.D., quotes Norman G. Bisset, Ph.D., of King's College at the University of London, as saying that lemon balm is helpful in treating migraine headaches. The German government has approved lemon balm as a sedative to relieve insomnia and as a stomach soother, probably because of the terpenes in the herb. Duke suggests a lemon balm tea consisting of 2 to 4 teaspoons of dried herb per cup of boiling water. Also, a lemon balm cream is useful in shortening the healing time of herpes sores within several days.[6]

Lemon balm is often used by aromatherapists for digestive and respiratory complaints of nervous origin, such as asthma, indigestion, and flatulence. It helps regulate the menstrual cycle and promote fertility, and is an effective remedy for wasp and bee stings. In low concentrations, lemon balm is used to treat eczema and other skin problems. The *British Herbal Pharmacopoeia* recommends the herb for gas, indigestion, psychological complaints, and depression.[7]

References

1. Woelbling, R. H., and K. Leonhardt, "Local Therapy of Herpes Simplex with Dried Extract from *Melissa officinalis*," *Phytomedicine* 1: 25–31, 1994.
2. Clayman, Charles B., medical ed., *The American Medical Association Home Medical Encyclopedia* (New York: Random House, 1989), 536–37.
3. Woelbling, R. H., and K. Leonhardt, ibid.
4. Mohrig, A., and R. G. Alken, "Melissa Extract in Comparison to Acyclovir," *Pharmazeutische Rundschaur,* 3–4, 1966.
5. Robbers, James E., and Varro E. Tyler, *Tyler's Herbs of Choice* (New York: The Haworth Herbal Press, 1999), 229.
6. Duke, James A., *The Green Pharmacy* (Emmaus, Pa.: Rodale Press, 1997), 236–37, 294–95, 387.
7. Lawless, Julia, *The Encyclopedia of Essential Oils* (Shaftesbury, Dorset, England: Element Books, 1992), 47–48.

59

Licorice

A member of the legume family, whose cousins include beans, peas, and the herb broom, licorice *(Glycyrrhiza glabra)* has been used for medicinal purposes for centuries. The Greek surgeon Dioscorides (A.D. 54–68) named the plant Glyrrhiza, from *glukos,* meaning "sweet," and *riza,* meaning "root." His research into medical botany resulted in a materia medica that included some 600 plants and their derivatives, which was the accepted reference for 16 centuries. Licorice was commonly used in Germany for medicinal purposes in the Middle Ages, and Saladinus, a writer of the mid-15th century, recorded that licorice extract was among the wares kept by Italian apothecaries.[1]

Research continues to explore the effectiveness of glycyrrhizin, a saponin from licorice root that has been shown to be an effective anti-inflammatory and antiallergenic agent. It also inhibits viral growth and is said to prevent and heal ulcers, as well as serve as a remedy for chronic hepatitis. Derivatives of glycyrrhetinic acid inhibit two enzymes that are involved in asthma, allergic diseases, and inflammation. Large amounts of licorice can deplete potassium stores, which could wreak havoc on the body's electrolyte balance.[2]

Licorice root seems to be an effective treatment for peptic ulcers, providing its glycyrrhetinic acid has been removed, reported Melvyn Werbach, M.D. Otherwise, it may elevate blood pressure.[3] "In a controlled study," Werbach said, "deglycyrrhizinated licorice (DGL) has been shown to be at least as effective as the newest class of antiulcer medications (the H2-receptor-histamine-blocking agents) in speeding healing of gastric and duodenal ulcerations. DGL also appears to protect against aspirin-induced damage to the gastric mucosa. Animal research suggests that it promotes regeneration of the ulcerated lining by increasing the number of mucus-secreting glands as well as the number of mucus-secreting cells in each gland."

For a nutritional healing plan using DGL licorice, Werbach recommends 760 to 1,520 mg of the chewable tablets three times daily between meals. As a maintenance dose, he suggests 760 mg two to three times a day.

A daily intake of more than 100 g of licorice—equivalent to 300 mg of glycyrrhetinic acid—is usually needed to raise blood pressure markedly, according to researchers at the University of Helsinki in Finland.[4] Susan J. Webber, M.D., who practices in Loveland, Colorado, recommends black licorice to treat canker sores. She insists that the herb speeds healing and reduces pain.[5]

Writing in *Family Practice News,* Gregory Maltz reported that about 400 compounds have been isolated from the licorice plant. Three key plants contain compounds—including licorice, soy, and garlic—that have pharmacologic activities. Maltz quoted a researcher at the University of California at San Diego as saying that there are similarities between steroid hormones and licorice-derived compounds called flavonoids, and that some of these compounds might benefit patients with depression. At dosages of 500 mcg/ml and lower, glycyrrhizin and related compounds in licorice inhibit the formation of giant cells by HIV. In HIV-positive patients, giant cells are one of the signals that the infection is moving from latency to active AIDS.[6]

"Licorice has a considerable reputation as an expectorant and cough suppressant, being frequently utilized in the treatment of symptoms associated with the common cold," reported James E. Robbers, Ph.D., and Varro E. Tyler, Ph.D., Sc.D. "Lozenges and candies containing licorice extract are especially suitable, but particularly in the United States, one must make certain that they do contain real licorice. Most 'licorice' candy manufactured in this country is simply flavored with anise oil."[7]

Peter Jaret, writing in *Hippocrates,* explained that glycyrrhizin is what gives licorice its intense sweetness. Purified glycyrrhizin protects lab animals from lethal doses of a flu virus. A substance called glabridin may reduce the risk of clogged arteries by blocking the oxidation of cholesterol. It is not advisable to drink more than three cups of licorice root tea daily, since large amounts of glycyrrhizin can elevate blood pressure.[8]

In a laboratory experiment, 200 mg/day of licorice, given to apolipoprotein-E–deficient mice for six weeks, protected LDL cholesterol from lipid peroxidation. The extract also reduced the lesions that might cause hardening of the arteries in the animals.[9]

Ronald L. Hoffman, M.D., who practices in New York City, recommends licorice tea to boost adrenal function. Since licorice is such a potent herb, however, its use should be monitored by a physician. That is because the herb has a powerful effect on the adrenal glands, slowing the breakdown of the mineralocorticoids and causing the body to retain sodium.[10]

Studies have shown that licorice extracts are effective against a variety of viral diseases, especially in lab glassware. These include HIV, hepatitis B, and Epstein-Barr. The extracts were also shown to inhibit tumor formation.[11]

Physicians have found that large amounts of licorice are associated with high blood pressure and sodium and water retention. At the VA Medical Center in Salt Lake City, Utah, physicians treated a 64-year-old healthy male who complained of shortness of breath, pulmonary distress, and fatigue. Prior to his admission, he had consumed four packages of black licorice, which contained 1,020 g of licorice, equal to about 3.6 g of glycyrrhizinic acid. After being given a diuretic to increase urine flow, there was a complete resolution of his case. Only three cases of congestive heart failure have previously been reported after ingestion of large amounts of licorice.[12]

Since glycyrrhizin is about 50 times sweeter than sugar, it is used as a remedy for coughs and as a flavoring for medicines with unpleasant tastes. In ancient Greece, licorice was used to treat dropsy, a swelling of the legs and ankles indicative of heart failure. Since the herb soothes inflamed mucous membranes, it was also used to treat irritated urinary, bowel, and respiratory passages.[13]

Licorice root is recommended for catarrhs of the upper respiratory tract and gastric and duodenal ulcers. It is not recommended for those with liver disorders such as cirrhosis, excessive salts in the blood, low blood pressure, or severe kidney insufficiency, or for pregnant women. Unless otherwise prescribed, the average daily dose of licorice is 5 to 15 g of root, equivalent to 200 to 600 mg of glycyrrhizin. As a liquid extract, the suggested dose is 0.5 to 1 g for catarrhs of the upper respiratory tract and 1.5 to 3 g for gastric and duodenal ulcers.[14]

A variety of formulas containing DGL licorice, licorice root supplements, and licorice tea and extracts are available over the counter. If you are using licorice for medicinal purposes, it is best to review your remedy with a physician.

References

1. Grieve, Maude, *A Modern Herbal* (New York: Dover Publications, 1971), 487ff.
2. "Licorice Effectiveness," *HerbalGram 11*, Winter 1987. Published by Herb Research Foundation and American Herbal Products Association.
3. Werbach, Melvyn, *Healing with Food* (New York: HarperPerennial, 1993), 317–18.
4. Nurminen, M. L., et al., "Dietary Factors in the Pathogenesis and Treatment of Hypertension," *Annals of Medicine* 30: 143–50, 1998.
5. Black, Joseph, and Susan J. Webber, "Oral Aphthous Ulcers: Salt, Licorice," *Cortlandt Forum* 44: 27–29, May 1990.

6. Maltz, Gregory, "Nutraceuticals: Commission Will Determine Their Regulatory Fate," *Family Practice News,* March 1, 1995.

7. Robbers, James E., and Varro E. Tyler, *Tyler's Herbs of Choice* (New York: The Haworth Herbal Press, 1999), 83.

8. Jaret, Peter, "Are Nutraceuticals Any Good?" *Hippocrates,* March 1998, 62–67.

9. Fuhrman, Bianca, et al., "Licorice Extract and Its Major Polyphenol Glabridin Protect Low-Density Lipoprotein Against Lipid Peroxidation in In Vitro and Ex Vivo Studies in Humans and in Atherosclerotic Apolipoprotein-E–Deficient Mice," *American Journal of Clinical Nutrition* 66: 267–75, 1997.

10. Hoffman, Ronald L., *Intelligent Medicine* (New York: Simon & Schuster, 1997), 239.

11. Badgley, Laurence, *Healing AIDS Naturally* (San Bruno, Calif.: Human Energy Press, 1986), 177.

12. Chamberlain, James J., and Igor Z. Abolnik, "Pulmonary Edema Following a Licorice Binge," *Western Journal of Medicine* 167(3): 184, Sept. 1997.

13. Weiner, Michael A., *Weiner's Herbal* (New York: Stein and Day, 1980), 118.

14. Blumenthal, Mark, ed., *The Complete German Commission E Monographs* (Boston: Integrative Medicine Communications and American Botanical Council [Austin, Texas], 1998), 161–62.

60

Lutein

According to the Alliance for Aging Research, it is estimated that approximately 13 million people in the United States, 30 years of age and older, show signs of macular degeneration, and that more than 1.2 million are in the later, vision-threatening stages of the disease. Age-related macular degeneration (AMD) is the major cause of irreversible loss of vision in those over age 65 in the United States. This slow, progressive, and painless condition affects the macula, the small central part of the retina that is responsible for distinguishing fine details.[1]

AMD occurs when the cells in the macula break down, causing loss of sight in the central field of vision. Although this breakdown may not become evident until age 60 or 70, it is never too early to be aware of the problem and take preventive measures.

There are two types of macular degeneration:

1. Dry AMD develops when small yellowish deposits known as drusen accumulate under the macula. The deposits gradually break down the light-sensing cells in the macula, often causing distorted vision in one eye. This normally does not cause total loss of reading vision, but the progression should be monitored to prevent it from developing into the more severe wet form.
2. Wet AMD occurs when small, new, abnormal blood vessels grow behind the retina toward the macula. They sometimes leak blood and fluid that can damage the macula, causing severe loss of vision. This condition often leads to legal blindness.

The fragile cells in the macula are highly susceptible to damage from oxygen-charged free radicals. Researchers have long assumed that people with a low intake of antioxidants are at risk for developing AMD. Alcohol, sunlight, and smoking also cause damage that can lead to AMD. Alcohol depletes the body of antioxidants, and cell damage from the sun results in deterioration of the macula. Those with light-colored eyes are more susceptible to damage from sunlight, as are those who are exposed to ultraviolet light for an extended period. Smoking, which reduces protective antioxidants in the eye, more than doubles the risk of AMD.

According to a number of studies, improving your diet can enhance your vision, reduce blurriness, and slow deterioration from AMD, possibly even preventing it. Two carotenoids that protect against AMD are lutein and zeaxanthin. They are the only pigments found in the macula. Beta-carotene, perhaps the best known carotenoid, is virtually absent in the eye.

At the Massachusetts Eye and Ear Infirmary in Boston, Johanna M. Seddon, M.D., and colleagues determined that patients with the highest intakes of lutein and zeaxanthin had the lowest risk for developing AMD. In fact, an intake of 6 mg/day of lutein led to a 43 percent lower prevalence of the disease than did lower amounts of lutein. A lower risk was also associated with those patients who frequently ate spinach and collard greens. The study involved 356 people with advanced stage I acute macular degeneration one year prior to their enrollment in the trial

and 520 controls. The participants ranged in age from 55 to 80.[2]

It is known that people who eat diets rich in lutein-containing foods—such as kale and spinach—generally have thick macular pigments and a low risk of developing AMD. To determine whether or not lutein supplements could increase the macular pigment, researchers gave 30 mg/day of lutein to two volunteers for 140 days. The results showed that the macular density in the two increased by 39 and 21 percent. This brought an estimated 30 to 40 percent decrease in the amount of damaging blue light reaching light receptors in the retina. It was concluded that the thicker macular pigment would reduce free radical damage to the retina and decrease the risk of AMD.[3]

In another study, scientists found that the prime risk factor for macular degeneration can be influenced by diet. For 15 weeks, 13 volunteers were asked to eat specific amounts of spinach and corn, rich in lutein and zeaxanthin, to determine whether large amounts of these nutrients would increase the density of the macular pigment. Eight of the 11 volunteers eating extra servings of spinach and corn had an average 33 percent increase in blood levels of lutein and an average 19 percent increase in macular pigment density.[4]

Specific dietary components such as lutein and zeaxanthin have shown promise in deterring AMD. Although stopping smoking, reducing alcohol consumption, wearing sunglasses, and other lifestyle modifications may reduce the risk of AMD, the consumption of specific dietary components containing carotenoids, vitamins, and so forth can reduce the risk even further. Lycopene, alpha-carotene, beta-carotene, and beta-cryptoxanthin also provide protection, in addition to vitamins A, C, and E, selenium, L-glutathione, zinc, and polyphenols.[5]

High concentrations of antioxidants, such as lutein and zeaxanthin, reduce damage from oxygen free radicals. When the retina is exposed to light and oxygen, free radicals are activated. It is also thought that the yellow pigment in the two carotenoids acts as an optical blue filter to reduce chromatic aberration and improve visual acuity.[6]

In a study in the United Kingdom, researchers reported that egg yolk and corn contained the highest percentages of lutein and zeaxanthin. Between 30 and 50 percent of the two carotenoids were found in kiwi, grapes, spinach, orange juice, zucchini, and various kinds of squash. Dark green leafy vegetables contain between 15 and 47 percent lutein but have very little zeaxanthin.[7]

In evaluating the dietary intakes of 8,191 adults in 1987 compared with 8,341 adults in 1992, researchers found that beta-carotene consumption was down 9.1 percent in white women and 5.7 percent in black women. Lutein consumption went down 18.3 percent in white women and 10.8 percent for black women. For men,

beta-carotene intake was up 16 percent for whites and 10.8 percent for blacks.[8]

At the Schepans Eye Research Institute in Boston, epidemiological data reveal that low blood levels of lutein and zeaxanthin, and other carotenoids, along with smoking, increase the risk of AMD. Carotenoids and antioxidant vitamins provide protection to the retina, which is damaged by oxidative stress caused by the absorption of light.[9]

In one study, men who consumed the largest amounts of lutein and zeaxanthin were 18 percent less likely to develop cataracts. The most protective foods were broccoli, corn, spinach, and tomato sauce. Free radical damage to proteins in the lens of the eye plays a key role in the development of cataracts.[10]

Lutein supplements can benefit people with retinitis pigmentosa, a degeneration of the rods and cones in the retina of both eyes. Twenty volunteers with this disorder and other degenerative retinal diseases were given 40 mg/day of lutein for two months, followed by 20 mg/day for an additional four months. Some of them also took other nutritional supplements. In 16 patients getting lutein supplements, 31 percent reported significant improvements in visual acuity, and 22 percent noted small improvements. Also, 20 percent reported significant improvements in visual field and 3 percent recorded small changes. Seventy-five percent experienced improvements in sensitivity to glare, adaptation to light and dark, color perception, or night vision. There were comparable results in those taking lutein alone and in those getting lutein and other supplements.[11]

In a cell-culture study, lutein halted the growth of breast cancer cells. Lutein and zeaxanthin act as antiproliferative agents toward breast cancer cells and may prevent the spread of breast cancer.[12]

A study involving 162 women and 145 men aged 40 to 60 found that higher levels of lutein and zeaxanthin in the blood were associated with a reduced risk of intima-media thickness and heart disease. Researchers studied the thickness of the carotid intima-media, which are layers of cells in a major blood vessel wall. A thicker carotid intima-media is associated with coronary heart disease. A mix of carotenoids, not just a single one, may be beneficial to health. Lutein from kale and broccoli, and beta-carotene from carrots are the most common carotenoids in the American diet.[13]

References

1. *Taking a Closer Look at Age-Related Macular Degeneration* (Washington, D.C.: Alliance for Aging Research, undated).

2. Seddon, Johanna M., et al., "Dietary Carotenoids, Vitamins A, C, and E, and Advanced Age-Related Macular Degeneration," *Journal of the American Medical Association* 272(18): 1413–20, Nov. 9, 1994.

3. Landrum, J. T., et al., "A One Year Study of the Macular Pigment: The Effect of 140 Days of a Lutein Supplement," *Experimental Eye Research* 65: 57–62, 1997.

4. Hammond, B. R., et al., "Dietary Modification of Human Macular Pigment Density," *Investigative Ophthalmology and Visual Science* 38: 1795–1801, 1997.

5. Pratt, Steven, "Dietary Prevention of Age-Related Macular Degeneration," *Journal of the American Optometric Association* 70(1): 39–47, Jan. 1999.

6. Schalch, Wolfgang, "Carotenoids in the Retina—A Review of Their Possible Role in Preventing or Limiting Damage Caused by Light and Oxygen," *Free Radicals and Aging*, 280–98, 1992.

7. Sommerburg, O., et al., "Fruits and Vegetables That Are Sources for Lutein and Zeaxanthin: The Macular Pigment in Human Eyes," *British Journal of Ophthalmology* 82: 907–10, 1998.

8. "Carotenoids and Consumption," *Nutrition Week* 27(37): 7, Sept. 26, 1997.

9. Snodderly, Max D., "Evidence for Protection Against Age-Related Macular Degeneration by Carotenoids and Antioxidant Vitamins," *American Journal of Clinical Nutrition* 62: 1448S–61S, 1995.

10. Brown, L., et al., "A Prospective Study of Carotenoid Intake and Cataracts Among U.S. Men," *American Journal of Epidemiology* 147: S54 (Abst. 213), 1998.

11. Zorge, I., et al., "Lutein Improves Visual Function in Some Patients with Congenital Retinal Degenerations—A Pilot Study via Internet," *Investigative Ophthalmology and Visual Science* 40: S697, (Abst. 3680-B538) 1997.

12. Milo, L., et al., "Lutein and Zeaxanthin Inhibit Human Breast Cancer Cell Proliferation," *FASEB Journal* 12: A830, 1998.

13. Dwyer, J. H., et al., "Plasma Carotenoids and Progression of Carotid Wall Thickness: The Los Angeles Atherosclerosis Study," *Circulation* 97: 829, (Abst. P61) 1998.

61

Lycopene

For men who want to protect themselves against prostate cancer, heart disease, lung cancer, and other health problems, lycopene, a natural carotenoid found in tomatoes, may be one of the best nutrients. Women can also benefit from a higher intake of lycopene, since it also protects against macular degeneration and other complications.

At the Barbara Ann Karamnos Center Institute in Detroit, Omer Kucuk reported that lycopene seems to shrink prostate tumors. A lycopene extract was given to 21 prostate cancer patients three weeks prior to surgery to remove the cancerous prostate. Twelve others did not receive the nutrient. Following surgery, the tumors were smaller and the cancer had spread less in those given lycopene.[1]

In a study by the American Health Foundation in Valhalla, New York, regular tomato consumption brought a 30 percent reduction in prostate cancer among 48,000 health professionals. Although there are more than 600 carotenoids known to science, the body utilizes only about 50. For protection against prostate cancer and other health problems, the researchers recommended eating more fruits and vegetables, especially tomato-based products.[2]

Lycopene, which accounts for 50 percent of all carotenoids in human blood, is concentrated especially in the testes, adrenal gland, and prostate. Unfortunately, lycopene stores are diminished with increasing age. Lycopene intake is associated with a reduction in cancers of the prostate, pancreas, and perhaps the stomach.[3]

In a review of the literature, Edward Giovannucci of Brigham and Women's Hospital and Harvard Medical School said there is evidence that the intake of tomatoes and tomato-based products may provide protection against prostate, lung, and stomach cancers. Lycopene may also provide protection against cancers of the pancreas, colon, rectum, esophagus, oral cavity, breast, and cervix. However, lycopene may not be the most important protective substance, since other beneficial compounds are present in tomatoes, and conceivably, complex interactions among multiple components may contribute to the anticancer properties in tomatoes. At any rate, the studies so far suggest that we can benefit by increasing our fruit and vegetable consumption.[4]

Researchers at Columbia University's Harlem Hospital Center in New York reported that low levels of lycopene may increase a person's susceptibility to lung cancer. Those who had the lowest levels of lycopene had a cancer risk about four times greater than smokers who had the highest intakes. It was also found that lung cancer patients who continued to smoke had the lowest lycopene levels of all the volunteers tested.[5]

Lycopene is apparently twice as powerful as beta-carotene. It is associated with a reduction in prostate and digestive tract cancers, and is apparently more resistant to the effects of alcohol and nicotine than beta-carotene.[6] Researchers at the Beltsville Human Nutrition Research Center, USDA, in Maryland reported that lycopene and lutein, found in fruits and vegetables as well as in human serum, have been shown to have strong antioxidant capabilities.[7]

In a German study, researchers found that lycopene blood levels were higher after volunteers had ingested heat-processed tomato products than after eating uncooked tomatoes. The heat seems to disrupt the cell structure of the tomato, making the lycopene more available.[8]

A study involving 1,379 European men found that those who consumed the most lycopene from foods were half as likely to suffer a heart attack as those who consumed little lycopene in their diets. The research team, headed by Lenore Kohlmeier, Ph.D., of the University of North Carolina at Chapel Hill, assessed lycopene concentrations and absorption by measuring its presence in body fat rather than by monitoring lycopene intake from the diet. Like beta-carotene, lycopene is fat soluble, and dietary fat is necessary for it to be absorbed in the intestines. But like a good antioxidant, lycopene provides protection against heart disease by preventing free radical damage to cells, genes, and molecules as it circulates through the blood.[9] "The protective association with lycopene was not seen in smokers," Kohlmeier said. "It did, however, interact with another major source of oxidative stress, stores of polyunsaturated fats, which are markers of consumption of high polyunsaturated fat diets. This suggests that lycopene may be operating under a tissue-specific antioxidant mechanism."

Laboratory studies have shown that lycopene has the highest antioxidant capacity of the carotenoids, and it has the ability to quench singlet oxygen and trap peroxyl radicals. It has also been shown that when skin is subjected to ultraviolet light stress, more lycopene is destroyed than beta-carotene, suggesting that lycopene may help mitigate oxidative damage in tissues. Singlet oxygen is a toxic by-product of many metabolic processes, and it is especially stimulated by smoking and sun exposure. Peroxyl radicals are a constituent found in smog, among other things.[10]

Using five volunteers, researchers determined the bioavailability of lycopene by giving them a serving of fresh tomatoes or tomato paste (23 g of lycopene), along with 15 g of corn oil. The bioavailability of lycopene was greater from tomato paste than from fresh tomatoes, suggesting that cooking and chopping seems to increase bioavailability by breaking down plant cell walls.[11]

From the available evidence, it seems prudent to increase our consumption of fruits and vegetables, especially cooked tomato products. As insurance against possible deficiencies of lycopene, supplements are available in health food stores and other outlets. Some of the formulas provide 5- and 10-mg potencies in softgel capsules.

References

1. Seppa, Nathan, "Tomato Compound Fights Cancer," *Science News* 155(17): 271, April 24, 1999.

2. "AHF Sponsors International Symposium on the Role of Lycopene and Tomato Products in Disease Prevention," *Primary Care and Cancer* 17(4): 30–32, April 1997.

3. Gerster, Helga, "The Potential Role of Lycopene in Human Health," *Journal of the American College of Nutrition* 16(2): 109–26, 1997.

4. Giovannucci, Edward, "Tomatoes, Tomato-Based Products, Lycopene, and Cancer: Review of the Epidemiologic Literature," *Journal of the National Cancer Institute* 91(4): 317–31, Feb. 17, 1999.

5. "Nutrient in Tomatoes Is Found to Lower an Individual's Risk of Lung Cancer," *Medical Tribune,* May 22, 1997, 33.

6. "Antioxidants and Lycopene," *Nutrition Week* 27(11): 7, March 21, 1997.

7. Khachik, Frederick, et al., "Lutein, Lycopene, and Their Oxidative Metabolites in Chemoprevention of Cancer," *Cellular Biochemistry* 22: 236–46, 1995.

8. "Tomato Research," *Nutrition Today* 34(2): 63, March/April 1999.

9. Kohlmeier, Lenore, et al., "Lycopene and Myocardial Infarction Risk in the EURAMIC Study," *American Journal of Epidemiology* 146: 618–26, 1997.

10. Riso, Patrizia, et al., "Does Tomato Consumption Effectively Increase the Resistance of Lymphocyte DNA to Oxidative Damage?" *American Journal of Clinical Nutrition* 69: 712–18, 1999.

11. Gartner, Christine, et al., "Lycopene Is More Bioavailable from Tomato Paste Than from Fresh Tomatoes," *American Journal of Clinical Nutrition* 66: 116–22, 1997.

62

Magnesium

Magnesium is involved in more than 300 enzyme systems in the body, and all enzymes utilizing adenosine triphosphate (ATP) require magnesium for substrate formation. ATP is a constituent containing "high energy" phosphate bonds that serve as energy activators in cells. Magnesium is necessary for potassium transport, calcium channel activity, and nerve conduction. The recommended dietary allowance (RDA) for magnesium is 320 mg/day for women and 420 mg/day for men.[1]

In a study involving 31 osteoporotic, postmenopausal women, magnesium supplements at 750 mg/day of six months, followed by a maintenance doses of 250 mg/day, increased radial bone mass. In another study, women taking 500 mg/day of calcium and 600 mg/day of magnesium along with a daily multivitamin experi-

enced an increase in bone mass in those postmenopausal women who were given estrogen replacement therapy. When there is a magnesium deficiency, the kidneys do not conserve potassium sufficiently, resulting in a potassium deficiency in the blood. Potassium therapy alone is not sufficient to correct the problem; magnesium therapy must be undertaken simultaneously.

Researchers have found that intracellular levels in the muscle (remember, the heart is a muscle), red blood cells, lymphocyte, and bone magnesium may be more accurate in assessing body magnesium stores. Six hundred milligrams of intravenous magnesium over a 24-hour period can help build up stores, but this therapy must be continued for three to seven days.

When Robert Rude, M.D., and colleagues at the University of Southern

California at Los Angeles examined more than 100 consecutive admissions to the hospital coronary care unit, they found that 53 percent had little or no magnesium in their bodies. Rude said, "I think hypomagnesmia certainly could be a contributing factor (in cardiovascular disorders). We know that magnesium depletion predisposes to high blood pressure and cardiac arrhythmias, and may predispose to coronary vasospasm and perhaps myocardial infarction (heart attack)."[2]

According to H. Alexander Heggtveit, M.D., of the University of Ottawa in Canada, there is strong evidence that lack of magnesium plays a decisive role in human heart ailments. When he examined heart muscle from victims of fatal heart attacks, he found that certain portions of the muscle contained up to 42 percent less magnesium than heart muscle from individuals who had died from other causes. He added that such a magnesium deficiency may predispose the human heart to fatal arrhythmias, or disturbances in the heart's beating rhythm.

Mildred S. Seelig, M.D., suggests that a magnesium deficiency accounts for the high incidence of heart disease in the United States and other Western countries. In one study, she reported on the magnesium levels of people around the world, including England and the United States, and found that only those living in the Orient—where hardening of the arteries is not common—have sufficient body reserves of magnesium. Magnesium has been declining in the American diet since 1900, partly because the milling of wheat strips away much of the magnesium, and certain chemicals used to keep vegetables a bright shade of green pull out essential minerals, including magnesium.

In evaluating more than 15,000 people aged 45 to 64, English researchers found that those with cardiovascular disease, high blood pressure, and diabetes had significantly lower blood levels of magnesium that those free of the disease.[3]

When researchers evaluated the diets of more than 41,000 female nurses ranging in age from 38 to 63, those who had lower blood pressure reported eating foods high in magnesium, such as chicken, mushrooms, spinach, and prunes.[4]

At the 1997 annual meeting of the American Diabetes Association, it was reported that low blood levels of magnesium may be a strong independent predictor of Type 2 diabetes in white individuals. In studying serum magnesium levels in 12,398 nondiabetic, middle-aged, African-American and white volunteers during a six-year period, researchers found no association between magnesium levels and diabetes in African Americans, but an inverse association was found in whites. At the end of the study, there were 807 new cases of Type 2 diabetes in whites. Researchers at Johns Hopkins University in Baltimore have shown that a magnesium deficiency adversely affects insulin metabolism.[5]

A study in Finland gave 56 diabetics 600 mg/day of magnesium for 90 days, and in another trial 2 g/day of vitamin C were administered. Those getting magnesium experienced a decrease in systolic and diastolic blood pressure in the insulin-dependent diabetics. Vitamin C brought lower cholesterol and triglyceride levels in non-insulin-dependent diabetics.[6]

Low magnesium levels may occur in about 25 percent of diabetic patients. Low blood levels of the mineral have been reported in childhood insulin-dependent diabetics and in adults with Type 1 and Type 2 diabetes. Magnesium deficiency can result from gastrointestinal loss, excess excretion by the kidneys, nutritional deficiencies, endocrine disorders, chronic alcoholism, major burns, and other causes.[7]

Giving pregnant women magnesium during pregnancy may help prevent severely underweight infants from developing cerebral palsy and mental retardation, according to Diana E. Schendel, Ph.D., of the Centers for Disease Control and Prevention in Atlanta, Georgia. It is generally believed that infants who are born weighing less than 3.3 pounds are 60 to 75 times more likely to develop cerebral palsy and 8 to 14 times more likely to be mentally retarded than children of normal birth weights.[8]

In a new study of 519 children who were followed for three to five years after birth, those with very low birth weights, whose mothers were given intravenous magnesium during pregnancy, were about 90 percent less likely to develop cerebral palsy and 70 percent less likely to show signs of mental retardation than other children born underweight. Pregnant women are often given magnesium sulfate either to prevent convulsions in those with preeclampsia or to stop preterm labor.

Israeli researchers evaluated 40 women with urinary problems who were given either 350 mg of magnesium twice daily or a placebo for four weeks. It was found that 11 of 20 patients given magnesium reported improvement in their urinary symptoms, compared with five given a placebo (55 versus 20 percent). No side effects were reported in the treatment group.[9]

At the University of Cukurova, Adana, Turkey, researchers reported that in evaluating 12 adult sickle cell patients, magnesium, zinc, and copper blood levels were significantly lower than in controls.[10]

Researchers at Linkoping University Hospital in Sweden studied 73 women with pregnancy-related leg cramps. The patients were given 122 mg of magnesium in the morning and 144 mg in the evening, or a placebo. Oral magnesium supplementation seems to be a valuable therapeutic tool in the treatment of pregnancy-related leg cramps.[11]

In two small trials, 360 mg of magnesium given three times daily from day 15 to the onset of menses can ease the severity of premenstrual syndrome (PMS) and reduce the duration of PMS-related migraine headaches. There is a strong association between migraine and estrogen.[12]

German researchers evaluated 81 patients between the ages of 18 and 65 who experienced 3.6 migraine headaches monthly.

The volunteers were given 600 mg/day of magnesium for 12 weeks, or a placebo. The researchers said that between weeks 9 and 12 the attack frequency was reduced by 41.6 percent in the magnesium group and 15.8 percent in the placebo group. High-dose magnesium is an effective treatment for migraine headaches.[13]

Researchers at the Magee-Women's Research Institute in Pittsburgh reported that magnesium has been used for more than 60 years for treating eclampsia in pregnant women. This condition brings on convulsions during pregnancy and the mineral is associated with a dramatic reduction of maternal and neonatal morbidity related to this problem. Magnesium is better than the drug phenytoin (Dilantin) in preventing eclamptic seizures, the researchers said.[14]

When 41 patients with rheumatoid arthritis were evaluated at the Albany Medical College in New York, their diets were deficient regarding the RDA for magnesium, zinc, and vitamin B_6. Folic acid and copper were deficient when compared to the typical American diet in both men and women. The researchers added that dietary supplementation with multivitamins and trace minerals is appropriate in this population.[15]

At Goteborg University in Sweden, the magnesium content was evaluated in 17 municipal water supplies. It was found that 854 people 50 to 60 years of age had died of acute myocardial infarction, and the deaths were related to the amount of magnesium in their drinking water. In males, at least, the data suggest that the mineral in drinking water (that is, "hard" water) is an important protective factor for death from acute myocardial infarction.[16]

Elderly people who rely heavily on over-the-counter medications that contain magnesium often ingest too much of the mineral. Too much magnesium can mimic other illnesses, such as muscle weakness, drowsiness, confusion, weakened reflexes, and other conditions. Products containing magnesium include milk of magnesia, Epsom salts, and magnesium-containing laxatives and antacids.[17]

The Adventist Health Study evaluated 31,208 non-Hispanic white Seventh-Day Adventists over a six-year period. Those who consumed nuts more than four times weekly had less fatal coronary heart disease and nonfatal myocardial infarctions when compared to those who ate nuts less than once per week. In addition, those who ate whole-wheat bread had lower rates of nonfatal myocardial infarction and fatal coronary heart disease when compared to those who ate white bread. Nuts are a rich source of monounsaturated fats and magnesium. A substudy of 147 patients from the same population study showed that 32 percent of the people ate peanuts; 29 percent, almonds; 16 percent, walnuts; and 32 percent, nuts such as hazelnuts and pecans. The fiber content in nuts is high, and there is no indication that frequent eating of nuts increases the risk of obesity, even though they are relatively high in calories.[18]

People don't necessarily need to become severely deficient in magnesium for the brain to become hyperactive, according to James G. Penland, Ph.D., and researchers at the Grand Forks Human Nutrition Research Center in North Dakota. Their study confirms earlier reports that a marginal magnesium intake overexcites the brain's neurons, resulting in less coherence—in other words, creating cacophony rather than symphony, according to electroencephalogram (EEG) measurements.[19] During half of the six-month study, 13 women were given 115 mg/day of magnesium, or about 40 percent of the RDA. During the remaining half of the study, they received 315 mg/day, or a little more than the recommendation for women. After only six weeks on the marginal intake, EEG readings showed significant differences in brain function.

Penland explained that magnesium is the fourth most abundant element in the brain and is essential for regulating central nervous system excitability. Clinical studies of those severely deficient in magnesium have reported epilepsy-type convulsions, dizziness, and muscle tremors or twitching, along with many psychological symptoms, including irritability, anxiety, confusion, depression, apathy, loss of appetite, and insomnia. Although the marginal intake did not produce such severe symptoms, it did hype brain activity. This was one of the first experimental studies in which magnesium intakes were tightly controlled and EEG measurements were analyzed by computer so that they could be statistically compared.

Magnesium deficiency may occur during long-distance running because of the increased demand by the skeletal muscles, according to a study that evaluated 26 runners who completed a 2- to 5½-hour marathon. While there were no changes in serum calcium, copper, or zinc levels, magnesium concentrations went down significantly.[20]

Many Americans are deficient in this mineral. In addition to nuts, magnesium is available in whole grains, peanut butter, nut butters, peanut and soybean flours, green leafy vegetables, and spices. Retail outlets carry a variety of magnesium supplements, including the mineral alone or with other nutrients. A good vitamin/mineral supplement is often excellent insurance against any possible deficiencies. Doctors often use magnesium intramuscularly or intravenously for treating many health complaints.

References

1. Rude, Robert K., "Magnesium Deficiency: A Cause of Heterogenous Disease in Humans," *Journal of Bone and Mineral Research* 13(4): 749–58, 1998.

2. Murray, Frank, *The Big Family Guide to All the Minerals* (New Canaan, Conn.: Keats Publishing, 1995), 149ff.

3. "Associations of Serum and Dietary Magnesium with Cardiovascular Disease, Hypertension, Diabetes, Insulin, and Carotid Artery Wall Thickness," *Journal of Clinical Epidemiology* 48: 927–40, 1995.

4. "Magnesium Lowers Blood Pressure," *Nutrition Week,* May 24, 1996, 7.

5. Kahn, Jason, "Magnesium Levels May Predict Risk of Type 2 Disease in Whites," *Medical Tribune,* July 17, 1997, 16.

6. Erikson, Johan, "Magnesium and Ascorbic Acid Supplementation in Diabetes Mellitus," *Annals of Nutrition and Metabolism* 39: 217–23, 1995.

7. Tosiello, Lorraine, "Hypomagnesemia and Diabetes Mellitus," *Archives of Internal Medicine* 156: 1143–48, June 10, 1996.

8. Christensen, Damaris, "Magnesium Sulfate Said to Benefit Low Birth Weight Babies," *Medical Tribune,* Feb. 6, 1997, 11.

9. Gordon, David, et al., "Double-Blind, Placebo-Controlled Study of Magnesium Hydroxide for Treatment of Sensory Urgency and Detrussor Instability: Preliminary Results," *British Journal of Obstetrics and Gynecology* 105: 667–69, June 1998.

10. Isbir, T., et al., "Zinc, Copper, Magnesium, and Sickle Cell Anemia," *Trace Elements and Electrolytes* 12(3): 161, 1995.

11. Dahle, Lars O., et al., "The Effect of Oral Magnesium Substitution on Pregnancy-Induced Leg Cramps," *American Journal of Obstetrics and Gynecology* 173(1): 175–80, 1995.

12. Boschert, Sherry, "Magnesium Can Curb Premenstrual Migraine," *Family Practice News,* March 1, 1996, 33.

13. Pelkert, A., et al., "Prophylaxis of Migraine with Oral Magnesium: Results from a Prospective, Multi-Center, Placebo-Controlled, and Double-Blind Randomized Study," *Cephalalgia* 16: 257–63, 1996.

14. Roberts, James N., et al., "Magnesium for Preeclampsia and Eclampsia," *New England Journal of Medicine* 333: 201–05, July 27, 1995.

15. Kremer, Joel M., and Jean Bigaouette, "Nutrient Intake of Patients with Rheumatoid Arthritis Is Deficient in Pyridoxine, Zinc, Copper, and Magnesium," *Journal of Rheumatology* 23(6): 990–94, 1996.

16. Rubenowitz, Eva, et al., "Magnesium in Drinking Water and Death from Acute Myocardial Infarction," *American Journal of Epidemiology* 143(5): 456–62, 1996.

17. Fung, Man C., et al., "Hyper-magnesemia: Elderly Over-the-Counter Drug Users at Risk," *Archives of Family Medicine* 4: 718–23, August 1995.

18. Durlach, Jean, ed., "Fatty Acid Profile, Fibre Content, and High Magnesium Density of Nuts May Protect Against Risk of Coronary Heart Disease Events," *Magnesium Research* 6(2): 191–92, 1993.

19. "Magnesium Calms the Brain," Food and Nutrition Research Briefs, Oct. 1995, 1.

20. Buchman, Alan L., "The Effect of a Marathon Run on Plasma and Urine Mineral and Metal Concentrations," *Journal of the American College of Nutrition* 17(2): 124–27, 1998.

63

Maitake

Grifola frondosa, the scientific name for maitake, is derived from a fungus found in Italy. The name is derived from the griffin, a mystical beast that was half lion and half eagle. The Japanese name, *maitake*, is associated with the mushroom's shape, which suggests a dancing nymph. The name is also derived from "dancing fungus," since it is believed that anyone lucky enough to find the mushroom dances with joy. The Chinese name for the mushroom is *Keisho*.[1] A culinary and medicinal mushroom popular in the Far East, maitake contains proteins, carbohydrates, fiber, vitamin B_1, vitamin B_2, vitamin D, potassium, and phosphorus. It also contains nucleotides, free sugars (tehalose, glucose, and mannitol), polysaccharides, enzymes, and organic acids.

In 1992, the National Cancer Institute confirmed the efficacy of maitake extract against HIV.[2] Researchers at the National Institute of Health in Japan made a similar discovery. Both teams reported that the extract not only prevents HIV-infected T cells from being destroyed, but also enhances the activity of the immune cells.[3]

At a pharmacological conference held at Kyushu Industrial College in Fukuoka, Japan, in 1992, Hiroaki Nanba, Ph.D., and colleagues reported that maitake mushroom contains potent anti-HIV and anticancer properties, as well as its use in reducing high blood pressure and controlling diabetes. After a person is infected with HIV, his helper T cells—the cells that recognize foreign matter in the body and help to destroy it—are themselves gradually destroyed. Nanba claimed that a polysaccharide (glucan) in maitake inhibits an HIV infection. In a lab glassware test, 97 percent of the 300,000 HIV-infected T cells remained alive after being subjected to 1/100,000 g of the maitake compound.[4]

Following a clinical trial, Nanba said that maitake D-fraction is effective against breast cancer, liver cancer, and lung cancer, although it is less effective against leukemia, stomach, and bone cancers. The tumor regression or reduction in symptoms was observed among 11 of 15 breast cancer patients; 12 out of 18 lung cancer patients; and 7 out of 15 liver cancer patients. When taken with chemotherapy, these response rates increased by 12 to 28 percent.[5] "A number of patients have been diagnosed as Stage I cancer, which had previously been Stage III," Nanba added. "Some drastic tumor reductions or remissions were also seen in many patients. A small chicken-egg-sized brain tumor of a 44-year-old male completely disappeared after taking D-fraction for four months."

Nanba said that various side effects from chemotherapy—loss of appetite, vomiting, nausea, hair loss, and leukopenia (deficiency of white blood cells)—were ameliorated among 90 percent of the patients. And 83 percent of the patients reported a lessening of pain.

Recent trials have indicated that maitake can control blood glucose levels by reducing insulin resistance and enhancing insulin sensitivity. One study used mice that have an obesity gene and are genetically diabetic. While being fed their regular diet, the blood glucose levels of the animals increased along with their body weight. However, when maitake was mixed with their chow, biomarkers such as blood glucose, insulin, triglycerides, and body weight were maintained at a significantly lower level.[6]

In a crossover test using the same animals, the feed for one group was switched at the beginning of the fifth week from maitake-enriched feed to normal feed and then switched back again. In the control group, which was not getting maitake, blood glucose had risen to 400 mg/dl. It went down to 230 mg/dl the week after the maitake feeding began. Two weeks later, it had gone down to 155 mg/dl. The researchers concluded that the changes in glucose values were brought about by the maitake feed prior to the change in body weight, and that the mushroom extract is effective in reducing glucose levels, insulin resistance, and triglycerides in diabetic mice. Further research is under way to determine maitake's effectiveness on humans.

In a laboratory experiment at Kobe Pharmaceutical University in Japan, maitake extract altered lipid metabolism by inhibiting the accumulation of fats in the liver and blood. Some uncontrolled human studies in Japan have found that the oral administration of maitake powder helps regulate levels of serum cholesterol and triglycerides.[7]

Harry G. Preuss, M.D., of Georgetown University Medical Center in Washington, D.C., is currently tabulating the results of his studies using ether-soluble fraction extracted from maitake against elevated blood pressure and Type 2 diabetes mellitus. So far the results are very encouraging.[8]

In an uncontrolled, nonrandomized study, Scott Gerson, M.D., evaluated the effects of maitake mushroom on blood pressure in 11 volunteers ranging in age from 46 to 68. The seven men and four women were documented to have mild to moderate hypertension. Each was given 500-mg caplets of maitake to be taken twice daily, in the morning and evening, at least 90 minutes before eating. The results of the six-week study showed that a mean decrease in systolic blood pressure was 14 mmHg, with a mean decrease in diastolic blood pressure of about 8mmHg.[9]

Since the mid-1980s, maitake's antitumor activity has undergone intensive study. Nanba has stated that polysaccharides in maitake, consisting of beta-1,6-linked glucan with 1,3-branches possess a strong ability to activate cellular immunity, resulting in superior antitumor activity when compared with other mushrooms. Maitake's acid-insoluble, alkali-soluble, hot-water extractable fraction, called D-fraction, has been found to be the most potent constituent when given orally.[10] In one trial, cancer metastasis was prevented by 91.3 percent after the administration of maitake D-fraction. The maitake-fed group also demonstrated an 81.3 percent prevention rate, suggesting that maitake is able to inhibit cancer metastasis.

In his book *8 Weeks to Optimum Health,* Andrew Weil, M.D., says he often recommends maitake to patients with cancer, AIDS, and other immune-deficiency states, chronic fatigue syndrome, chronic hepatitis, and environmental illnesses that may represent toxic overloads.[11] "My tonic of choice at the moment is a liquid extract called maitake D-fraction, which concentrates the immune-boosting constituents," Weil wrote. "I take five drops in water three times a day, and since I've been doing so, I almost never get colds, even though my children and their friends are constantly bringing colds into our house."

Maitake products are readily available in health food stores and other outlets. In addition to 500-mg caplets and extracts, maitake is available in a caffeine-free tea containing Siberian ginseng and other herbs such as rosemary, licorice root, echinacea, and lavender. The extract is also available in capsules. Another tea contains maitake and green tea. Also available is a prostate formula containing maitake, saw palmetto berry, tomato lycopene, green tea extract, and pumpkin seed powder. Follow the directions on the labels.

References

1. Mizuno, Takashi, and Cun Zhuang, "Maitake, *Grifola Frondosa:* Pharmacological Effects," *Food Reviews International* 11(1): 135–49, 1995.

2. "In Vitro Anti-HIV Drug Screening Results, Developmental Therapeutics Program," National Institutes of Health, Jan. 17, 1992, unpublished.

3. Ishikawa, K., "Anti-HIV Activity in Cytopathic Effect of Proteoglucan Extracted from Maitake Mushroom,"

National Institutes of Health, Jan. 23, 1991, unpublished.

4. "Anti-HIV Activity Found in Maitake Mushroom," *Explore More!,* Nov. 2, 1993, 25.

5. Nanba, Hiroaki, "Maitake D-Fraction: Healing and Preventing Potentials for Cancer," *Townsend Letter for Doctors and Patients,* Feb.–March 1996, 84–85.

6. Lieberman, Shari, and Ken Babal, *Maitake: King of Mushrooms* (New Canaan, Conn.: Keats Publishing, 1997), 31–32.

7. Kubo, Keiko, and Hiroaki Nanba, "The Effect of Maitake Mushroom on Liver and Serum Lipids," *Alternative Therapies* 2(5): 62–66, September 1996.

8. Preuss, Harry G., "Preliminary Studies," 1998, unpublished.

9. Gerson, Scott, "Blood Pressure–Lowering Effect of *Grifola Fondosa* (Maitake)," July 6, 1994, unpublished.

10. Nanba, Hiroaki, "Activity of Maitake D-Fraction to Inhibit Carcinogenesis and Metastasis," *Cancer Prevention,* Vol. 768, *Annals of the New York Academy of Sciences,* Sept. 30, 1995.

11. Weil, Andrew, *8 Weeks to Optimum Health* (New York: Alfred A. Knopf, 1997), 137–38.

64

Manganese

Sometimes confused with magnesium, manganese was initially recognized as an element in 1774 by Swedish chemist Carl W. Scheele, and was isolated that same year by his colleague, Johann G. Ghan. Its name is a somewhat corrupted form of *magnesia,* the Latin word for "magnetic stone."[1]

The mineral is poorly absorbed, some 45 percent, mostly in the small intestine, with the rest being excreted in the feces. Absorption is inhibited by excessive amounts of calcium, phosphorus, or iron in the diet. Manganese is necessary for the formation of bone and the growth of other connective tissues; for blood clotting; in insulin action; in cholesterol synthesis; and as an instigator of various enzymes in the metabolism of carbohydrates, fats, proteins, and nucleic acids (DNA and RNA).

Manganese deficiency is associated with growth impairment, bone abnormalities, diabetic-like carbohydrate changes, incoordination, and increased susceptibility to convulsions, according to Abram Hoffer, M.D., Ph.D. Approximately one-third of children with epilepsy have low blood levels of manganese.[2] He went on to say that a deficiency in manganese caused by tranquilizers can result in tardive dyskinesia. He referred to work by Kunin that theorized that because phenothiazines can bind manganese, and because the mineral is found in high amounts in the extrapyramidal system, this was the cause of tardive dyskinesia. Using 20 to 60 mg/day of manganese, Kunin found that in 15 schizophrenics with tardive dyskinesia, seven were completely cured; only one did not respond. Vitamin B_3 (niacin) is also an important addition to this therapy.

"In general," Hoffer said, "I have seen similar dramatic responses. Tardive dyskinesia has not been any problem in my large schizophrenia practice. The disorder will almost disappear when vitamin therapy is used, and, if it should appear, it can be easily treated with manganese supplementation. Ideally, each tranquilizer tablet should contain enough manganese to prevent chelation of the body's manganese. My guess is that 1 to 3 mg/day in these tablets would prevent tardive dyskinesia."

In *Nutrition Today,* Jeanne Freeland-Graves, Ph.D., R.N., of the University of Texas at Austin reviewed the many attributes of manganese in human health. Deficiencies in the mineral have been involved with abnormalities in brain function, glucose tolerance, reproduction, and skeletal and cartilage formation. The mineral is involved in over a dozen enzyme systems, including arginase, superoxide dismutase, and aminopeptidase. A manganese deficiency causes the rash miliaria crystallina, in which sweat cannot be excreted, causing small, clear blisters to fill with fluid.[3]

Manganese deficiency is also associated with high cholesterol levels, Freeland-Graves continued. Blood concentrations of the mineral in osteoporotic women have been shown to be some 25 percent of that found in normal women. Sugar intake has been related to manganese deficiency, along with other trace minerals. While manganese has a low toxicity level, extreme amounts can result in dementia, psychiatric disorders resembling schizophrenia, and neurologic disorders similar to Parkinson's disease. Dietary levels as high as 18 mg/day (found in India in those eating bran muffins) have not produced any side effects, so the suggested upper limit of 5 mg/day seems to be conservative. Low dietary intakes of manganese are probably due to high intakes of meat and refined and fast foods, which are poor sources of the mineral.

In his book *Mental and Elemental Nutrients,* Carl C. Pfeiffer, Ph.D., M.D., reported that a high level of copper in many schizophrenics can be reduced by dietary intakes of zinc and manganese. This combination is more effective than either mineral alone. He added that high copper levels in the schizophrenics have been ignored by the medical establishment, and that there is little dispute over the biochemical fact that zinc and manganese may replace copper and thus reduce high copper levels in the blood. In oral doses, manganese is never harmful, but in those over age 40 it has occasionally elevated blood pressure.[4]

Pfeiffer added that since levels of spermine (which is important in cell and tissue growth and also found in sperm) in the blood decrease with age, young patients with Tourette's syndrome (swearing, motor tics, etc.) are also especially low in spermine for their ages. Spermine levels can be raised with trace elements and diet, with manganese appearing to be the most important. Copper is high in many neoplastic diseases and, as mentioned, the combination of zinc and manganese is most effective in mobilizing copper from the tissues.

Although little is known about the many functions of spermine in the body, consistently low levels found in patients with senility warrants further study. Trace elements and vitamin supplements are beneficial and should be used to relieve confusion and memory loss. Some confused geriatric patients become rational when Theragran-M is stopped and a source of zinc and manganese is administered.

Patients with rheumatoid arthritis should have supplements of zinc, manganese, vitamin B_3, vitamin C, and two eggs daily, Pfeiffer said. If they cannot eat eggs, elemental sulfur should be supplied at 200 mg/day. Roger Williams, Ph.D., also recommended various nutrients for rheumatoid arthritis, including vitamin B_3, pantothenic acid (B_5), folic acid, vitamin B_6, zinc, and manganese, since many of these patients are often deficient in these nutrients.

Manganese is a necessary constituent of metalloproteins such as superoxide dismutase, pyruvate carboxylase, and glutamine synthetase. Since it is one of the least toxic heavy metals, it readily crosses the blood-brain barrier in adults and the developing fetus. However, it can be toxic for those exposed to the metal, such as miners and ore plant workers. Several countries have replaced the lead in gasoline with a manganese antiknock compound, and further research is needed to determine any long-term neurodegenerative disorders that might be associated with gasoline.[5]

Manganese, copper, and zinc are critical components for a number of processes, especially in the production of the antioxidant superoxide dismutase. The three minerals play an active role in cellular defense against free radical damage.[6]

Since manganese is associated with the biosynthesis of the bone matrix, a long-term deficiency in the mineral creates calcium loss from bone. Women with osteoporosis have lower levels of manganese in their blood, lower bone mineral content, and lower bone mineral density than women without the disease. However, manganese, copper, and zinc supplements slow bone loss in postmenopausal women.[7]

Women at risk of osteoporosis are encouraged to include calcium, copper, zinc, and manganese in their diets. A two-year, double-blind study involved 200 postmenopausal women and used these dosages: calcium, 1,000 mg/day; zinc, 15 mg/day; copper, 2.5 mg/day; and manganese, 5 mg/day.[8]

Manganese, which is needed to activate the key enzymes in the body's ability to use sugar for energy, is often depressed in diabetics, according to Melvyn Werbach, M.D. Although routine manganese supplementation is not always recommended, Type 1 (insulin-dependent) diabetics with low blood levels of the mineral may find their insulin needs are reduced with manganese supplements. For these patients, Werbach recommends 3 to 5 mg/day.[9]

Researchers at the Grand Forks Human Nutrition Research Center in North Dakota have confirmed that dietary calcium and manganese have a functional role in symptoms occurring during menstrual distress. During the double-blind study, 10 women were treated with 587 to 1,336 mg/day of calcium and 1 to 5.6 mg/day of manganese. The increase in calcium reduced mood swings, concentration, behavioral symptoms, and pain during the menstrual phase of the cycle. In addition, water retention was reduced during the premenstrual phase. With increased calcium intake, lowered dietary manganese increased mood swings during the premenstrual phase.[10]

Irregular exhaustive exercise, such as jogging on sultry days, might cause tissue damage aggravated by poor dietary intakes of important antioxidants. Defense mechanisms in the body to protect against free radical damage include the antioxidant systems that contain enzymes such as superoxide dismutase and xanthine oxidase, and scavenger nutrients such as beta-carotene, vitamin C, vitamin E, selenium, manganese, and zinc.[11]

Major food sources of manganese include brown rice, rice bran and polish, nuts, spices, whole grains, molasses, beans, soybeans, sunflower seeds, potatoes, lettuce, and blueberries.

Although there is no recommended dietary allowance for manganese, the trace mineral is essential for good health. Ask your physician about using manganese.

References

1. Ensminger, A., et al., *Foods and Nutrition Encyclopedia* (Clovis, Calif.: Pegus Press, 1983), 1370–72.

2. Hoffer, Abram, *Orthomolecular Medicine for Physicians* (New Canaan, Conn.: Keats Publishing, 1989), 87–88.

3. Freeland-Graves, Jeanne, "Manganese: An Essential Nutrient for Humans," *Nutrition Today,* Nov.–Dec. 1988, 13–19.

4. Pfeiffer, Carl C., *Mental and Elemental Nutrients* (New Canaan, Conn.: Keats Publishing, 1975), 253ff., 449, 454ff.

5. Aschner, Michael, "Manganese Neurotoxicity and Oxidative Damage," *Metals and Oxidative Damage in Neurological Disorders,* chapter 5, 77–93, 1997.

6. Zidenberg-Cherr, Sheri, and Carl L. Keen, "Essential Trace Elements in Antioxidant Processes," *Trace Elements, Micronutrients, and Free Radicals,* 107–27, 1992.

7. Garrison, Robert, Jr., and Elizabeth Somer, *The Nutrition Desk Reference* (New Canaan, Conn.: Keats Publishing, 1995), 501.

8. Saltman, P., "The Role of Minerals and Osteoporosis," *Journal of the American College of Nutrition* 11(5): 599/Abst. 7, 1992.

9. Werbach, Melvyn, *Healing with Food* (New York: HarperPerennial, 1993), 117–18.

10. Penland, James G., and Phyllis E. Johnson, "The Dietary Calcium and Manganese Effects on Menstrual Cycle Symptoms," *American Journal of Obstetrics and Gynecology* 168(5): 1417–23, May 1993.

11. Reddan, R., "Vitamin E and Selenium in Exercise-Induced Tissue Damage," *The Nutrition Report* 11(2): 10, 16, Feb. 1993.

65

Melatonin

The pineal gland, a small cone-shaped structure in the brain, secretes the hormone melatonin after dark, reaching its peak around midnight. Researchers have learned that exposure to light, even in minute amounts, depresses melatonin secretion, and that carefully timed exposure to light can have a dramatic effect on jet lag, according to Richard Dawood, M.D.[1]

"In studies, the best results have been attained when a small dose of melatonin is given approximately two hours before bedtime on the first night in the new time zone and for several nights thereafter, depending on the distance that has been traveled," Dawood said. "The number of doses is roughly the same as the number of time zones crossed. Thus, when traveling between New York and London, one would take melatonin for five nights upon arrival and upon return—to accommodate for the five-hour time difference."

Military aviation missions involve rapid deployment and night operations, which disrupt sleep. At Fort Rucker, Alabama, physicians gave 10 mg of melatonin or a placebo to 29 male air crew members prior to travel, on the day of travel, and for five days after arrival at their destination. It was reported that melatonin helped to readjust the sleep/wake cycle and reduced jet lag after traveling across time zones. The placebo group reported a significant reduction in sleep patterns.[2]

Studies have shown that melatonin can improve jet lag symptoms and may replace conventional treatments such as short-acting hypnotics. Melatonin can be taken at 5 mg/day three or four days before traveling, especially in an eastward direction, and continued for three or four days after arrival.[3]

In *The Experts Speak* in 1997, Byung P. Yu, Ph.D., of the University of Texas Health Science Center at San Antonio said that the unique nature of melatonin comes from its various attributes: (1) It is a natural product biosynthesized by the body; (2) it is a hormone that declines with age; (3) unlike other antioxidants that have limited accessibility to scavenging activity due to poor distribution in the cell, melatonin is quite easily scattered; and (4) it is known to be a scavenger of hydroxyl radicals, the most reactive and destructive free radicals.[4]

Melatonin is apparently quite safe and can induce sleep, prevent jet lag, and assist night-shift workers with sleep irregularities at doses of 3 mg/day, reported *Family Practice News*.[5] At the National Hospital for Neurology and Neurosurgery in London, physicians evaluated a 24-year-old woman who had had her pineal gland surgically removed and who spent most of the day sleeping. Since there was a variation in her melatonin levels, she was given 2 mg of melatonin at night. After eight weeks of therapy, she slept normally during the night and needed only a 20-minute nap during the day.[6]

Melatonin was effective in alleviating sleep disturbances in nine girls with Rett syndrome. The girls, with a mean age of 10.1 years, were given from 2.5 to 7.5 mg/day, which improved sleep patterns during the first three weeks of treatment.[7] Rett syndrome, named after Andreas Rett, an Austrian pediatrician, is a rare, genetic brain disorder that affects only girls. The child appears normal until about 12 to 18 months of age, when autism, writhing movements, and other side effects surface.

At the Community Mental Health Center in Maastricht, The Netherlands, researchers studied a 44-year-old woman who was depressed and could sleep only two to three hours nightly. After giving her 5 mg of melatonin, there was sleep improvement the second night. During seven days of melatonin therapy at 5 mg/day, her sleep pattern increased from two to three hours to six or eight hours per night, and she reported that her clinical condition had improved.[8]

Untreated sleep disturbances can have a significant adverse effect on the intellectual development of children, according to researchers at Children's Hospital in Vancouver, Canada. Melatonin should be given shortly before bedtime. It is quickly absorbed and patients are usually asleep within 30 minutes. The half-life of melatonin is only one hour; within three or four hours it is excreted by the body. The most effective dose of fast-release melatonin in some studies is between 5 and 10 mg/day.[9]

Melatonin, in conjunction with routine chemotherapy, may be useful as a treatment for osteosarcoma, or bone cancer. It seems there is a concurrent decrease in melatonin levels with the exponential increase in bone growth during puberty, which could be a key factor in the development of osteosarcoma.[10]

In a double-blind study at Instituto Neurologico in Milan, researchers gave 10 mg of melatonin to 10 patients with cluster headaches, while 10 others received a placebo for two weeks. The melatonin therapy brought a significant reduction in headache frequency, as well as the need for fewer headache medications. Five of the 10 patients in the treatment group reported that the frequency of their attacks declined three to five days after treatment began, and they experienced no further headaches until melatonin was discontinued. There was no response in those with chronic cluster headaches or those in the placebo group. One theory about the effectiveness of melatonin is that it may modulate calcium's entry into the cells. Melatonin also inhibits the synthesis of prostaglandin E2, which can activate inflammation surrounding a blood vessel or lymph vessel.[11]

Researchers at Oregon Health Sciences University in Portland found that a daily 10-mg dose of melatonin successfully "entrained" the free-running rhythms of six out of seven totally blind people, returning them to a normal, 24-hour sleep pattern. In an earlier study, a 5-mg dose of melatonin was not effective. Charmane Eastman, M.D., of Rush Presbyterian–St. Luke's Medical Center in Chicago, commenting on the Oregon study, said that the study has implications not only for the blind, who often list sleep problems as one of the most difficult aspects of their disability, but also for sighted people, whose circadian rhythms can be altered by jet lag or shift work.[12]

Melatonin or treatments preserving the rhythm of melatonin formation can retard the rate of aging and the time of onset of age-related diseases, according to studies at the University of Texas Health Science Center at San Antonio. That is because aged animals and humans are melatonin deficient and more sensitive to oxidative stress. New therapies involving the effect of certain amino acid antagonists and stimulants of melatonin synthesis—such as magnesium—may lead to therapeutic approaches for the prevention of diseases related to premature aging.[13]

Since melatonin in over-the-counter supplements is a hormone, its use should be monitored carefully. However, in the dosages recommended in the studies just mentioned, there seems to be no cause for alarm.

References

1. Dawood, Richard, "Bon Voyage . . . but Beware," *Medical and Health Annual* (Chicago: Encyclopaedia Britannica, 1995), 33–34.
2. Comperatore, Carlos A., et al., "Melatonin Efficacy in Aviation Missions Requiring Rapid Deployment and Night Operations," *Aviation, Space, and Environmental Medicine* 67(6): 520–24, June 1996.
3. Croughs, R. J. M., and T. W. A. de Bruin, "Melatonin and Jet Lag," *The Netherlands Journal of Medicine* 49: 164–66, 1996.
4. Hamilton, Kirk, "Aging, Antioxidant Defense, and Melatonin," *The Experts*

Speak (Sacramento, Calif.: Health Associates Medical Group, 1997), 1. Also, Byung P. Yu, "A New Outlook for Antioxidant Defense System," *Aging and Clinical Experimental Research* 7: 338–39, 1995.

5. "Is Melatonin a Dream Drug for Insomnia?" *Family Practice News,* Sept. 1, 1995, 17.

6. Lehmann, E. D., et al., "Somnolence Associated with Melatonin Deficiency After Pinealectomy," *The Lancet* 347: 323, Feb. 3, 1996.

7. McArthur, Angela J., and Sarojinim S. Budden, "Sleep Dysfunction in Rett Syndrome: A Trial of Exogenous Melatonin Treatment," *Developmental Medicine & Child Neurology* 40: 186–92, 1998.

8. de Vries, Marten W., "Melatonin as a Therapeutic Agent in the Treatment of Sleep Disturbance in Depression,"

Journal of Nervous and Mental Disease 185(3): 201–2, 1997.

9. Jan, James E., et al., "Melatonin Treatment of Chronic Sleep Disorders," *Journal of Child Neurology* 13(2): 98, 1998.

10. "Melatonin in Osteosarcoma: An Effective Drug?" *Medical Hypotheses* 48: 523–25, 1997.

11. Leone, M., et al., "Melatonin versus Placebo in the Prophylaxis of Cluster Headache: A Double-Blind Study with Parallel Groups," *Cephalgia* 16: 494–96, 1996.

12. Goode, Erica, "Melatonin Used to Restore Sleep Patterns in Blind People," *New York Times,* June 22, 1999, F6.

13. Poeggeler, B., et al., "Melatonin, Hydroxyl Radical-Mediated Oxidative Damage, and Aging: A Hypothesis," *Journal of Pineal Research* 14: 151–68, 1993.

66

Milk Thistle

Situated under the right side of the diaphragm and underneath the lower ribs, the liver is the largest gland in the human body (the skin is the largest organ in the body). Weighing about 1,500 g, the liver is supplied with blood by the hepatic artery, a branch of the abdominal aorta, and the portal vein, which transfers blood to the liver from the intestines. The main functions of the liver include the formation and breakdown of proteins, fats, and carbohydrates and their storage. Inside the liver, various hormones are broken down; drugs are changed and excreted; amino acids are converted into urea (the end product of protein decomposition) and excreted; bile is secreted; and the fat-soluble vitamins (A, D, E, and K) are stored. Since the liver plays such a significant role in keeping us healthy, it is subject to a variety of diseases (hepatitis, cancer, cirrhosis, etc.). Unlike other tissues, however, the liver can regenerate itself.[1]

The herb milk thistle *(Silybum marianum)* and its main constituent, silymarin, are of great benefit to the liver. The active constituent of silymarin is silybum, which is said to work as an antioxidant by scavenging free radicals and inhibiting lipid peroxidation. Other active ingredients in silymarin are flavonolignans, silydianin, and silychristine, according to Kenneth Flora, M.D., et al., of Oregon Health Sciences University in Portland.[2]

Double-blind studies using silymarin in acute viral hepatitis suggests that it reduces complications, hastens recovery, and shortens hospital stays, Flora said. A typical dosage of silymarin is 140 mg three times daily. In one double-blind trial, 60 patients given psychotropic medications received either 800 mg/day of silymarin or a placebo for 90 days. The researchers reported that silymarin therapy brought improved liver function, regardless of whether the psychotropic drugs were discontinued. In a six-month, double-blind study, researchers evaluated patients who abused alcohol and had histologic documentation of chronic alcoholic hepatitis. Seventeen patients were given either 140 mg of silymarin two times daily or a placebo for six months. This brought positive effects on histology, lymphocyte proliferation, and lipid peroxidation.

In another study, 170 cirrhosis patients who abstained from alcohol greatly improved when treated with silymarin. The treated group received 140 mg of silymarin three times a day. In still another study, 2,600 patients with chronic liver diseases were given 560 mg/day of silymarin for eight weeks; 63 percent reported a resolution in their individual symptoms. No adverse side effects were reported.

Silymarin may be effective in preventing cirrhosis of the liver. When bound to phosphatidylcholine (silibin phytosome), silymarin has a higher bioavailability and thus may have a greater effect than unbound silymarin in preventing the development of alcoholic cirrhosis of the liver. A treatment group was given 450 mg/day of silymarin. While the results versus placebo were not what researchers expected, many in the study group had a coexisting hepatitis C virus infection. Of the patients with hepatitis C who were given silymarin, none died. Of those with hepatitis C who were given a placebo, however, 4 out of 16 died.[3]

In a 12-month study involving 60 insulin-treated diabetics with cirrhosis, silymarin improved not only liver function but also blood sugar control. During the trial, researchers gave the patients either 600 mg/day of silymarin, insulin therapy, or standard therapy alone.[4]

Researchers at University Hospitals of Cleveland in Ohio and Case Western Reserve University, also in Cleveland, found that silymarin protected hairless mice from ultraviolet-B radiation-induced nonmelanoma skin cancer. After exposing the animals to UVB-radiation, 9 mg of silymarin were applied topically; controls received a placebo treatment. At the end of 30 weeks, the silymarin-treated animals showed a 20 percent reduction in the number of tumors compared to the controls. The number of tumors went down by 67 percent. The size of the tumors in the silymarin-treated group went down by 66 percent, compared to the controls. Based on this research, clinical trials exploring the usefulness of silymarin as a protective agent against solar radiation–induced nonmelanoma skin cancers in humans are warranted.[5]

Milk thistle is an antidote to death-cap mushroom poisoning, lanthanides, carbon tetrachloride, and other liver-damaging agents. Silymarin alters the structure of the outer cell membrane of the toxin in such a way as to prevent its penetration into the interior of the cell, and it stimulates the regeneration of the liver and formation of new hepatocytes.[6]

References

1. Brown, J. A. C., *The Stein and Day International Medical Encyclopedia* (New York: Stein and Day, 1971), 278–79.

2. Flora, Kenneth, et al., "Milk Thistle *(Silybum marianum)* for the Therapy of Liver Disease," *American Journal of Gastroenterology* 93(2): 139–43, Feb. 1998.

3. Pares, A., et al., "Effects of Silymarin in Alcoholic Patients with Cirrhosis of the Liver: Results of a Controlled, Double-blind, Randomized, and Multicenter Trial," *Journal of Hepatology* 28: 615–21, 1998.

4. Velussi, M., et al., "Long-Term (12 Months) Treatment with an Antioxidant Drug (Silymarin) Is Effective on Hyperinsulinemia, Exogenous Insulin Need, and Malondialdehyde Levels in Cirrhotic Diabetic Patients," *Journal of Hepatology* 26: 871–79, 1997.

5. Katiyar, Santosh, K., et al., "Protective Effects of Silymarin Against Photo-carcinogenesis in a Mouse Skin Model," *Journal of the National Cancer Institute* 89(8): 556–66, April 16, 1997.

6. Blumenthal, Mark, ed., *The Complete German Commission E Monographs* (Boston: Integrative Medicine Communications and American Botanical Council [Austin, Texas], 1998), 169–70.

67

MSM

Methylsulfonylmethane (MSM) is a naturally occurring sulfur compound found in fruit, vegetables, meat, fish, and milk. Stanley W. Jacob, M.D., who has researched MSM for more than 20 years, has stated that MSM and its related compounds, DMSO (dimethyl sulfoxide) and DMS (dimethyl sulfide), are the sources of 85 percent of the sulfur found in living organisms. The natural level of MSM in the circulatory system of an adult male is about 0.2 ppm, and adults excrete from 4 to 11 mg of MSM daily in urine.

MSM is extracted from DMSO, which has been used since the 1940s as an industrial solvent. In the 1960s, it was promoted as a topical application for strains, sprains, bruises, and arthritis. At one time DMSO was banned by the FDA but was later approved for the treatment of interstitial cystitis (fibrosis of the bladder wall, occurring in women over age 40).[1]

DMSO was initially synthesized in 1866 by Alexander M. Saytzeff, a Russian researcher. He found the substance, a wood-pulp derivative, to be colorless and clear, similar to water. The medical applications for DMSO have been the subject of a number of international conferences, the first in 1965 in West Berlin. Other conferences have been held under the auspices of the New York Academy of Sciences, University of Vienna Medical School, and others. Many years ago it was featured on the TV newsmagazine *60 Minutes*, and has since had a host of proponents and detractors.[2]

Chauncey D. Leake, the famous pharmacologist, stated in 1966 at the New York Academy of Sciences conference, "Rarely has a new drug come so quickly to the judgment of the members of the health profession with so much verifiable data from so many parts of the world, both experimentally and clinically, as to safety and efficacy."

Sulfur is a necessary component of the sulfur-continuing amino acids methionine, cystine, and cysteine. The mineral is found in keratin, the tough protein substance in skin, nails, and hair. It is apparently necessary for the synthesis of collagen. As a component of biotin, the B vitamin, sulfur is required for fat metabolism and as a component of thiamine (B_1) and insulin. It is required for carbohydrate metabolism, and as a component of coenzyme A, it is important in energy metabolism. Sulfur is found in various connective tissues and in glutathione.[3]

Stanley W. Jacob, M.D., and coauthors Ronald M. Lawrence, M.D., Ph.D., and Martin Zucker wrote that MSM is often so effective for pain relief that doctors are able to lower the dosage of medications they prescribe for patients. Occasionally, they are even able to discontinue the medications. MSM is said to bring relief without the many side effects that often result from prescription pain medications.[4]

The authors added, "Clinical experience involving thousands of cases had demonstrated that MSM provides relief in about 70 percent of patients with pain. Given the massive incidence of pain problems in our society, this suggests a huge role for MSM if it were to be recommended by physicians as an addition to their regular treatment for pain. MSM certainly fits the growing demand of patients seeking alternative remedies that do not cause adverse side effects."

MSM is said to relieve many types of pain, including: degenerative wear-and-tear arthritis, rheumatoid arthritis, chronic back pain, chronic headaches, muscle pain, fibromyalgia, tendinitis and bursitis, carpal tunnel syndrome, temporomandibular joint syndrome (TMJ), posttraumatic pain and inflammation, and heartburn.

At Oregon Health Sciences University in Portland, Stanley W. Jacob, M.D., has used both DMSO and MSM for athletic injuries, strained or cramped muscles, and overextended joints, reported Martin Zucker in *Physical*. Because of DMSO's oysterlike odor, many athletes have switched to MSM. According to one personal trainer and former collegiate baseball coach, MSM is "beneficial in a big way." He added, "I have trained with weights since 1979 at a very intense level, and there has never been a time after doing heavy leg work that there wasn't some stiffness and soreness the next day . . . until MSM came along. After only a day or two, I experienced a significant decrease in muscle soreness. This effect has continued ever since I began using MSM daily more than a year and a half ago."[5]

Also in *Physical,* a former champion bodybuilder said, "If you are not taking something like MSM, you often have to take aspirin, ibuprofen, anti-inflammatories, or assorted muscle rubs and creams that only give temporary relief. With MSM, you have a new and important aid against the inevitable muscle soreness that comes with peak intensity training." He finds that 3 to

5 g of MSM works well for him and reduces muscle soreness by about 40 percent.

Steven J. Bock, M.D., codirector of Rhinebeck Health Center for Progressive Medicine in New York and a clinical instructor at Albany Medical College, often prescribes MSM for patients with arthritis, reported Deborah Mitchell. He also gives those patients ginger extracts, glucosamine sulfate, and chondroitin sulfate, suggesting that the right combination of natural remedies is key to successful therapy. Hunter Yost, M.D., an orthomolecular physician in Tucson, Arizona, uses MSM to treat patients with allergies, autoimmune disorders, chronic fatigue syndrome, and arthritis. After testing patients for various nutrients, if he detects a need for sulfur, he prescribes MSM and other nutrients.[6]

The usual dosage for MSM is around 1 or 2 g/day. Consult your health care practitioner. MSM supplements are readily available over the counter in capsules, capsules with glucosamine and vitamin C, lotion with aloe vera, eyedrops, moisturizing cream, shampoo and conditioner, lip balm, toothpaste, medicinal powder, liquids, and other formulations.

References

1. Hendler, Sheldon Saul, *The Doctors' Vitamin and Mineral Encyclopedia* (New York: Simon & Schuster, 1990), 371–72.

2. Halstead, Bruce W., and Sylvia A. Youngberg, *The DMSO Handbook* (Colton, Calif.: Golden Quill Publishers, 1981), 9–11.

3. Ensminger, A., et al., *Foods and Nutrition Encyclopedia* (Clovis, Calif: Pegus Press, 1983), 2071–72.

4. Jacob, Stanley W., Ronald M. Lawrence, and Marin Zucker, *The Miracle of MSM* (New York: G. P. Putnam's Sons, 1999), 3ff.

5. Zucker, Martin, "Blast Muscle Pain with MSM," *Physical,* June/July 1999, 44–48.

6. Mitchell, Deborah, *MSM: The Natural Pain Relief Remedy* (New York: Avon Books, 1999), 129–30.

68

N-Acetylcysteine (NAC)

An amino acid derivative, N-Acetyl-cysteine (NAC) is used in clinical practice to treat acetaminophen overdosing, strengthen the immune system, lower cholesterol, extend the lives of AIDS patients, counteract liver toxicity, and fight infections.

N-Acetylcysteine is the antidote of choice for treating poisoning caused by paracetamol (acetaminophen, such as Tylenol in the U.S.), a drug used to reduce pain and fever. It protects against liver damage by replenishing intracellular glutathione stores and decreasing the binding of acetaminophen to liver proteins. The usual dosage is 10 ml ampoules, which contain 2 g of NAC. It is given as an infusion of 150 mg/kg in 200 ml of 5 percent dextrose water for 15 minutes, and 50 mg/kg in 500 ml of 5 percent dextrose water over four hours, then 100 mg/kg in 1 L of 5 percent dextrose water over 16 hours. This amounts to about 300 mg/kg of NAC over a 20-hour period. Few side effects have been reported. Oral methionine is a glutathione precursor, but it is not as effective as NAC because of vomiting and other complaints. Supportive therapy includes fluids, electrolytes, and vitamin replacement.[1]

Fifty-two hours of intravenous NAC is as effective as 72 hours of oral NAC, reported the *Journal of Pediatrics*. The study involved 25 pediatric patients suffering from acetaminophen poisoning, compared to 29 controls.[2]

Early treatment of acetaminophen overdose with oral or intravenous NAC is highly effective in preventing severe liver damage, according to researchers in England. Oral doses have ranged from 70 to 140 mg/kg, while intravenous doses are usually 50 to 100 mg/kg. Vitamin K is also given to patients with blood-clotting abnormalities caused by liver damage.[3]

NAC may still be of benefit to patients when administered 24 hours after they have swallowed too much acetaminophen. This was determined while New Jersey researchers were evaluating 58 patients who had taken too much of the drug.[4]

A 13-year-old female was admitted to the University of Massachusetts Medical Center in Worcester 19 hours after ingesting two handfuls of Tylenol Extended Relief, a formulation containing 650 mg of time-release acetaminophen per tablet. She was given an oral dose of 140 mg of NAC per kg of body weight, followed by six doses of 70 mg/kg and 11 doses of 100 mg/kg. The patient was sent home clinically well on the fourth day of therapy. The physicians had decided to give larger than usual doses of NAC, since they determined that she had taken a massive overdose.[5]

A study in The Netherlands reported that 600 mg/day of NAC is safe and can be recommended for chemoprevention against lung cancer due to its ability to enhance glutathione, its antioxidant property, its ability to repair DNA, and other modalities.[6]

German researchers gave 600 mg/day of NAC three times daily for five days to 17 nonsmoking patients with severe lung inflammation. Following the therapy, glutathione levels significantly increased in the bronchial fluid. The researchers concluded that NAC supplementation may augment antioxidant protection for patients with pulmonary fibrosis.[7]

In Switzerland, researchers studied 61 patients with mild to moderate acute lung injury and other factors relating to acute respiratory distress, giving them 40 mg/kg/day of NAC or a placebo intravenously for three days. The one-month mortality rate for the NAC group was 22 percent, compared to 35 percent in the controls. At the end of the treatment period, 5 of 29 in the NAC group and 12 of 25 in the placebo group were being given ventilatory support. The lung injury index showed a significant regression in the NAC patients, and no adverse side effects were reported.[8]

Researchers in Munich evaluated 18 patients with fibrosing alveolitis. Inflammation of the alveoli (tiny air sacs in the lungs), often caused by inhaling dust of animal or plant origin, reduces the elasticity of the lungs and impairs breathing. The patients were given 600 mg of NAC three times daily for 12 weeks, along with immunosuppressive therapy. Pulmonary function tests improved significantly with the NAC therapy. NAC should be considered as adjunctive therapy for this condition. One of the patients withdrew from the study due to diarrhea.[9]

NAC has shown protective effects in a variety of cancer experiments, according to researchers at the University of Genoa in Italy. They found that NAC may detoxify carcinogenic compounds, have antioxidant properties, inhibit cancer-causing products, and enhance the thiol concentration in intestinal bacteria. Also, pharmacological amounts of NAC may reduce urinary excretion of mutagens in smokers.[10]

A 45-year-old woman was admitted to the General Infirmary in Leeds, England, suffering from malaise, jaundice, and an enlarged liver. She was diagnosed as having viral myocarditis due to liver dysfunction and was placed on a ventilator. The woman received 150 mg/kg of NAC in 100 ml of 5 percent dextrose by infusion. She continued to get 6.25 mg/kg/hour and was subsequently weaned from the ventilator. After getting an ACE inhibitor, she made a full recovery.[11]

At the University of Milan, researchers reported that in 10 patients with high cholesterol levels, 1,200 to 3,600 mg/day of NAC increased HDL cholesterol by 10 mg/dl, or 16.2 percent. There were no changes in total cholesterol, triglycerides, or lipoprotein-a.[12]

Using a laboratory animal model, researchers at the University of Miami School of Medicine in Florida suggested that NAC should be studied as a possible treatment for hair loss due to chemotherapy.[13]

It is possible that treatment with NAC of HIV-infected patients in the early stages of the infection may help prevent the progression of the disease to full-blown AIDS, according to a research team in Germany. Because 90 percent of the patients they evaluated were in pre-AIDS stages, the supplement is a safe and inexpensive drug that should be considered acceptable therapy.[14]

Since NAC can stimulate glutathione production, supplementation with the nutrient may help AIDS patients to live longer, according to Leonard Herzenberg, Ph.D., and Leonore Herzenberg, Ph.D., of the Stanford University Medical Center in California. They studied 204 HIV-infected patients with no outward signs of illness in the beginning. Those with normal levels of glutathione outlived those with low levels during the three-year follow-up. Glutathione levels and CD4 cell (helper cell) counts can give a more accurate indication of survival than CD4 cell counts alone. When NAC supplements were administered to HIV-positive patients, five deaths occurred by the end of a two- to three-year period, compared to 12 of 19 HIV patients who were not given NAC.[15]

At UCLA Medical Center, researchers reported that NAC may be of benefit to AIDS patients, both adults and children, whose defects in leukocytoxicity may be due to glutathione depletion.[16] With so much valuable research to commend it, it is surprising that N-Acetylcysteine is not more widely used by the medical profession.

References

1. Spearman, C. W., et al., "Paracetamol Poisoning," *South African Medical Journal* 83: 825–26, Nov. 1993.
2. Perry, Holoy, E., and Michael W. Shannon, "Efficacy of Oral Versus N-Acetylcysteine in Acetaminophen Overdose: Results of an Open-Label, Clinical Trial," *Journal of Pediatrics* 132: 149–52, 1998.

3. Thomas, S. H. L., "Paracetamol (Acetaminophen) Poisoning," *Pharmacy Therapy* 60: 91–120, 1993.

4. "Hepatic Transaminase Levels in Acetaminophen Toxicity," *Emergency Medicine,* 1996, 91.

5. Grandins, Andis, et al., "Overdose of Extended-Release Acetaminophen," *New England Journal of Medicine,* July 20, 1995, 196.

6. Zandwijk, Nico van, "N-Acetylcysteine (NAC) and Glutathione (GSH): Antioxidant and Chemopreventive Properties with Special Reference to Lung Cancer," *Journal of Cellular Biochemistry* S22: 24–32, 1995.

7. Meyer, A., et al., "The Effect of Oral N-Acetylcysteine on Long Glutathione Levels in Idiopathic Pulmonary Fibrosis," *European Respiratory Journal* 7: 431–36, 1994.

8. Suter, Peter M., "N-Acetylcysteine Enhances Recovery from Acute Lung Injury in Man: Randomized, Double-Blind, Placebo-Controlled Clinical Study," *Chest* 105: 190–94, 1994.

9. Behr, Jurgen, et al., "Antioxidative and Clinical Effects of High-Dose N-Acetylcysteine in Fibrosing Alveolitis," *American Journal of Respiratory and Critical Care Medicine* 156: 1897–1901, 1997.

10. De Flora, Silvio, et al., "Chemopreventive Properties and Mechanisms of N-Acetylcysteine. The Experimental Background," *Journal of Cellular Biochemistry* S22: 33–41, 1995.

11. Rowbotham, David S., et al., "N-Acetylcysteine Infusion in Viral Myocarditis: A Case Report," *International Journal of Cardiology* 60: 315–16, 1997.

12. Franceschini, G., et al., "Dose-Related Increase of HDL-Cholesterol Levels After N-Acetylcysteine in Man," *Pharmacological Research* 28(3): 213–18, 1993.

13. Jimenez, Joaquin, et al., "Treatment with ImuVert/N-Acetylcysteine Protects Rats from Cyclophosphamide/Cytarabine-Induced Alopecia," *Cancer Investigation* 10(4): 271–76, 1992.

14. Droge, W., et al., "HIV-Induced Cysteine Deficiency and T-Cell Dysfunction—a Rationale for Treatment with N-Acetylcysteine," *Immunology Today* 13(6): 211–14, 1992.

15. "Glutathione May Hold Key to HIV Survival," *Medical Tribune,* March 20, 1997, 25.

16. Roberts, Robert L., et al., "N-Acetylcysteine Enhances Antibody-Depleted Cellular Cytotoxicity in Neutrophils and Mononuclear Cells from Healthy Adults and Human Immunodeficiency Virus–Infected Patients," *Journal of Infectious Diseases* 172: 1492–1503, 1995.

69

NADH

A naturally occurring coenzyme in every living cell, NADH (nicotinamide adenine dinucleotide) is found in meat, poultry, and fish. It is a potent antioxidant form of vitamin B_3 (niacin) and serves as a coenzyme necessary for cellular development and energy production. NADH stimulates cellular production of the neurotransmitters dopamine, noradrenaline, and serotonin and is believed to enhance mental clarity, alertness, and concentration. It is recommended for depression, Alzheimer's disease, Parkinson's disease, chronic fatigue syndrome, and other illnesses.

In 1993, J. G. D. Birkmayer, M.D., Ph.D., of the Birkmayer Institute for Parkinson Therapy in Vienna and a professor at the University of Graz in Austria, isolated the first and only stable oral tablet form of NADH. In an open trial in Austria, 17 patients with dementia of the Alzheimer's type were given 10 mg (2 tablets) of NADH 30 minutes before the first meal. This brought an improvement in cognitive dysfunction in all of the patients. The therapy continued between 8 and 12 weeks, and no side effects were reported.[1] The same researchers, in an open trial of 205 patients suffering from depression, gave the volunteers NADH orally at a dose of 5 mg or intramuscularly or intravenously at a dose of 12.5 mg. The therapy was given from 5 to 310 days. The patients showed a beneficial clinical effect.[2]

In still another study, 885 patients with Parkinson's disease were enrolled in the trial. Half of the volunteers were given NADH by intravenous infusion over 30 minutes, while the others received 5 mg of NADH orally in capsules. Either therapy was given every other day for 14 days.

There was a beneficial clinical effect in about 80 percent of the patients—19.3 percent showed a very good improvement in their disability; 58.8 percent showed a moderate improvement; and 21.8 percent did not respond to NADH therapy. The oral dose of NADH brought an overall improvement in disability, which was similar to that brought by the intravenous form. It was reported that younger patients and patients with a shorter duration of the disease are more likely to respond, compared with older patients or those with a longer duration of the disease.[3]

Researchers at Georgetown University School of Medicine in Washington, D.C., conducted a study involving 26 females ranging in age from 26 to 57 who had suffered from chronic fatigue syndrome from 1 to 16 years. The volunteers were randomly assigned to receive either 10 mg of NADH or a placebo for a four-week trial. Following a four-week break in the protocol, the so-called wash-out period, the women were crossed over to the alternate regimen for the final four weeks.[4]

Eight of the 26 (31 percent) taking NADH achieved significant improvement in the relief of their symptoms. This contrasts with 2 of 26 (8 percent) in the placebo group. No serious side effects were reported by those taking the supplement.

The researchers concluded, "Collectively, the results of this pilot study indicate that NADH may be valuable adjunctive therapy in the management of the chronic fatigue syndrome, and suggest that further clinical trials be performed to establish its efficacy in this clinically perplexing disorder which afflicts 3 out of every 1,000 people."

A study in 1995 among cyclists and long-distance runners found that NADH increased oxygen capacity, decreased reaction time, and improved mental acuity and alertness. Each participant received 5 mg/day of NADH for one month. Five athletes reported improved reaction time by up to 10 percent; eight athletes improved 10 to 20 percent; and three athletes experienced over 20 percent improvement. In a later study, European champion soccer players were given the same amount of NADH for one month. L-dopa levels increased in the blood from 30 to 100 percent. L-dopa is converted to the neurotransmitter dopamine, which is necessary for muscle strength, instinct movements, spontaneous reactions, libido, and emotional drive.[5]

Using spontaneously hypertensive rats, Harry G. Preuss, M.D., and colleagues at Georgetown University Medical Center reported that 5 mg of NADH brought a reduction in blood pressure of 15 mmHg below the control group. The researchers believe NADH can also lower lipid peroxidation in the kidney, which may decrease the rate of progressive kidney failure.[6] Lipids/fats are very susceptible to oxidation, and an antioxidant is necessary to counteract the free radical generation known as peroxidation.

NADH supplements are available over the counter in 2.5 and 5 mg dosages. Studies are continuing on the effectiveness of this versatile supplement. If you are experiencing chronic fatigue syndrome, depression, Alzheimer's disease, Parkinson's disease, or other illnesses, ask your doctor about using NADH. It is also beneficial for athletes.

References

1. Birkmayer, J. G. D., "Coenzyme Nicotinamide Adenine Dinucleotide: New Therapeutic Approach for Improving Dementia of the Alzheimer Type," *Annals of Clinical and Laboratory Science* 26(1): 1–9, 1996.

2. Birkmayer, J. G. D., "The Coenzyme Nicotinamide Adenine Dinucleotide (NADH) as Biological Antidepressive Agent: Experience with 205 Patients," *New Trends in Clinical Neuro-pharmacology,* 1992, 1–7.

3. Birkmayer, J. G. D., et al., "Nicotinamide Adenine Dinucleotide (NADH)— A New Therapeutic Approach to Parkinson's Disease: Comparison of Oral and Parenteral Application," *Acta Neurologica Scand.* 87(Suppl.) 146: 32–35, 1993.

4. Forsyth, Linda M., et al., "Therapeutic Effects of Oral NADH on the Symptoms of Patients with Chronic Fatigue Syndrome," *Annals of Allergy, Asthma, and Immunology* 82(2): 185–91, Feb. 1999.

5. Birkmayer, Georg, *NADH: The Energizing Coenzyme* (New Canaan, Conn.: Keats Publishing, 1998), 25.

6. Preuss, Harry G., et al., "Nutrients and Trace Elements as They Affect Blood Pressure in the Elderly," *Geriatric Nephrology and Urology* 6: 169–79, 1997.

70

Olive Leaf Extract

According to ancient Greek legend, Athena, goddess of war, and Poseidon, god of the sea, were in dispute over a small settlement on a rock in eastern Greece. A jury of gods said they would rule in favor of the one who could most benefit the settlement's inhabitants. Poseidon caused a salt spring to rise from the rock, while Athena produced an olive tree, the first one to be grown. The gods ruled in favor of Athena and her gift of agriculture.[1]

The olive *(Olea europea)* is one of the oldest fruit crops on the planet. Ancient records indicate the limestone hills of Attica, the Greek peninsula, as the location of the tree's first cultivation. In 1769, the Spanish introduced the olive tree to California, where Franciscan missionaries pressed the fruit into oil for cooking and eating and into fuel for lamps.

An extract from olive leaves has been used medicinally for thousands of years, according to Earl Mindell, R.Ph., Ph.D. The leaf contains a biologically active compound, elenolic acid, known for its antibacterial and antiviral constituents. Animal studies have shown that olive leaf extract can lower blood pressure and prevent the oxidation of LDL cholesterol. The extract can be used by those suffering from chronic infections, notably those who have not responded to other therapies, Mindell said.[2]

Robert C. Atkins, M.D., reported that doctors used olive leaf extract as long ago as 1927 to treat malaria. Calcium enolate, one of its constituents, is effective in dispatching viruses and bacteria, and it keeps latent viruses from reappearing. In addition, olive leaf brings relief to those with pneumonia, gonorrhea, tuberculosis, influenza, viral encephalitis, viral meningitis, hepatitis B, shingles, herpes, and Epstein-Barr virus. Olive leaf is also used for treating urinary infections, surgical infections, and yeast infections.[3]

Atkins went on to say that large doses of olive leaf initially may make the patient feel more ill before he feels better, since the killing of microorganisms such as yeast inundates the body with toxins from dying organisms, and the liver has problems dispatching these quickly. When the reaction passes, and the dosage is reduced, the problem usually abates. Atkins minimizes the problem by keeping the dosage to 500 mg/day. He may later increase the amount to 2,000 mg/day, which is usually sufficient. When the infection abates, he reduces the dosage to one or two capsules daily.

In animal experiments, olive leaf has been used as a bronchodilator, to dilate coronary arteries, and as a diuretic for reducing high blood pressure, low blood sugar, and heart irregularities.[4]

Morton Walker, D.P.M., recounted numerous anecdotal cases in which physicians and other health care providers prescribed olive leaf for psoriasis, fibromyalgia, chronic fatigue syndrome, Lyme disease, AIDS, and many other illnesses. He quotes Joseph J. Territo, M.D., of Elmwood Park, New Jersey, as saying, "My experience in using olive leaf extract capsules indicates that patients exhibit an improvement in their psoriasis of up to 70 percent. I've witnessed improvement not only in the reduction of psoriatic scales but also in the skin's redness related to them, and also in a lessening of the inflammatory response."[5]

Territo added, "With the olive leaf capsules taken internally and the olive leaf gel applied topically, my patients have an even greater improvement in their psoriasis lesions—as much as a 75 percent success ratio."

At the Volcani Institute of Agriculture Research, Rehovot, Israel, a research team tested oleuropein, a constituent in olive leaf, and found that the substance effectively killed a bacterium similar to *Streptococcus*. They theorized that oleuropein damaged the bacterial cell membrane, which caused intracellular components like phosphorus, potassium, and glutamate to leak out and damage the cell.[6]

Because of its antioxidant activity, olive leaf extract may offer protection against coronary heart disease, according to a research team at the University of Milan. When LDL cholesterol is exposed to oxygen, it leads to atherosclerotic plaque that contributes to hardening of the arteries and heart disease. The researchers believe that oleuropein blocks LDL cholesterol, thereby protecting vitamin E, which is beneficial in preventing a heart attack.[7]

Walker reported on an anecdotal case in which Bernard Friedlander, D.C., of California used olive leaf extract as a preventive treatment for a 34-year-old woman exposed to genital herpes. The therapy was administered before any lesions appeared. A year later, no herpes lesions had developed and she remained symptom free.[8]

Although olive leaf extract has been used medicinally for thousands of years, it has been only fairly recently that holistic physicians have discovered this beneficial substance. While much of the evidence is anecdotal, there is considerable support for using olive leaf extract for many health problems. Various supplements are available over the counter, so ask your health care provider about this unusual product.

References

1. Ensminger, A., et al., *Foods and Nutrition Encyclopedia* (Clovis, Calif.: Pegus Press, 1983), 1681ff.

2. Mindell, Earl, *Earl Mindell's Supplement Bible* (New York: Simon & Schuster, 1998), 114–15.

3. Atkins, Robert C., *Dr. Atkins' Vita-Nutrient Solution* (New York: Simon & Schuster, 1998), 298–99.

4. Blumenthal, Mark, ed., *The Complete German Commission E Monographs* (Boston, MA: Integrative Medicine Communications and American Botanical Council [Austin, Texas], 1998), 357.

5. Walker, Morton, *Olive Leaf Extract* (New York: Kensington Books, 1997), 84.

6. Juven, B., et al., "Studies on the Mechanism of the Antimicrobial Action of Oleuropein," *Journal of Applied Bacteriology* 35: 559–67, 1972.

7. Visioli, F., and C. Galli, "Oleuropein Protects Low-Density Lipoprotein from Oxidation," *Life Sciences* 55: 1965–71, 1994.

8. Walker, Morton, "Antimicrobial Attributes of Olive Leaf Extract," *Townsend Letter for Doctors and Patients,* July 1996, 80–85.

71

Pantothenic Acid (B$_5$)

Little has been written about pantothenic acid since the death of Roger Williams, Ph.D., of the University of Texas at Austin, the man who discovered it. Sometimes referred to as vitamin B$_5$, pantothenic acid is a constituent of coenzyme A and plays an active role in metabolic processes. Coenzyme A serves in the formation and breakdown of fatty acids and in the entry of fat and carbohydrates into the citric acid cycle, a series of chemical reactions that provide energy for the body.

Won O. Song, Ph.D., of Michigan State University at East Lansing stated that coenzyme A is used by the body to detoxify harmful chemicals found in drugs, herbicides, insecticides, and so forth. She added that pantothenic acid is involved in many different metabolic pathways, including the conversion of food to energy, the synthesis of important hormones, and the body's utilization of body fat and cholesterol. B$_5$ deficiencies are often found in the elderly, in those with a drinking problem, and in people who are taking cholesterol-lowering drugs. Deficiencies include burning feet, loss of appetite, depression, fatigue, insomnia, vomiting, and muscular cramping and weakness.[1]

At Central Hospital, Hong Kong, People's Republic of China, Lit-Hung Leung, M.D., has found pantothenic acid useful in treating both acne vulgaris and obesity. Forty-five males and 55 females with acne were given 10 g (10,000 mg) of pantothenic acid daily plus a cream containing 20 percent by weight of the vitamin, which was applied to the lesions four to six times daily. A noticeable decrease in sebum secretion on the face was evident following two or three days of therapy. After about two weeks, the lesions began

276

to fade in many of the patients. For those with severe acne, it might take six months or longer to control the problem, Leung said. The dosage might have to be increased to 15 to 20 g/day. The vitamin is valuable in this instance because it is related to fat metabolism.

As for obesity, Leung said that the B vitamin may mobilize fatty acids and convert them to fully utilized energy. The study involved 40 males and 60 females ranging in age from 15 to 55 who were confined to a diet of 1,000 calories per day. The volunteers were given 10 g of pantothenic acid in four divided doses, which brought the average weight loss to 1.2 kg per week. Researchers often prescribe vitamin C and the B complex in divided doses, since they are water soluble and readily pass out of the system during the day in urine and feces. The divided doses permit more of the vitamin to do its work before being excreted. The patients experienced no weakness or other side effects while on megadoses of the vitamin. When one's ideal body weight is reached, Leung recommends 2 to 3 g/day of pantothenic acid as a maintenance dose to allow the body to freely mobilize fat into energy.[2]

Pantothenic acid and vitamin C may be the treatment of choice for open wounds, according to a Swiss study of 27 patients undergoing surgery for removal of tattoos. Seventeen of the patients were given 1 g/day of vitamin C and 200 mg/day of pantothenic acid. A control group of 10 received 3 g/day of vitamin C and 900 mg/day of pantothenic acid. The breakdown of scars was higher in those getting the larger amounts of supplements.[3]

Blood levels of pantothenic acid seem to be lower in those with rheumatoid arthritis than in those without the disease, according to Melvyn Werbach, M.D. The more severe the disease, the lower the amounts of the vitamin. In one double-blind study, pantothenic acid supplements brought significant reductions in pain, disability, and the duration of morning stiffness, compared to those getting a placebo. As therapy for rheumatoid arthritis, Werbach recommends a beginning dose of 500 mg/day, increasing to 500 mg four times daily by day 10. Discontinue after two months if no improvement is noticed.[4]

Some time ago, English physicians injected pantothenic acid and royal jelly (the larval food of the queen bee) into 20 patients with rheumatoid arthritis. The patients reported an improvement in their symptoms as long as they took the injections. Royal jelly is the richest natural source of pantothenic acid, as well as a substance called 10-hydroxy-delta 2-decenoic acid. The researchers were later able to combine the two substances so that the patients could take the supplement by mouth.[5]

Hay fever, an allergic reaction to grass, pollen, molds, spores, fumes, and other substances, can sometimes be relieved with nutritional supplements, reported Ralph Golan, M.D. He recommends 500 to 1,000 mg of pantothenic acid two or three times daily; 1,000 to 2,000 mg of vitamin C three times daily; and up to 25,000 IU of vitamin A daily.[6]

Food sources of pantothenic acid include liver, eggs, broccoli, cauliflower, lean beef, skim milk, white and sweet potatoes, tomatoes, and molasses. While there is no recommended dietary allowance for pantothenic acid, the intake recommended by some health care practitioners ranges from 4 to 7 mg/day for adults.

References

1. Feinstein, Alice, ed., *Healing with Vitamins* (Emmaus, Pa.: Rodale Press, 1996, 14–15.

2. Leung, Lit-Hung, "A Stone That Kills Two Birds: Pantothenic Acid in the Treatment of Acne Vulgaris and Obesity," *Journal of Orthomolecular Medicine* 12(2): 99–114, 1997.

3. Vaxman, F., et al., "Can the Wound Healing Process Be Improved by Vitamin Supplementation?—Experimental Study on Humans," *European Surgical Research* 28(4): 306–14, 1996.

4. Werbach, Melvyn, *Healing with Food* (New York: HarperPerennial, 1993), 344–45.

5. Adams, Ruth, and Frank Murray, *Body, Mind, and the B Vitamins* (New York: Larchmont Books, 1981), 145–46.

6. Golan, Ralph, *Optimal Wellness* (New York: Ballantine Books, 1995), 370.

72

Phosphatidylcholine (PC)

Consumers are often confused when buying phosphatidylcholine (PC) supplements, since phosphatidylcholine is the official name for lecithin, and lecithin supplements are also sold over the counter. To further complicate matters, choline, a relative of the B complex of vitamins, is also available in supplement form. To chemists and biochemists, phosphatidylcholine refers to lecithin. PC, the key ingredient in lecithin, is a molecule composed of saturated, unsaturated, and/or polyunsaturated acids, and also contains glycerin, phosphorus, and choline. However, the lecithin sold over the counter is not pure PC, but rather a mixture of phospholipids containing only about 10 to 20 percent pure lecithin. PC is now available as a supplement containing up to 55 percent PC. To avoid further confusion, Sheldon Saul Hendler, M.D., Ph.D., uses the term *phosphatidylcholine*

when referring to pure lecithin, and to the name lecithin when he is discussing the products typically sold in health food stores.[1]

Most commercial lecithin products contain between 10 and 20 percent PC, depending on the manufacturer. It would normally take at least 10 lecithin capsules to provide the amount of PC used in many controlled studies. One commercially available PC product contains 35 percent PC, and is sold in 650-mg softgel capsules. The suggested dosage is six capsules (three in the morning and three in the evening).

Researchers at the University of Frankfurt conducted a double-blind study in which 20 dialysis patients, in two different groups, received either 450 mg of PC tablets morning and evening, for a total dose of 2.7 g/day in six capsules, or a placebo. PC brought a 37.8 mg/dl decrease in total cholesterol within two weeks after therapy began. This decrease remained constant during the treatment period. A 32 mg/dl decrease in LDL cholesterol was also found when compared with controls. After four weeks, triglyceride levels went down by 58.2 mg/dl, and after six weeks, by 43.4 mg/dl.[2]

At United Parma Hospitals in Italy, researchers suggested that PC should be considered as an important support treatment for lipid disorders. In their study, 29 diabetic patients were divided into two groups. In the treatment group, PC was given at a dose of 1,200 mg/day in the form of three 200-mg capsules with two main meals. The PC therapy led to a rapid fall in blood cholesterol, which was apparent after 30 days and statistically significant after 90 days, bringing a 15.1 percent reduction in cholesterol. At 90 days, there was a 13 percent increase in HDL cholesterol, and beginning at 60 days and onward, there was a drop in LDL cholesterol of 20 percent, compared to the controls.[3]

As a building block of cell membranes, PC is an unusually versatile nutrient. Sine alcohol is perhaps the most significant cause of liver damage. Charles Lieber, M.D., of Mount Sinai School of Medicine and the Bronx Veterans Affairs Medical Center in New York, and colleagues studied a group of baboons who were fed sufficient amounts of alcohol to cause liver damage. Half of the animals were then given PC, while the other baboons served as controls. Several years into the study, the PC group had developed early stages of cirrhosis of the liver, but the disorder did not progress further and remained stable for more than six years. Three of the animals developed fatty liver and were taken off the supplement, although they continued to consume alcohol. They soon developed advanced liver damage. Lieber and his associates concluded that PC supplements are an effective deterrent in halting the progression of early-stage alcoholic liver damage to severe cirrhosis.[4]

An Indonesian research team evaluated 101 patients with tuberculosis who had suffered liver damage from rifampicin, an antitubercular agent, and other drugs. The patients were divided into two groups. The treatment group was given 1,350 mg/day of PC, while the control group got a placebo. The PC patients improved considerably with regard to various liver function measures when compared with the control group.[5]

In a double-blind study researchers studied 50 volunteers suffering from hepatitis-B virus and severe liver damage. The treatment group was given 1,350 mg/day of PC, while the controls were given a placebo. After a year, the patients given PC had experienced considerably greater benefits than the controls. That is, 20 of 25 in the PC group were judged to have experienced good to moderately good results, while 6 of 25 in the control group had only moderate improvement. Nineteen patients did not respond. In the treatment group, improvements continued after the trial had ended.[6]

A Japanese study found that a combination of PC and vitamin B_{12} increased acetylcholine concentrations and improved memory as well as learning abilities. In another study, 80 college students were given 25 grams of PC or a placebo. Ninety minutes after ingesting the supplement, there was a significant improvement in learning among the PC-treated students. Since PC improves overall health of the brain, heart, and central nervous and immune systems, it also holds great promise as a supplement for athletes.[7]

For more information on lecithin, see the entry on lecithin in this book.

References

1. Hendler, Sheldon Saul, *The Doctors' Vitamin and Mineral Encyclopedia* (New York: Simon & Schuster, 1990), 258–59.

2. Kirsten, R., et al., "Reduction of Hyperlipidemia with 3-sn-Polyenyl-Phosphatidylchole in Dialysis Patients," *International Journal of Clinical Pharmacology, Therapy, and Toxicology* 27(3): 129–34, 1989.

3. Arsenio, L., et al., "An Investigation into the Therapeutic Effects of Phosphatidylchole in Diabetes with Dyslipidemia," *La Clinica Therapeutics* 114(2): 117–27, July 31, 1985.

4. Lieber, C. S., et al., "Hepatic Phosphatidylethanolamine Methyltransferase Activity is Decreased by Ethanol and Increased by Phosphatidylcholine," *Alcoholism: Clinical and Experimental Research* 18: 592–95, 1994. Also, C. S. Lieber, et al., "Phosphatidylcholine Protects Against Fibrosis and Cirrhosis in the Baboon," *Gastroenterology* 106: 152–59, 1994.

5. Marpaung, B., et al., "Tuberkulostatische Kombinations—Therapie Aus INH, RMP, and EMB," *Therapiewoche* 38: 734–40, 1988. (In German)

6. Ilic, V., and A. Begic-Jamev, "Therapy for HBsAG-Positive Chronically Active Hepatitis: Effect of 'Essential' Phospholipids," *Medical Welt* 85: 523–25, 1991. (In German)

7. Martinez, Carolyn, "PC Helps Athletes Stay Sharp," *Physical*, June/July 1999, 38–42.

73

Phosphatidylserine (PS)

Derived from soy phospholipids, phosphatidylserine (PS) is believed to play a key role in the function of brain cells, helping to maintain or improve cognitive functions. It is also being tested for use on attention deficit disorder (ADD) and attention deficit hyperactivity disorder (ADHD).

T. H. Crook, Ph.D., of the Memory Assessment Clinics in Bethesda, Maryland, in conjunction with researchers from Vanderbilt University School of Medicine, Nashville, Tennessee; Stanford University School of Medicine, Palo Alto, California; and a pharmaceutical company in Italy conducted a study involving 149 volunteers ranging in age from 50 to 75.[1] The participants were given 300 mg/day of PS (100 mg in three equal doses), versus a placebo group, for 12 weeks. Assessments were made periodically during the study as well as during a four-week follow-up after the study ended. PS was well tolerated, and after three weeks of PS therapy, improvements had been made in learning names and faces, recalling names and faces, and recognizing faces. Since this progress was not maintained throughout the 12 weeks of the study, the researchers segregated 57 people into a subgroup who were considerably more memory impaired. Their average age was 64.3 years. While improving in the just-named variables, they also exhibited a significant improvement with PS therapy in telephone number recall, misplaced objects recall, paragraph recall (Wechsler Memory Scale–Logical Memory Subtest), and ability to concentrate while reading, conversing, and performing tasks.

The researchers reported that PS had improved the subgroup's performance by an average of two points in their ability to learn names and faces, essentially "rolling back the clock" roughly 12 years. In other words, from being a cognitive age equivalent to a person of 64, these volunteers were restored, on average, to a cognitive age of 52.

Later, researchers conducted a test involving 51 people ranging in age from 55 to 85, with an average age of 71. A placebo group was also included.[2] In the double-blind, randomized trial, those assigned to the PS group were given 300 mg/day for 12 weeks. At the conclusion of the study, the research team said that the PS-treated volunteers had improved in the following categories: memory of names of familiar people and names of interviewers or clinic staff, recall of the location of frequently misplaced objects, recall of details of events from the previous day, and recall of details of events during the past week.

C. Villardita and colleagues in Italy conducted a double-blind study involving 170 volunteers ranging in age from 55 to 80 years of age, with an average age of 65.7 years. The PS group received 100 mg three times daily, while the controls were given a look-alike pill. The study ran for three months, and a number of neuropsychological tests were administered at 45 days into the study and at the end of the trial.[3] At the end of the 90-day period, 12 of 24 test batteries had reached statistical significance in favor of PS. Also, improvements on the tests for attention and vigilance were said to be significant. PS also considerably improved the participants'

performance on the Rey Auditory Verbal Learning test, which determines immediate recall, and on the Semantic Memory Test, which evaluates immediate and delayed recall.

One of the largest and longest-running studies involved 425 volunteers ranging in age from 65 to 93. They were selected from 23 institutions in northern Italy, and all of the participants had moderate to severe cognitive atrophy.[4] The volunteers were divided into groups. The treatment group received 300 mg/day of PS, and the placebo group got a "nothing" pill for six months. Memory and learning scores were much improved in the PS group, the researchers said.

At the Geriatric Institute for Education and Research and the Department of Geriatrics, Kaplan Hospital, Rehovot, Israel, researchers confirmed that soy-based PS can improve both memory and cognition in healthy seniors.[5] The Israeli researchers established that at the end of the three-month study, the PS group had improved considerably over the placebo group in manipulating information, in visual and number recall, and in mood. The 72 seniors, ranging in age from 60 to 80, had been given 300 mg/day of PS, while the controls received 500 mg/day of lecithin.

Similar results were reported by P. Masturzo and colleagues. They conducted an open, placebo-controlled study involving men who had disturbances in their daily "clocks" (the 24-hour circadian rhythm).

Because of this, some people suffer from depression and the "winter blues" during the dark winter months. PS restored the daily rhythm of thyrotropin hormone secretion, thereby correcting the problem.[6]

Richard A. Kunin, M.D., a physician in private practice in San Francisco, has been conducting a pilot study to determine the efficacy of using PS for ADD and the related ADHD, which involve impaired attention, memory, and behavioral control. Early reports have been encouraging.

"PS is proven compatible with many commonly used drugs," according to Parris Kidd, Ph.D. "It has the potential to safely stimulate a rebalancing of brain functions in ADD/ADHD children, and thereby to provide meaningful clinical benefits for these troublesome disorders."

In 23 published clinical studies, of which 12 were double-blind, there is apparently no danger from long-term use of PS. In a few cases, taking over 200 mg or more as a single dose can lead to nausea in susceptible people because of PS's stimulation of dopamine release. This effect is minimized by taking PS with meals.

PS is available in a variety of potencies in health food stores and other outlets. If you are experiencing memory problems, why not give PS a try? The recommended dose is 300 mg/day for one month and then a maintenance dose of 100 mg/day.

References

1. Crook, T. H., et al., "Effects of Phosphatidylserine in Age-Associated Memory Impairment," *Neurology* 41: 644–49, 1991.
2. Crook, T. H., et al., "Effects of Phosphatidylserine in Alzheimer's Disease," *Psychopharmacology Bulletin* 28: 61–66, 1992.
3. Villardita, C., et al., "Multicentre Clinical Trial of Brain Phosphatidylserine in Elderly Subjects with Mental Deterioration," *Clinical Trials Journal* 24: 84–93, 1987.
4. Cenacchi, B., et al., "Cognitive Decline in the Elderly: A Double-Blind, Placebo-Controlled Multicenter Study on Efficacy of Phosphatidylserine Administration," *Aging and Clinical Experimental Research* 5: 123–33, 1993.
5. Gindin, J., et al., "The Effect of Plant Phosphatidylserine on Age-Associated Memory Impairment and Mood in the Functioning Elderly," *Geriatric Institute for Education and Research*, Rehovot, Israel, unpublished, 1995.
6. Masturzo, P., et al., "TSH Circadian Secretions in Aged Men and Effect of Phosphatidylserine Dosing," *Chronobiologia* 17: 267–74, 1990.

74

Pine Bark Extract

Derived from French maritime pine bark extract, pycnogenol is a versatile supplement containing a rich complex of more than 40 water-soluble antioxidants, including a number of procyanidin compounds and organic acids. Its most notable constituents are proanthocyanidins, a potent subclass of antioxidant flavonoids. It also contains a number of other related organic acids, along with other polyphenols, such as hydroxycinnamic acids, caffeic acid, ferulic acid, gallic acid, and taxifolin. Clinical research has shown that pine bark extract provides protection against heart disease and cancer, jump-starts sperm in subfertile patients, neutralizes free radicals, and contributes a variety of other health-giving properties.

Researchers from the United States and Germany reported at a press briefing during the American Society for Biochemistry and Molecular Biology Annual Meeting, May 19, 1998, in Washington, D.C., that pycnogenol significantly reduced platelet aggregation, a condition in which the smallest blood cells tend to stick together, form clumps, and pave the way for a possible heart attack or stroke.[1]

"Pycnogenol serves as a natural shield, helping to prevent cell aggregation which would restrict the blood supply struggling to move through the narrow arteries," explained Ronald Watson, Ph.D., of the University of Arizona Medical School at Tucson. "Here's a completely natural substance with remarkable activity, producing effects within minutes. It may have enormous health implications for an aging population."

In the study, whose coauthor was Peter Rohdewald, Ph.D., of the University of Muenster in Germany, 39 healthy smokers

(22 in Muenster and 17 in Arizona) were given a single dose of 100 to 120 mg of pycnogenol or 500 mg of aspirin. During the two hours prior to having their blood drawn, the volunteers were allowed to smoke to increase platelet aggregation and blood clumping. The study focused on smokers, since it is easier to measure their dramatically increased clumping of platelets. The results showed that both pine bark extract and aspirin significantly reduced platelet aggregation, but a single, smaller dose of pycnogenol was as effective as a five-times-larger amount of aspirin. This study is of interest to those who are considering taking aspirin to possibly prevent a heart attack but cannot cope with its side effects, such as internal bleeding and stomach problems. While pycnogenol did not increase bleeding, aspirin did.

At the University of South Florida at Tampa, David F. Fitzpatrick, Ph.D., and colleagues conducted a lab experiment in which they determined that French maritime pine bark may accelerate blood flow and thus reduce the risks associated with coronary heart disease. The researchers used rings of the aorta from rats and found that pycnogenol aids in dilating blood vessels, thereby expanding them so that they can transport blood more efficiently. The study also suggested that pine bark extract may well decrease the clumping of platelets that clog arteries, as well as decrease oxidation of low-density lipoprotein cholesterol.[2]

"In our experiments," Fitzpatrick said, "when the aortic ring was placed in a solution with stress hormones, the muscle contracted. But when pycnogenol was added, the contracted muscle relaxed. A series of experiments demonstrated that this was due to an effect of pycnogenol on the endothelial cell layer. Pycnogenol directly stimulates endothelial cells to produce nitric oxide, which is an important blood vessel protective substance."

Ironically, about the time of the Florida experiments, three American pharmacologists were awarded the Nobel Prize in medicine for discovering how nitric oxide can widen blood vessels and help regulate blood pressure.

At the Fourth Annual International Pycnogenol Symposium in 1997, Anthony W. Martin, D.C., Ph.D., of LaSalle University in Canada said that pycnogenol is of great help to those with chronic fatigue syndrome (CFS). The immune disjunction that occurs in CFS, he said, is consistent with free radial damage at the cellular level. As an antioxidant, pycnogenol protects the cell wall from free radical damage. In addition, it strengthens capillaries, which results in improved blood flow to the major organs often affected in CFS patients. It also relieves fibromyalgia symptoms that often debilitate CFS patients. Finally, it reduces histamine secretion, which relieves allergy symptoms common among those with CFS.[3]

Another speaker at the symposium, Lester Packer, Ph.D., of the University of California at Berkeley, said that his studies have shown that pycnogenol can regulate and even inhibit nitric oxide production. Although nitric oxide is essential for some cellular and physiological functions, it can be deleterious in large amounts in the wrong tissue. Nitric oxide has been linked to inflammation, rheumatoid arthritis, and Alzheimer's disease. Pycnogenol provides a sparing effect on vitamin E while undergoing oxidative stress. As a flavonoid complex, pycnogenol provides additional benefits by recycling and regenerating important antioxidants.

Other researchers have demonstrated that nitric oxide can help the body destroy pathogenic bacteria. But as we have seen, excessive amounts can be harmful and lead to heart disease, diabetes, arthritis, stroke, and other illnesses.[4]

Speaking at the 1998 annual meeting of the Oxygen Club of California, Packer stated that pycnogenol can help the immune system fight off infections such as colds and flu by affecting cellular production of nitric oxide. Strict regulation of nitric oxide production is essential to health, including immune defenses against viruses, bacteria, and other parasites.[5]

"Studies have shown that pycnogenol serves two significant functions as both an antioxidant and as a circulation enhancer," Packer said. "As an antioxidant, it protects against free radicals, boosts defenses against disease, and safeguards from environmental stress. As a circulation enhancer, it helps improve circulation, strengthens blood vessels, and delivers oxygen and nutrients throughout the body. And it appears to act in the redox antioxidant network at the interface between vitamin C and vitamin E. In fact, pycnogenol was found to be remarkably effective in extending the effectiveness of vitamin C and to regenerate vitamin E."

Using new analytical technologies, scientists decided to determine whether or not pycnogenol, *ginkgo biloba* extract, green tea, and several other antioxidants would extend the effectiveness of vitamin C. In this experiment, pycnogenol was considerably more effective in delaying the breakdown of vitamin C and helping to "refresh" it.[6]

At the Oxygen Club of California World Congress in 1999, C. Saliou et al. reported that pycnogenol provides protection against ultraviolet radiation in sunlight, which causes undesirable changes in the skin. Free radicals produced from UV radiation can increase the risk of cancer.[7]

Speaking at the 54th Annual Meeting of the American Society for Reproductive Medicine/16th World Congress on Fertility and Sterility in 1998, Scott J. Roseff, M.D., of the West Essex Center for Advanced Reproductive Endocrinology in West Orange, New Jersey, gave a daily supplement of pycnogenol to four subfertile men who had a relatively high number of deformed sperm, as well as low sperm counts and activity, which limited their ability to fertilize an egg. After 90 days of supplementation, the percentage of nondeformed sperm increased by an average of 99 percent in the men. Sperm count and activity remained unchanged.[8] "The increase in structurally normal sperm is significant, although this is just a preliminary study. But pycnogenol could enable some couples to forego expensive in vitro fertilization in favor of simpler and less expensive intrauterine insemination," Roseff said.

Pycnogenol increases endurance time by 21 percent in both men and women during exercise, according to Paul Pavlovic, M.D., Ph.D., of Paradise, California, who addressed the Fifth Annual Meeting of the Oxygen Society in 1998. Pine bark extract protects against damage caused by free radicals during periods of exertion, much like lemon juice prevents a cut apple from turning brown after it is exposed to air. Therefore, athletes, whether professionals or weekend warriors, may improve their performance because the key components in the body are protected and can function more efficiently.[9]

"We need oxygen to survive, but too much can be harmful," Pavlovic continued. "The same can be said for exercise. While physical exercise is necessary in maintaining good health, we must manage the increased production of free radicals created during exercise. This increase often leads to oxidative damage in muscle, blood, liver, and other tissues, and this damage could conceivably counter the effect of even a moderate training program by reducing the muscle's ability to repair itself."

In the study, codirected by David Swanson, Ph.D., of California State University at Chico, 24 healthy men and women were assigned to a double-blind, crossover study. Group 1 received 100 mg of pycnogenol twice daily for four weeks, followed by a placebo for four weeks. Group 2 was given a placebo for four weeks and then the same amount of pycnogenol for four weeks. Analyzing the data after the study ended, the researchers found that pycnogenol significantly increased endurance by 21 percent when compared to controls.

A. W. Martin, D.C., Ph.D., wrote that pycnogenol is an antioxidant that is 50 times more powerful than vitamin E and 20 times more potent than vitamin C. As a "saturation dose," he recommends 25 mg for every 25 pounds of body weight. A 100-pound person would take four tablets daily; a 150-pound person would need six tablets a day. As a maintenance dose, he suggests 50 mg/day.[10]

As a chiropractor and practicing nutritionist, Martin uses varying amounts of pycnogenol in his practice. For attention deficit disorder, saturation dose for 7 to 10 days, then 50 mg/day; for asthma and allergies, saturation dose for 7 to 10 days (for asthma, extend to six weeks), then 50 to 100 mg/day; for arthritis, saturation dose for six weeks, then 100 mg/day; for colds and flu, 200 to 300 mg/day at first sign of infection, then return to maintenance dose; for chronic fatigue syndrome and fibromyalgia, saturation dose for six weeks, followed by the same therapy for one to two years; for cardiovascular disease, saturation dose for six weeks, then maintenance dose of 100 mg/day; for leg cramps, saturation dose for 10 days, then maintenance dose of 50 mg/day; for premenstrual syndrome, saturation dose for six weeks, then maintenance dose of 100 mg/day; for varicose veins, saturation dose for 10 days, followed by maintenance dose of 100 mg/day.

References

1. Watson, Ronald, et al., "Pycnogenol Inhibits Platelet Aggregation In Vivo," paper presented at American Society for Biochemistry and Molecular Biology Annual Meeting, Washington, D.C., May 20, 1998.

2. Fitzpatrick, David F., et al., "Endothelium-Dependent Vascular Effects of Pycnogenol," *Journal of Cardiovascular Pharmacology* 33(4): 509–15, 1998. Also, Michael Hoad, "Nutritional Supplement Extracted from French Maritime Pine Bark May Reduce Risks Associated with Heart Disease," USF News Release, University of South Florida, Tampa, Oct. 1998.

3. Martin, Anthony W., "Pycnogenol—Chronic Fatigue Syndrome," paper presented at Fourth Annual International Pycnogenol Symposium, May 4–7, 1997, Biarritz, France. Also, Lester Packer, "Nitric Oxide and Pycnogenol," ibid.

4. Virgili, F., et al., "Pyrocyanidins Extracted from Pinus Maritima (Pycnogenol): Scavengers of Free Radical Species and Modulators of Nitrogen Monoxide Metabolism in Activated Murine Raw 264.7 Macrophages," *Free Radical Biology and Medicine* 24: 1120–29, 1998.

5. Packer, Lester, "Cold and Flu Sufferers Take Note: Pycnogenol May Help Immune System," paper presented at Oxygen Club of California/1998 World Congress, Santa Barbara, California, Feb. 5–8, 1998.

6. Cossins, E., et al., "ESR Studies of Vitamin C Regeneration, Order of Reactivity of Natural Source Phyto-chemical Preparation," *Biochemistry and Molecular Biology International* 45: 583–97, 1998.

7. Saliou, C., et al., "French Pinus Maritima Bark Extract Prevents Ultraviolet-Induced NF-kB-Dependent Gene Expression in a Human Keratinocyte Cell Line," paper presented at Oxidants and Antioxidants in Biology/Oxygen Club of California World Congress, Santa Barbara, California, March 3–6, 1999.

8. Roseff, Scott J., et al., "Pycnogenol May Keep Sperm from Getting Bent Out of Shape," paper presented at 54th Annual Meeting of the American Society for Reproductive Medicine/16th World Congress on Fertility and Sterility, San Francisco, California, Nov. 11, 1998.

9. Pavlovic, Paul, "Pycnogenol Increases Endurance During Exercise by 21 Percent," paper presented at Fifth Annual Meeting of the Oxygen Society, Washington, D.C., Nov. 17, 1998.

10. Martin, A. W., *The Truth About Pycnogenol* (Timmins, Ontario, Canada: R&T Press, 1996), 100ff.

75

Pyruvate

Pyruvic acid/pyruvate, an organic three-carbon acid that is a key intermediate in carbohydrate, fat, and protein metabolism, is involved in a number of metabolic processes in the body. For example, it can complete oxidation to water and carbon dioxide in the Krebs cycle; serve in the formation of a fatty acid; aid in the conversion of the amino acid alanine; and help in the formation of glucose by reversing the enzymatic sequence that normally breaks down glucose. Named after Sir Hans Adolph Krebs, a German biochemist working in England, the Krebs cycle supports energy production by the mitochondria, the cell's powerhouses. Also called citric acid cycle, it provides energy for storage in phosphate bonds such as adenosine triphosphate (ATP).[1]

Pyruvic acid is essentially a by-product of energy metabolism of a sugar or starch. Since pyruvic acid is usually not suitable as a supplement, it is often stabilized in combination with calcium, magnesium, sodium, or potassium to form a salt called pyruvate. Clinical studies have shown that pyruvate can promote weight loss, enhance fat loss, increase exercise endurance, decrease fatigue, inhibit the formation of free radicals, and possibly increase muscle mass.[2]

Earl Mindell, R.Ph., Ph.D., reported that in one study, obese women were placed on a low-fat diet and then given either pyruvate supplements or a placebo. After three weeks of therapy, women in the treatment group had lost 37 percent more weight and almost 50 percent more fat than the controls. In another study, athletes using pyruvate were less tired and were able to increase their performance by 20 percent compared to those not taking the supplement. As a sports supplement,

Mindell recommends six to eight 500-mg tablets daily before exercise or eating. For weight loss, he suggests at least 4,000 mg/day.[3]

Although pyruvate supplementation increases the natural body levels by about 5 to 10 times, it is a natural supplement found in the body's heart, brain, and liver, according to Ronald T. Stanko, M.D. Since it has no side effects and is found in our bodies and diets at all times, it should be considered an enhancing, rather than a doping, agent. Gymnastic champion Shannon Miller trained with pyruvate supplements prior to winning a gold medal in the 1996 Olympic Games in Atlanta. She reportedly could train harder and longer with the supplement, but did not use it during competition.[4]

Stanko went on to say that preliminary trials and many anecdotal reports suggest an improved capacity for exercise in the untrained, "normal" population using pyruvate. Reports have shown that pyruvate increases the ability to lift weights, run, and do sit-ups.

A research team in Greenwich, Connecticut, conducted a six-week, double-blind study involving 28 men and 25 women. The volunteers received 6 g of pyruvate per day in a proprietary weight-loss supplement while consuming a 2,000-calorie diet. The participants also were given zinc, vitamin B_6, herbs, and dihydroxyacetone, a substance that pyruvate was paired with in prior studies. The volunteers exercised for 30 minutes, five days a week. A second group followed the same procedure but took a placebo. A third group received no additional supplements. In the pyruvate-treated group, there was a drop in percentage of body fat from 21 to 18 percent. Participants lost almost 5 pounds during the trial, and there was a 3.4-pound gain in lean body mass. No change regarding fat was observed in the control or placebo groups.[5]

At the University of Pittsburgh Medical Center, researchers evaluated 34 volunteers with high cholesterol levels. After consuming a low-cholesterol, low-fat diet for four weeks, the participants were given daily doses of either 22 to 44 g of pyruvate or 18 to 35 g of polyglucose as a placebo. Seventeen volunteers were in each study group. Results showed that there was no difference in blood levels of cholesterol, LDL cholesterol, HDL cholesterol, and triglycerides between the two groups. While the pyruvate supplement did not have any effect on plasma lipid concentrations, it did enhance body weight and fat losses.[6]

In an earlier study, the same researchers, this time at Montefiore University Hospital in Pittsburgh, found that pyruvate supplementation of a high-fat, high-cholesterol, anabolic diet does decrease blood levels of total cholesterol and LDL-cholesterol concentrations. The study involved 40 people with high cholesterol levels who were randomly given either 36 or 53 g of pyruvate or 21 or 37 g of polyglucose, the placebo, for six weeks as a portion of carbohydrate energy. There was no change in the placebo group, but there was a 4 to 5 percent respective reduction in the pyruvate group in total cholesterol and LDL cholesterol. No change was found in HDL cholesterol or triglyceride levels in either group. Resting heart rate, diastolic blood pressure, and rate-pressure product were reduced by 9, 6, and 12 percent, respectively, in the pyruvate volunteers.[7]

Pyruvate triggers the release of ATP, the fuel that energizes the body. It has also been found to lower blood pressure and cholesterol levels in the body. Dosages as low as 5 g/day have been beneficial. Few side effects have been reported, but it is not recommended for children or pregnant women.[8]

Retail outlets have a variety of pyruvate supplements available over the counter. Some foods contain rather high levels of pyruvate, including fruits, vegetables, cheeses, beer, wines, and fermented foods. Most foods have less than 25 mg per serving, however.

References

1. Ensminger, A., et al., *Foods and Nutrition Encyclopedia* (Clovis, Calif: Pegus Press, 1983), 1892.

2. "Pyruvate," *Whole Foods Magazine*, Aug. 1998, section II.

3. Mindell, Earl, R.Ph., *Earl Mindell's Supplement Bible* (New York: Simon & Schuster, 1998), 130–31.

4. Stanko, Ronald T., and Laura O'Hare, *The Power of Pyruvate* (Los Angeles: Keats Publishing, 1999), 53–54.

5. Antonio, Jose, "Pyruvate Update," *Physical/Let's Live*, May 1998, 2–3.

6. Stanko, Ronald T., et al., "Pyruvate Supplementation of a Low-Cholesterol, Low-Fat Diet: Effects on Plasma Lipid Concentrations and Body Composition in Hyperlipidemic Patients," *American Journal of Clinical Nutrition* 59: 423–27, 1994.

7. Stanko, Ronald T., et al., "Plasma Lipid Concentrations in Hyperlipidemic Patients Consuming a High-Fat Diet Supplemented with Pyruvate for Six Weeks," *American Journal of Clinical Nutrition* 56: 950–54, 1992.

8. Mindell, Earl, *Earl Mindell's Vitamin Bible for the 21st Century* (New York: Warner Books, 1999), 341.

76

Quercetin

Quercetin, a bioflavonoid, is a jack-of-all-trades: it functions as an antioxidant to destroy free radicals while protecting us in many other ways.

According to Bozidar Stavric, intensive studies of quercetin in a variety of disciplines have found that it is antimicrobial and inhibits tumor promotion by chemical cancer-causing agents. In addition, it decreases capillary fragility, protects against diabetic cataracts, has antiviral and antiallergic activity, inhibits platelet aggregation and thrombotic activity, and has been used as an anti-inflammatory agent. Some studies have suggested quercetin's benefit in the treatment of squamous cell cancers and acute leukemia. Quercetin and its glycoside, rutin, have been used to treat a number of medical problems throughout the world. Together, they have sometimes been referred to as vitamin P. Stavric added that the consumption of quercetin as part of a regular diet does not induce any health problems and may in fact contribute to the reduction of risk for cancers and other chronic diseases.[1]

At the National Institute of Public Health and Environmental Protection in Bilthoven, The Netherlands, a research team followed 552 men, 50 to 69 years of age, for up to 15 years. During that time, 42 cases of first fatal or nonfatal stroke were documented. Dietary flavonoids, predominantly quercetin, were inversely associated with stroke incidence. The researchers suggested that regular flavonoid consumption may protect against stroke. About 70 percent of the flavonoid intake in the study came from black tea.[2]

In a laboratory setting, Japanese researchers found that quercetin, along with tumor necrosis factor, enhanced antiviral activity against vesicular stomatitis virus, which originates in animals, and encephalo-myocarditis virus, a viral disease characterized by degeneration and inflammation of skeletal and cardiac muscle and lesions of the central nervous system. Tumor necrosis factor is a protein that activates leukocytes (white blood cells) and has antitumor activity.[3]

Researchers in Canada, in a lab experiment, evaluated the effects of three plant polyphenols—quercetin, ellagic acid, and chlorogenic acid—against two carcinogens, benzo(a)pyrene and 2-amino-3-methylimidazol quinoline. The flavonoids had a protective effect against the cancer-causing agents not only at a cellular level, but also by reducing their bioavailability. Animal studies have demonstrated that polyphenols such as quercetin can hinder the uptake of some cancer-causing agents from the gastrointestinal tract.[4]

An in vitro study at the School of Medicine and Biomedical Sciences in Buffalo, New York, found that two flavonoids—quercetin and fisetin—along with vitamin C, significantly impaired the growth of human squamous cancer cells. Although vitamin C had no effect on cellular proliferation in this study, the antiproliferative effect may be due to the vitamin's ability to protect the two flavonoids against oxidative destruction.[5] The flavonoids and vitamin C are closely related and are often found together in nature.

As a dietary antioxidant flavonoid, quercetin has properties that inhibit cancer-causing substances. In evaluating the absorption of quercetin in the small intestine after the ingestion of onions, quercetin rutinoside (rutin), and quercetin aglycone, researchers found absorption was 52, 17, and 24 percent, respectively. The bioavailability from apples and rutinoside was one-third that of onions.[6]

In a laboratory experiment, quercetin was shown to reduce the bioactivation of certain pro-carcinogens. The flavonoid detoxified reactive oxygen species in cells, and some of its other characteristics contributed to its anticarcinogenic effects.[7]

Fruits and vegetables, all rich sources of flavonoids and antioxidants, provide a defense against free radicals, which are implicated in cancer, heart disease, and other health problems. Writing in *Clinical Biochemistry*, Stavric reviewed the many chemoprevention substances in the human diet, particularly the flavonoids quercetin and myrecetin in *ginkgo biloba*.[8]

Because quercetin and other flavonoids are scavengers of free radicals and other deleterious substances, they inhibit the oxidation of LDL cholesterol. Researchers have long suggested that an increase in flavonoid consumption will reduce the risk of cardiovascular disease.[9]

Quercetin supplements stabilize the membranes of cells that release histamine, the mediator of many allergic reactions, according to Andrew Weil, M.D. He recommends a dosage of 400 mg twice daily between meals. Since quercetin is a preventive and not a symptomatic treatment, it is best to use it regularly, Weil said. If you have seasonal allergies, start taking the flavonoid several weeks before you expect the onset of symptoms. Otherwise, take it for two or three months and then gradually reduce the dose to see if the improvements are maintained.[10]

Diabetics are prone to cataracts at an early age because the disease accelerates free radical damage, wrote Ronald L. Hoffman, M.D. Elevated insulin levels are associated with free radical production and with lipid peroxidation, which is a measure of free radical activity in the blood. One form of diabetes-specific-type cataracts is caused by the deposition of sorbitol, a sugar, in the eye. In diabetics, both sorbitol and fructose can be deposited in the eyes, causing nerve and lens damage. Scientists have been searching for a substance that could act as an aldose-reductase inhibitor and inhibit the conversion from glucose to sorbitol. Such a substance is the bioflavonoid quercetin. Designer drugs have been tested, but so far quercetin, a natural agent, is the best recommendation. Hoffman recommends 1,000 to 5,000 mg/day of quercetin to protect diabetics.[11]

Quercetin is available from a variety of sources in the diet, including onions, buckwheat, tea, apples, red cabbage, grapes, green beans, citrus fruits, red wine, kale, and cherries. The average diet probably contains only about 25 mg/day of quercetin.

References

1. Stavric, Bozidar, "Quercetin in Our Diet: From Potent Mutagen to Probable Anticarcinogen," *Clinical Biochemistry* 27: 245–47, Aug. 1994.

2. Keli, Sirving O., "Dietary Flavonoids, Antioxidant Vitamins and Incidence of Stroke: The Zupthen Study," *Archives of Internal Medicine* 157: 637–42, March 25, 1996.

3. Ohnoshi, Eiko, and Hisaichi Bannai, "Quercetin Potentiates Tumor Necrosis Factor–Induced Antiviral Activity," *Antiviral Research* 22: 327–31, 1993.

4. Stavric, B., and T. I. Matula, "Flavonoids in Foods; Their Significance for Nutrition and Health," *Lipid Soluble Antioxidants: Biochemistry and Clinical Applications,* 1992, 274–94.

5. Kandaswami, Chithan, et al., "Ascorbic Acid–Enhanced Antiproliferative Effect of Flavonoids on Squamous Cell Carcinoma In Vitro," *Anticancer Drugs* 4(1): 91–96, Feb. 1993.

6. Hollman, Peter C. H., et al., "Bioavailability of the Dietary Antioxidant Flavonol Quercetin in Man," *Cancer Letters* 114: 139–40, 1997.

7. Musonda, C. A., et al., "Effects of Quercetin on Drug Metabolizing Enzymes and Oxidation of 2, 7-Dichlorofluroscin in HepG2 Cells," *Human and Experimental Toxicology* 16: 700–08, 1997.

8. Stavric, Bozidar, "Role of Chemopreventers in Human Diet," *Clinical Biochemistry* 27(5): 319–32, 1994.

9. Alberico, L., "Antioxidant Effect of Flavonoids," *Angiology* 48(1): 39–44, Jan. 1997.

10. Weil, Andrew, *Spontaneous Healing* (New York: Alfred A. Knopf, 1995), 254.

11. Hoffman, Ronald L., *Intelligent Medicine* (New York: Simon & Schuster, 1997), 359, 366.

77

Red Clover

In the early part of the 20th century, a variety of "Trifolium compounds" were sold to treat venereal disease and other health problems. One of these extracts, from red clover *(Trifolium pratense),* was marketed by the Wm. S. Merrell Chemical Company in Cincinnati, Ohio. Although the American Medical Association remained skeptical about the use of red clover for medicinal purposes, the herb remained in the *National Formulary* until 1946. Red clover was one of the many herbs included in the notorious Huxley Clinic cancer treatment.[1]

Although red clover has remained a favorite of many herbalists over the years, renewed interest in the herb surfaced in the 1940s, when researchers in Australia detected a condition known as clover disease in sheep. The animals were essentially infertile because of the large amounts of estrogenic isoflavones in their diet. Since estrogens and estrogenlike compounds can stop ovulation in very high doses (as in oral contraceptives), the animals could not become pregnant.[2]

Tracing the problem to subterranean clovers, scientists then found that other members of the clover family, including red clover, contained the isoflavones, as do soy, chickpeas, lentils, and other plants. Isoflavones are the most important type of phytoestrogen in the diet. Of the 1,000 or so isoflavones found in plants, four have estrogenic effects: genistein, biochanin, daidzein, and formononetin. Soy contains two of these (genistein and daidzein), and red clover contains all four.

It has been known for some time that plant estrogens function in the body like steroidal estrogens. Although plant estrogens are weaker than the steroidal estrogens produced by the ovaries, they are found in the body at levels hundreds of times greater than those of steroidal estrogens. Many researchers believe that the plant estrogens, such as those found in red clover, hold the key to the riddle of the lower incidence of menopausal symptoms in various countries around the world compared to Western countries. Plant estrogens provide a supplementary source of estrogens, which help to soften the beginning of menopause and lead to fewer short-term problems like hot flashes and fewer long-term problems such as heart disease and osteoporosis.[3]

Red clover contains between 1 and 2.5 percent isoflavones. Since the herb is rich in phytoestrogens, which act in the body in the same way as the female hormone estrogen, its constituents minimize menstrual cramps by bringing the body's hormone levels into better balance.[4]

In a study at the Royal Hospital for Women in Sydney, researchers evaluated three groups of women consisting of 12 women each, who received either a placebo; one tablet of red clover isoflavone extract; or four tablets of the extract daily. The treatment period was three months. In a second study at Royal North Shore Hospital in Sydney, 86 women were allocated to two groups of 43 women each. Group 1 was given a placebo, while Group 2 got one tablet of red clover extract daily. The study lasted for three months.[5] In all groups in both trials, there was a significant improvement in both incidence and severity of hot flashes. There was no significant difference between placebo and treatment groups in terms of clinical response in hot flash incidence and severity, but there was a very strong correlation between clinical response in the incidence of hot flashes and urinary levels of isoflavones. In other words, increasing urinary levels of isoflavones meant a strong alleviation of hot-flash symptoms. The women getting only one red clover tablet had a significant increase of 18.1 percent in HDL cholesterol.

Another study at Royal North Shore Hospital evaluated 43 menopausal women who were given either a placebo or a red clover supplement. While there were no discernible differences between the two groups, there was a positive correlation between increasing levels of urinary daidzein and menopausal symptoms. This indicated that daidzein is the active isoflavone metabolite in alleviating menopausal symptoms.[6]

All isoflavonoids are weak estrogens, and these amounts could have biological effects, especially in postmenopausal women with low estrogen levels. High levels of isoflavonoid phytoestrogens may partly explain why hot flashes and other menopausal symptoms are so infrequent in Japanese women due to their high intake of soy (tofu, miso, etc.).[7]

Red clover is being tested for a variety of health conditions. Researchers at the Baker Medical Institute and Latrobe University in Melbourne, Australia, conducted a test in which menopausal women were given 40 mg/day and later 80 mg/day of isoflavones from red clover. Arterial compliance, as measured by ultrasound on the carotid artery and blood flow into the aorta rose by 23 percent with the 80-mg dose of red clover and slightly less with the 40-mg dose. An important cardiovascular risk factor that diminishes with menopause, arterial compliance was significantly improved with red clover isoflavones.[8]

Lignans and isoflavones from dietary sources seem to play a role in the prevention of several types of cancer. By inhibiting the effect of growth factors and angiogenesis, genistein—found in red clover and soy, among other products—may be a more important inhibitor of cancer growth. Lignans and isoflavones may also provide protection against cardiovascular diseases and osteoporosis due to their estrogenic and antioxidative effects.[9]

At Queen Elizabeth II Medical Centre, Perth, Western Australia, David Ingram, M.D., and associates stated that there is a substantial reduction in breast cancer risk among women with a high intake (as measured by excretion) of phytoestrogens, especially the isoflavonoic phytoestrogen equol and the lignan enterolactone.[10]

Frederick O. Stephens, M.D., and colleagues at the Royal Prince Alfred Hospital in Sydney stated that concentrated phytoestrogens taken by a 66-year-old male for one week prior to a prostate operation resulted in certain changes in prostate cancer typical of those seen in patients treated with estrogens and regarded as histological evidence of tumor regression. These and other findings suggest that dietary phytoestrogens may be at least partly responsible for the lower incidence of prostate cancer in areas with high dietary phytoestrogen content. Stephens suggested that adding phytoestrogen products to a Western diet may provide protection against prostate cancer.[11]

A study at the University of Sydney found that phytoestrogens are precursors of biologically active, hormonelike compounds. These phytoestrogens are converted by intestinal bacteria into compounds with weak estrogenic activity and some antiestrogen and antioxidative activity, with the two most active components being genistein and daidzein. These compounds influence not only sex hormone metabolism, but also intracellular enzyme protein synthesis growth factors and malignant cell proliferation, differentiation, and angiogenesis. Thus, they perhaps have an overall anticancer protective function with a special role in preventing breast cancer.[12]

For menopausal complaints, the suggested dosage of red clover extract is one 40-mg tablet daily. It is available over the counter. Each tablet contains 40 mg of isoflavones, including genistein and daidzein. Another 40-mg tablet of red clover is available over the counter for treating prostate problems.

References

1. Foster, Steven, and Varro E. Tyler, *Tyler's Honest Herbal* (New York: Haworth Press, 1999), 315–17.

2. Kelly, Graham, *Isoflavones* (North Ryde, NSW, Australia: Novogen, Nov. 1997).

3. Brown, Donald, et al., *Clinical Applications of Natural Medicine: Menopause.*, monograph (Seattle: Natural Product Research Consultants, 1997).

4. Duke, James A., *The Green Pharmacy* (Emmaus, Pa.: Rodale Press, 1997), 325, 328.

5. Kelly, Graham, op. cit.

6. Baber, Rod, et al., "A Study of Clover Extract as a Treatment of Menopausal Symptoms," paper presented at the First Australian Menopause Society Congress, Oct. 26–29, 1997, Perth, Australia.

7. Adlercreutz, Herman, et al., "Dietary Phyto-Oestrogens and the Menopause in Japan," *The Lancet* 339(8803): 1233, May 16, 1992.

8. Nestel, Paul J., et al., "Isoflavones from Red Clover Improve Systemic Arterial Compliance but Not Plasma Lipids in Menopausal Women," *Journal of Clinical Endocrinology and Metabolism* 84(3): 895–98, 1999.

9. Adlercreutz, Herman, "Phytoestrogens: Epidemiology and a Possible Role in Cancer Protection," *Environmental Health Perspectives* 103(Suppl. 7): 103–12, 1995.

10. Ingram, David, et al., "Case-Control Study of Phyto-Oestrogens and Breast Cancer," *The Lancet* 350(9083): 990–94, Oct. 4, 1997.

11. Stephens, Frederick O., "Phytoestrogens and Prostate Cancer: Possible Preventive Role," *Medical Journal of Australia* 167(3): 138–39, Aug. 4, 1997.

12. Stephens, F. O., "Breast Cancer: Aetiological Factors and Associations (A Possible Protective Role of Phytoestrogens)," *Australian and New Zealand Journal of Surgery* 67(11): 755–60, Nov. 1997.

78

Red Wine

Researchers have long attempted to explain the "French paradox": why the French have a lower-than-expected rate of mortality from coronary heart disease (CHD) in a society that enjoys a diet rich in fats and saturated fats. It has been suggested that the low prevalence of ischemic heart disease in France resembles that of the Mediterranean countries, where the amount of fats in the diet is much lower. Epidemiologists say the low disease rates in France may be linked to the consumption of certain foods. Thus far, the French paradox has been linked with the consumption of the phenolic compounds in red wine, monounsaturated olive oil, and foie gras.[1]

At California State University at Fresno, researchers attempted to explain the French paradox as it relates to the consumption of wine. They suggested that the antioxidants in wine, such as resveratrol, quercetin, and epicatechin, reduce LDL cholesterol and provide protection against cardiovascular disease. Wine and grape components also contain vasorelaxants, which reduce tension in blood vessel walls. Moderate alcohol consumption may reduce LDL cholesterol and also cut the risk of CHD.[2]

The California researchers also reported that both red and white wine are excellent sources of salicylic acid and its metabolites, which contain vasodilators as well as several anti-inflammatory properties. Salicylic acid is a crystalline phenolic compound found in aspirin. However, white wine, which has less salicylic acid than red wine, has double the widely recommended daily dose of 30 mg of aspirin to provide cardiovascular protection. There may be synergistic effects from the antioxidants and the wine's salicylic acid constituents, and the alcohol in the wine may actually enhance antioxidant absorption from the intestinal tract.

Two plant scientists at Cornell University in Ithaca, New York, have identified resveratrol as the chemical in wine that is responsible for lowering levels of cholesterol in wine drinkers. Resveratrol is the same natural compound that grapes use to fight fungal diseases, according to Leroy Creasy and Evan Siemann, who published their findings in the February 1992 issue of the *American Journal of Enology and Viticulture*. Creasy and Siemann zeroed in on resveratrol based on Japanese studies they had read. One Japanese article, written nearly 10 years ago, described how resveratrol had been identified as an active ingredient in Chinese and Japanese folk medicine. In fact, resveratrol was responsible for the medicinal effects of Japanese knotweed, a folk remedy used since ancient times to lower high levels of fatty substances in the blood.[3]

The Cornell scientists found that red wines from Bordeaux were very high in resveratrol, whereas white Bordeaux wines were low in the substance. After analyzing some 30 wines, they found that some have almost 200 times more resveratrol, with red wines tending to have higher levels. Chardonnay wines from New York had, on average, three times more resveratrol than Chardonnay wines from California. Higher levels are expected in red wine because it comes primarily from the grape skins, which

remain during the fermenting process. White wines are fermented without grape skins.

"We suspect the New York wines have higher levels of resveratrol because the grapes are under much more disease pressure than in California," Creasy said. "That means that the New York plants have to produce more resveratrol to fight off fungal infections."

At Universita degli Studi di Padova in Italy, researchers reported that some wines contain more resveratrol than others. The phenolic substance may increase the production of HDL cholesterol.[4] Resveratrol, found in peanuts as well, may be the antioxidant substance that reduces the biological processes that are risk factors for cardiovascular disease, according to scientists at Banting Institute at Toronto.[5]

Using the Lyon Diet Heart Study, researchers in the United Kingdom investigated whether a Mediterranean diet might be better than a prudent Western diet. They found that platelet aggregation, which might provoke a heart attack, was low in the Mediterranean group based on diet and in the Western group based on intake of wine. Thus, populations in the south of France may be protected by the Mediterranean diet, while the rate of heart disease in the northern part of the country may be reduced by intake of wine.[6]

A study in Israel found that red wine was more effective in lowering LDL cholesterol than white wine, probably because it enhanced the polyphenol concentration in the blood plasma. The study involved 17 volunteers who were divided into two groups. One group of eight was given 400 ml of red wine daily for two weeks, while the remaining nine got a similar amount of white wine. Red wine resulted in a 20 percent reduction in the likelihood of blood plasma undergoing lipid peroxidation, as well as reducing the propensity of LDL oxidation. White wine ingested for two weeks brought a 34 percent increase in the likelihood of lipid peroxidation in plasma, and a 41 percent increase in the propensity of LDL to undergo lipid peroxidation.[7]

While red wine and grape juice may provide protection against cardiovascular disease, red wine may provide more protection, since its flavonoid content is primarily quercetin. The flavonoids in grape juice are diffused by other flavonoids and are bound to a variety of sugars, which might reduce bioavailability.[8]

Speaking at an annual meeting of the American Heart Association in Dallas, Masayoshi Hashimoto, M.D., of the University of Tokyo said that polyphenols in red wine may provide beneficial vasodilatory effects and therefore protect against heart disease. Vasodilators allow the blood vessels to expand, thereby allowing more blood to go through. In a Japanese study, vasodilation improved by 30 percent after a small group of healthy men drank red wine.[9]

Researchers at Papworth Hospital, University of Surrey, and other facilities in the United Kingdom concurred that moderate consumption of red wine may reduce the risk of heart disease. The polyphenols in red wine inhibit the oxidation of LDL, and it is believed that the oxidation of the polyunsaturated fat components of LDL may play a role in hardening of the arteries, which could lead to heart disease. Although some scientists do not believe wine consumption prevents coronary heart disease, the intake of flavonoids has been shown to be inversely correlated with mortality from coronary artery disease.[10]

Resveratrol has anticancer, anti-inflammatory, and antiaggregating properties after it is absorbed and enters the bloodstream, according to Maria Elena Ferraro and colleagues in Italy. However, their study revealed a role for resveratrol that is not linked to its antioxidant activity. They found that resveratrol provides a preventive effect on the endothelial cells that line internal body cavities. Earlier studies showed resveratrol to be useful in reducing atherosclerotic processes and consequent coronary artery disease through the inhibition of platelet aggregation.[11]

Small amounts of wine may help to prevent age-related macular degeneration (AMD), the leading cause of blindness in people over age 65, according to Thomas O. Obisesan, M.D., of the Howard University School of Medicine in Washington, D.C. Those who consumed 2 to 12 glasses of red or white wine per year cut their chances of developing AMD almost in half, when compared to those who abstained from alcohol.[12] Obisesan told a meeting of the

American Geriatrics Society in Atlanta, Georgia, in 1997 that the macula, which lies at the center of the retina and is responsible for sharp vision, may become damaged through oxidation and that phenols may provide protection. The pathway concerns the tendency of platelets to accumulate among blood vessel walls. Wine, with its high phenolic content, tends to decrease platelet aggregation.

Depending on who is doing the research, researchers have found resveratrol in wines, grape juice, peanuts, olives, and green tea to be very beneficial.

References

1. Drewnowki, Adam, et al., "Diet Quality and Dietary Diversity in France: Implications for the French Paradox," *Journal of the American Dietetic Association* 96: 663–69, 1996.

2. Muller, C. J., and K. C. Fugelsang, "Take Two Glasses of Wine and See Me in the Morning," *The Lancet* 343: 1428–29, June 4, 1994.

3. Lang, Susan, "Cornell Researchers Identify Substance in Wines That Reduces Cholesterol," *Cornell News,* Aug. 2, 1991.

4. Celotti, Emilio, et al., "Resveratrol Content of Some Wines Obtained from Dried Valpolicella Grapes: Recioto and Amarone," *Journal of Chromatography* 730: 47–52, 1996.

5. Goldberg, David M., "More on Anti-oxidant Activity of Resveratrol in Red Wine," *Clinical Chemistry* 42(1): 113–14, 1996.

6. Logeril, Michel de, and Patricia Salen, "Wine Ethanol, Platelets, and Mediterranean Diet," *The Lancet* 353: 1067, March 27, 1999.

7. Fuhrman, Bianca, et al., "Consumption of Red Wine with Meals Reduces the Susceptibility of Human Plasma and Low-Density Lipoprotein to Lipid Peroxidation," *American Journal of Clinical Nutrition* 61: 549–54, 1995.

8. Miyagi, Y., et al., "Inhibition of Human Low-Density Lipoprotein Oxidation by Flavonoids in Red Wine and Grape Juice," *American Journal of Cardiology* 80: 1627–31, 1997.

9. Kahn, Jason, "Benefits of Red Wine May Not Be Due to Alcohol Content," *Medical Tribune* 40(1): 24, Jan. 7, 1999.

10. Nigdikar, Shailja V., et al., "Consumption of Red Wine Polyphenols Reduces the Susceptibility of Low-Density Lipoproteins to Oxidation In Vivo," *American Journal of Clinical Nutrition* 68: 258–65, Aug. 1998.

11. Ferrero, Maria Elena, et al., "Activity in Vitro of Resveratrol on Granulocyte and Monocyte Adhesion to Endothelium," *American Journal of Clinical Nutrition* 68: 1208–14, 1998.

12. Watson, Virginia, "Wine Consumption Decreases Risk of Age-Related Blindness," *Medical Tribune* 38(11): 7, June 5, 1997.

79

Red Yeast Rice Extract

R ed yeast rice, a fermented product of rice on which red yeast *(Monascus purpureus)* has been grown, has been used for thousands of years in the Far East to ferment rice into wine, as a spice, and as a preservative. In 1996, the rice extract was introduced into the United States as Cholestin to help treat the estimated 58 million Americans with "moderately elevated" cholesterol counts of between 200 and 239.

The FDA later banned the Chinese product because its active ingredient, lovostatin, was believed to be similar to the cholesterol-lowering drug Mevacor. That made the dietary supplement an unapproved drug. The manufacturer maintained that the cholesterol-lowering product was simply ground-up rice sold in capsule form, and that it was the same natural product consumed as a food yeast for

thousands of years. The company added that more than 50 studies had proven that the supplement does lower cholesterol.[1] For a time the FDA attempted to intercept incoming shipments of raw Chinese red rice yeast in port. Merck, which produces Mevacor, stated that if Cholestin were allowed to stay on the market, it would "undermine" the entire drug regulatory process and eliminate incentives for pharmaceutical companies to develop new drugs.[2] A federal judge in Utah later overturned the FDA ruling, and the food supplement was allowed to remain on the market for the time being.

The use of red yeast rice in China was originally documented in the Tang dynasty in A.D. 800, according to David Heber and colleagues at UCLA School of Medicine. In addition to being used to make wine, the rice has been used as a food preservative for maintaining the color and taste of fish and meat and for medicinal purposes. A description of its manufacture is found in the ancient Chinese pharmacopoeia *Ben Cao Gang Mu-Dan Shi Bu Yi,* published during the Ming dynasty (1368–1644). Chinese researchers have reported that red yeast rice has been studied in animals and humans and has been found to reduce cholesterol levels by between 11 and 32 percent and triglyceride concentrations by 12 to 19 percent. Red yeast rice is a staple in many Asian countries, notably China and Japan, where daily consumption ranges from 14 to 55 g per person. Several large prospective clinical trials have shown that the supplement is useful in the primary and secondary prevention of heart disease and other complications of hardening of the arteries.[3]

With this information as background, the UCLA researchers examined the efficacy and safety of red yeast rice in lowering cholesterol levels in an American population consuming a diet similar to the American Heart Association Step I diet. The researchers recruited 83 healthy volunteers, 46 men and 37 women ranging in age from 34 to 78 who were not being treated with lipid-lowering drugs. Total cholesterol in the participants ranged from 204 to 338 mg/dl; LDL cholesterol, 128 to 277 mg/dl; and triglycerides, 55 to 246 mg/dl. The volunteers were treated with 2.4 g/day of red yeast rice or a placebo during the 12-week trial. They were instructed to consume a diet providing 30 percent of energy from fat, not more than 10 percent from saturated fat, and not more than 300 mg of cholesterol daily.

Red yeast rice was found to significantly reduce total cholesterol, LDL cholesterol, and triglyceride concentrations, compared to placebo. It provides a new, novel, food-based approach to lowering cholesterol levels in the general population. The California researchers reported on two studies from China. In one, 324 patients with high cholesterol levels were given 1.2 g/day of red yeast rice for eight weeks. Serum cholesterol levels decreased by 23 percent, triglyceride levels went down by 36.5 percent, and HDL cholesterol increased by 19.6 percent. In the second study, a red yeast rice supplement was given to 101 patients with high cholesterol levels. Total cholesterol decreased by 19.5 percent and triglyceride levels went down by 36.1 percent in the treated group. HDL cholesterol increased by 16.7 percent.

The UCLA researchers suggested a need to reassess national Cholesterol Education Program guidelines concerning pharmacological intervention. The Chinese red yeast rice supplement used in their study costs between $20 and $30 a month, whereas cholesterol-lowering drugs cost between $120 and $300 monthly, with an average of $187/month.

A study conducted at Tufts University Medical School in Boston reported that the red yeast rice supplement reduced cholesterol levels by 16.4 percent following an eight-week study.[4]

Red yeast rice supplements are available over the counter in health food and other stores. If you are concerned about your cholesterol, ask your doctor about this interesting product.

References

1. Stolberg, Sheryl Gay, "Drug Agency Moves Against an Anti-Cholesterol Product," *New York Times,* May 21, 1998, A17.

2. Childs, N. D., "Herbal Statin Violates Merck's Mevacor Patent," *Family Practice News,* June 15, 1998, 20.

3. Heber, David, et al., "Cholesterol-Lowering Effects of a Proprietary Chinese Red-Yeast-Rice Dietary Supplement," *American Journal of Clinical Nutrition* 69: 231–36, 1999.

4. *SciMed News,* March 26, 1999.

80

SAM-e

Discovered in 1952 and available in Europe since 1976, S-adenosyl-methionine is produced naturally in the body from the sulfur-containing essential amino acid methionine and the energy-yielding compound adenosine triphosphate (ATP). It is sold as an over-the-counter supplement called SAM-e for a variety of health conditions, including depression, osteoarthritis, Alzheimer's disease, cirrhosis of the liver, Parkinson's disease, and fibromyalgia.

SAM-e is necessary for more than 35 biochemical reactions in the body. It is found in all tissues of plants and animals, where it contributes to the synthesis, activation, and metabolism of various biological compounds, such as hormones, neurotransmitters, nucleic acids (found in DNA), proteins, and phospholipids (a component of cell membranes), and to the detoxification of harmful compounds in the body.

During the last 20 years, numerous studies in the United States and Europe have confirmed that SAM-e is effective in treating depression and osteoarthritis, according to Teodoro Bottiglieri, Ph.D., of Baylor University Medical Center Institute of Metabolic Disease in Dallas. In fact, the effect of SAM-e on mood and joint health has been shown in clinical trials to be comparable to prescription drugs such as imipramine and clomipramine for depression, and better than placebo.[1]

"SAM-e has been shown to enhance brain dopamine and serotonin neurotransmitter metabolism and receptor function," Bottiglieri said. "It may also aid in the repair of the myelin sheath that surrounds nerve cells. These mechanisms are likely to be responsible for the antidepressant effects of SAM-e. Concerning osteoarthritis, SAM-e is said to stop and reverse degenerative joint disease by promoting cartilage formation and enhancing repair."

Depression, a serious mood disease with far-reaching health implications, will affect about 20 percent of the population during their lifetimes, said Richard Brown, M.D., of Columbia University College of Physicians and Surgeons in New York. Fifty percent of depressed people who are successfully treated undergo a relapse within one year and within 10 years, almost 90 percent will have a relapse. Current treatments for depression, including tricyclics (TCAs) and serotonin reuptake inhibitors, are effective in managing depression, but have significant side effects, including sexual dysfunction, weight gain, dry mouth, blurred vision, constipation, bladder problems, dizziness, headache, drowsiness, nausea, insomnia, and agitation.[2]

"Clinical studies and patient experience have shown that SAM-e is effective in treating people with mild to severe depression," Brown said. "A meta analysis (a compilation of studies) of more than 1,000 patients showed that the effect size (effect of antidepressant over placebo) in patients getting SAM-e was 17 to 38 percent better than placebo. That is significant, since standard antidepressants generally show an average effect size of about 20 percent. Also, SAM-e appears to have a faster action than TCAs such as imipramine. When used in combination with imipramine, SAM-e induced a faster response than imipramine

alone. And SAM-e is well tolerated with side effects similar to placebo."

SAM-e is a significant compound for long-term maintenance of joint health, and for prevention of osteoarthritis, a degenerative joint disease characterized by loss of joint cartilage and excessive development of adjacent bone, stated Peter W. Billigmann, M.D., of the University of Landau in Germany. The loss of compressibility of cartilage seems to be a central feature in the development of osteoarthritis.[3] "SAM-e is useful therapy because it exerts anti-inflammatory and analgesic effects," Billigmann continued. "We see similar effects with nonsteroidal, anti-inflammatory drugs (NSAIDs)—diclofenac, piroxicam, ibuprofen—by inhibiting prostaglandin synthesis. But NSAIDs have a number of potential side effects (gastrointestinal complaints and central nervous system, kidney, and liver problems)."

He went on to say that SAM-e is well tolerated by the gastric mucosa as well as by other organs. In addition, SAM-e acts synergistically with locally applied hyaluronic acid, a gelatinous material that acts as a lubricant and shock absorbant. Thus, the effect is much faster and the therapy lasts longer.

In their book, *Stop Depression Now*, Brown and Bottiglieri review the clinical trials and their own observations about SAM-e:[4]

1. In Spain, Italy, Russia, and Germany, SAM-e outsells the antidepressant Prozac.

2. Folic acid and vitamin B_{12} can reduce homocysteine levels by converting it to methionine, the building block of SAM-e. SAM-e helps to remove homocysteine by increasing the activity of an enzyme that converts this potentially harmful amino acid into beneficial glutathione.

3. For mild to moderate depression, the recommended dosage of SAM-e is 400 mg/day. If this doesn't bring results in two weeks, increase to 800 mg/day.

4. Along with SAM-e, the researchers recommend 800 mcg/day of folic acid and 1,000 mcg (1 g)/day of vitamin B_{12}.

5. SAM-e is valuable for menopausal women with or without depression, since it reduces sleep disturbances.

6. A German study found SAM-e beneficial in treating patients with osteoarthritis. The study involved 20,621 patients with osteoarthritis of the knee, hip, spine, and fingers. They were given 600 mg/day of SAM-e for the first two weeks; 400 mg/day for the second two weeks; and 200 mg/day thereafter. Eighty percent of the patients said that they had a reduction in severity of symptoms in all arthritic sites.

7. SAM-e is useful in treating depression related to Parkinson's disease. In the New York study, treatment began with 800 mg/day and was increased to 3,300 mg/day. The standard depression-rating test (Hamilton Rating Scale) was used, in which a score of 18 is considered severe depression. At the beginning of the test, the mean Hamilton score for the patients was 28.3. After two months of SAM-e therapy, the score fell to 8.

SAM-e was effective in treating 40 alcoholic patients with major depression who were given 200 mg intravenously daily, followed by 400 mg twice a day orally. Significant improvements were noted in most psychometric testing on day 14 and continued throughout the study. There were no adverse side effects.[5]

Researchers in Italy studied 20 patients 35 to 65 years of age with nonalcoholic cirrhosis, and 11 healthy volunteers 25 to 60 years of age who served as controls. Following a 12-hour fast, the study group received 1.5 mg/kg of body weight of nicotinamide (B_3). This brought a significantly higher production of SAM-e in the cirrhosis patients when compared to controls. The authors concluded that SAM-e may be expended in the metabolism of nicotinamide, and thus is a rational adjuvant therapy for patients with cirrhosis of the liver.[6]

In a hospital trial in Barcelona, rats given carbon tetrachloride developed cirrhosis of the liver. However, in the animals given SAM-e for six weeks, only one of the six rats developed the disease. Early administration of SAM-e in a rat model of carbon tetrachloride–induced liver injury restored glutathione levels and reduced lipid peroxidation, thereby decreasing the possibility of cirrhosis.[7]

Forty-seven Italian patients with primary fibromyalgia were given 200 mg of SAM-e intramuscularly daily plus 400 mg orally twice daily for six weeks. The supplement significantly reduced tenderness and mean scores for depression and anxiety. SAM-e was well tolerated, with very few side effects reported. The supplement's benefits for fibromyalgia patients derive from its antidepressant action and antiinflammatory and analgesic effects.[8]

Researchers at the University of Pisa have reported that SAM-e may be an ideal candidate for treating secondary fibromyalgia syndrome due to its antidepressive effect. SAM-e has been shown to be a methyl donor in many methylation processes in the brain. Thirty patients with fibromyalgia were given 400 mg/day for 15 days by intravenous injection or a placebo. All patients completed the study, and all in the treatment group reported a significant decrease in pain.[9]

Bottiglieri reported that SAM-e is an important methyl donor in psychological, neurologic, and metabolic disorders and is involved in more than 35 methylation reactions involving DNA, proteins, phospholipids, catechol, and indole-amines. Some trials have shown low cerebrospinal fluid SAM-e levels in people with neurologic disorders, such as Alzheimer's disease, degeneration of the spinal cord, and HIV-related problems among others. He suggested that oral or intravenous amounts of SAM-e may be a possible treatment for some of these disorders.[10]

An Italian study evaluated 48 depressed patients treated for a month with SAM-e. Inpatients were given 400 mg/day intravenously or intramuscularly, while outpatients received 800 mg/day orally. Progress was monitored using the Beck's Depression Inventory, based on scores at the beginning and end of the study. It was concluded that SAM-e acts as an antidepressant and is effective and relatively safe in depressed patients who have associated internal illnesses.[11]

SAM-e was beneficial in treating seven patients ranging in age from 29 to 43 with spherocytosis, an inherited disorder in which sphere-shaped red blood cells cause anemia, jaundice, and other health problems. The patients were given 400 mg/day intravenously for two weeks, followed by 200 mg/day for 10 weeks. The supplement was instrumental in inducing statistically significant differences in various laboratory parameters after 12 weeks of therapy.[12]

SAM-e appears to be a breakthrough supplement in the treatment of a variety of disorders such as depression and low mood, which is believed to affect about 17.6 million adult Americans annually.

References

1. Bottiglieri, Teodoro, "Biochemistry of SAM-e," paper presented at the Science of SAM-e Symposium, New York Academy of Sciences, Feb. 24, 1999.

2. Brown, Richard D., "SAM-e and Mood Enhancement: Observations and Findings," ibid.

3. Billigmann, Peter W., "SAM-e and Joint Mobility," ibid.

4. Brown, Richard, Theodoro Bottiglieri, and Carol Colman, *Stop Depression Now* (New York: G.P. Putnam's Sons, 1999), 5, 70, 122, 129, 219, 233.

5. Agricola, R., et al., "S-Adenosyl-Methionine in the Treatment of Major Depression Complicating Chronic Alcoholism," *Current Therapeutic Research* 55(1): 83–91, Jan. 1994.

6. Cuomo, R., et al., "S-Adenosyl-L-Methionine (SAM-e)–Dependent Nicotinamide Methylation: A Marker of Hepatic Damage," *Fat-Storing Cells and Liver Fibrosis,* 71st Falk Symposium, Florence, Italy, July 1, 1993, 348–53.

7. Gasso, Marta, et al., "Effects of S-Adenosylmethionine on Lipid Peroxidation and Liver Fibrogenesis in Carbon Tetrachloride-Induced Cirrhosis," *Journal of Hepatology* 25: 200–05, 1996.

8. Grassetto, Maurizio, and Antonella Varotto, "Primary Fibromyalgia Is Responsive to S-Adenosyl-L-Methionine," *Current Therapeutic Research* 55(7): 797–806, July 1994.

9. Tavoni, A., et al., "Evaluation of S-Adenosylmethionine in Secondary Fibromyalgia: A Double-Blind Study," *Clinical and Experimental Rheumatology,* 106–7, 1998.

10. Bottiglieri, T., et al., "S-Adenosylmethionine Levels in Psychiatric and Neurological Disorders: A Review," *Acta Neurologica Scandinavia* 154S: 19–26, 1994.

11. Criconia, Anna Marie, et al., "Results of Treatment with S-Adenosyl-L-Methionine in Patients with Major Depression and Internal Illnesses," *Current Therapeutic Research* 55(6): 666–74, June 1994.

12. Maggio, A., et al., "Effects of S-Adenosyl-L-Methionine on Hereditary Spherocytosis: A Tentative Therapeutic Approach," *Drug Investigation* 8(2): 118–21, 1994.

81

Saw Palmetto

In 1990, Americans made an estimated 425 million visits to providers of unconventional therapies, compared to 338 million visits to primary care physicians. Three of these alternative therapies could save up to 20 percent of each dollar spent annually on health care. One of these, an extract from saw palmetto *(Serenoa repens),* has been shown in double-blind studies to be as effective as conventional drugs in treating enlarged prostate. The herbal extract is nontoxic and costs 60 percent less than regular medications. Western medicine doesn't always provide what patients want, and that is one of the reasons why many have turned to alternative medicine.[1] Saw palmetto is a native American palm tree growing 6 to 10 feet tall, found from the Carolinas to Texas. Florida is a major producer of the reddish brown berries from which the extract is made.

Benign prostatic hyperplasia (BPH) is a noncancerous enlargement of the prostate gland. The gland surrounds the urethra in men, the tube that expels urine from the body. When the prostate becomes enlarged, it squeezes the urethra, thereby restricting the flow of urine. BPH often contributes to bladder problems, urinary tract infections, and urinary retention.[2]

Some studies have suggested that a high-fat, high-cholesterol diet contributes to BPH, since the body converts cholesterol into male hormones. Obesity is another risk factor, and it has been suggested that men who have a waist size over 43 inches are twice as likely to develop BPH when compared to those who have a waist size of 35 inches or smaller.

Typical symptoms of BPH include the inability to empty the bladder, a frequent urge to urinate, the need to make numerous trips to the bathroom at night (nocturia), inability to urinate, difficulty in starting and stopping the flow of urine, a weak flow of urine, and dribbling of urine following urination.

BPH can appear in men as young as age 40, according to Donald J. Brown, N.D. Statistics indicate that the incidence in men 40 to 59 years of age is 50 to 60 percent, and the annual tab for treating the condition is pegged at $1 billion annually.[3]

It is thought that dihydrotestosterone (DHT), an active form of the male hormone testosterone, causes prostate enlargement, since high levels of the substance have been found in the prostate tissue of those with BPH. Abnormal levels of DHT are associated with an increased risk of prostate cancer, Brown said. An enzyme, 5 alpha-reductase (5-AR) converts testosterone to DHT, and 5-AR increases as men age. This is thought to play a major role in the development of BPH. Saw palmetto extract reduces DHT in prostate tissue by blocking the action of 5-AR. It also halts the binding of DHT to prostate cells.

Proscar, an FDA-approved drug for the treatment of enlarged prostate due to BPH, is less than 50 percent effective after patients have taken it for one year, reported Julian Whitaker, M.D. By contrast, saw palmetto extract is effective in nearly 90 percent of patients, with benefits usually surfacing after four to six weeks of therapy. Instead of spending $75 a month for Proscar, men could be spending $15 monthly for saw palmetto

extract and getting better results, Whitaker emphasized.[4]

At the 1988 International Saw Palmetto Symposium, Dietmar Bach, M.D., of St. Agnes Hospital, in Bocholt, Germany, discussed a study supporting saw palmetto's effectiveness against BPH. The study evaluated 315 men with BPH who were treated with saw palmetto for three years. The percentage of volunteers reporting better or symptom-free results were: nocturia, 73 percent; reduced daytime frequency of urination, 53 percent; complete voiding of the bladder, 75 percent; reduction in prostate size, 28 percent. In addition, 46 percent of the men experienced an increase in the flow of urine; 15 percent had an increase in the amount of urine expelled; and 50 to 60 percent had a decrease in the amount of residual urine left in the bladder.[5]

An extract from saw palmetto is prescribed up to 10 times more often than Proscar or Hytrin in Europe for treating BPH. In one study involving 46 men who completed the trial, an improvement in the symptom score of 50 percent or more was recorded after treatment with the herb for two, four, and six months in 21 percent (10 of 48); 30 percent (14 of 47); and 46 percent (21 of 46) of the patients, respectively. No important change was noted in peak urinary flow rate, and no side effects were noted.[6]

After viewing data from a double-blind study involving 35 patients with BPH, an Italian researcher said that saw palmetto extract is able to inhibit the nuclear estrogen receptors and prostatic tissue samples of BPH patients. The treatment group received 160 mg/day of the extract for three months. The therapy was well tolerated and there was a low incidence of side effects.[7]

Belgian researchers evaluated 305 out of 505 patients with mild to moderate symptoms of BPH who were given 160 mg twice daily of saw palmetto extract during a three-month study. The extract improved several parameters after 45 days of therapy, including International Prostate Symptom scores, quality-of-life scores, urinary flow rates, residual urinary volume, and size of prostate. Following 90 days of treatment, 88 percent of the patients and 88 percent of the participating physicians considered the therapy effective. The incidence of side effects was only 5 percent, and the treatment did not mask the possible development of prostate cancer. Saw palmetto extract appears to be an effective and well-tolerated pharmacologic agent in the treatment of BPH, and it compares favorably with existing medical therapies for treating the disorder.[8]

Approximately 30 phytotherapeutic substances are currently available in Europe for treating BPH, and most are derived from eight plant sources. The most common and potent active ingredient is from saw palmetto. The plants are rich sources of flavonoids and are useful in inhibiting prostaglandin synthesis, lowering cholesterol, inhibiting 5 alpha-reductase, blocking androgen binding to receptors, and acting as an alpha-adrenergic blocking agent. A review of the literature shows significant benefit with these plant compounds over placebo in more than 70 percent of the patients.[9]

Saw palmetto supplements are readily available in various outlets. The usually recommended dosage of the standardized extract is 160 mg twice daily.

References

1. Gerber, Paul C., "Alternative Medicine: All Eyes on NIH's Office of Alternative Medicine," *Physician Management,* March 1994, 30–42.

2. Inlander, Charles B., and the Staff of People's Medical Society, *The Men's Health and Wellness Encyclopedia* (New York: Macmillan, 1998), 336.

3. Brown, Donald J., *Herbal Prescriptions for Better Health* (Rocklin, Calif.: Prima Publishing, 1996), 167ff.

4. Whitaker, Julian, *Dr. Whitaker's Guide to Natural Healing* (Rocklin, Calif.: Prima Publishing, 1995), 21ff.

5. Bach, Dietmar, paper presented at the International Saw Palmetto Symposium, Naples, Florida, Aug. 20–22, 1998.

6. Gerber, G. S., et al., "Saw Palmetto *(Serenoa repens)* in Men with Lower Urinary Tract Symptoms: Effects on Eurodynamic Parameters and Voiding Symptoms," *Urology* 51: 1003–07, 1998.

7. Sciarra, F., et al., "Evidence of *Serenoa repens* Extract Displays an Antisterogenic Activity in Prostatic Tissue of Benign Prostatic Hypertrophy Patients," *European Urology* 21: 309–14, 1992.

8. Braeckman, Johann, "The Extract of *Serenoa repens* in the Treatment of Benign Prostatic Hyperplasia: A Multi-Center Open Study," *Current Therapeutic Research* 55(7): 776–85, 1994.

9. Buck, A. C., "Phytotherapy for the Prostate," *British Journal of Urology,* 78: 325–36, 1996.

82

Selenium

In various parts of the United States, the soil contains only small amounts of the trace mineral selenium. People who eat foods cultivated in these soils are often deficient in the mineral. This is most apparent in the Pacific Northwest, the northeastern states, Florida, Michigan, Indiana, Ohio, Pennsylvania, West Virginia, and parts of Illinois. Ingested selenium is absorbed in the intestine, mostly in the duodenum, where it is bound to a protein and transported in the blood to tissues. Selenium deficiencies are somewhat difficult to detect, since vitamin E and the sulfur-containing amino acids cysteine and methionine may serve as substitutes for some of selenium's functions.[1]

One of selenium's biochemical functions is its role as part of the enzyme glutathione peroxidase, which protects cells against oxidative damage. Glutathione peroxidase is present in the liver, heart, lung, pancreas, skeletal muscles, lens of the eye, white blood cells, and blood plasma, where it breaks down toxic peroxides formed during metabolism before they cause damage to the vital membranes in cells. Inorganic forms of selenium bind with toxic minerals such as arsenic, cadmium, and mercury and render them less harmful. In the process, however, the toxic substances may tie up some of the selenium.

In 1966, Raymond Shamberger, M.D., revealed that cancer patients had reduced levels of selenium in their blood. This was related to crops grown in selenium-poor soils. In 1977, Gerhard Schrauzer et al. reported that in 27 countries, cancer deaths were inversely associated with the amount of selenium in the national diets. In 1978, Schrauzer stated that selenium supplements could cut cancer deaths in the

United States by 80 to 90 percent, saving 200,000 to 225,000 lives.[2]

At the Arizona Cancer Center at Tucson, Larry C. Clark, M.P.H., Ph.D., and colleagues studied 1,312 patients with a mean age of 63 who had a history of basal cell or squamous cell carcinoma (skin cancers) from 1983 to 1991. Volunteers were given either 200 mcg/day of selenium or a placebo. Although the mineral did not protect against the development of basal or squamous cell cancers, there was a 49 percent decrease in death from lung, prostate, and colorectal cancers.[3]

Researchers at the University of Georgia at Athens found evidence that 200 mcg/day of selenium provides protection against several forms of cancer, with a 50 percent reduction in total cancer deaths. Selenium is necessary for antioxidant defenses; thyroid hormone function, especially the formation of T3 lymphocyte cells; sperm formation; and immune function associated with cellular immunity. A progressive decline in selenium levels parallels T-cell loss, which has been widely documented in HIV patients. A selenium deficiency has been associated with muscle weakness, cardiomyopathy, and immune dysfunction, including candidiasis, impaired phagocytosis, and decreased CD4 T cells.[4]

Another study at the University of Georgia evaluated 81 institutionalized elderly French volunteers who were given daily a placebo; 20 mg of zinc and 100 mcg of selenium; or 120 mg of vitamin C, 15 mg of vitamin E, and 6 mcg of beta-carotene. After two years of therapy, there was a significant drop in the mean number of infections in the volunteers who took the minerals, but not those who took the vitamins.[5]

Researchers in Miami have reported that dietary supplements of selenium may lower the risk of prostate, lung, and colorectal cancers. In the study, which began in 1983, volunteers ranging in age from 18 to 80 were given 200 mcg/day of selenium or a placebo. All of the patients had previously had skin cancer. Although additional studies were needed, this study indicated the possibility of preventing cancer with a nutritional supplement.[6]

In a randomized intervention trial by researchers at the Harvard School of Public Health and other facilities in the Boston area, it was determined that the risk of prostate cancer for men receiving a daily supplement of 200 mcg of selenium was one-third that of men given a look-alike pill. The volunteers provided questionnaires to ascertain their daily food intake, along with toenail clippings, which are often used to determine long-term selenium intake. The researchers concluded, "The findings of our study provide further support for the hypothesis that a higher intake of selenium may reduce the risk of advanced prostate cancer."[7]

In evaluating 974 men with a history of skin cancer, Clark and colleagues randomly assigned the volunteers to take either 200 mcg/day of selenium or a placebo. The patients were treated for 4.5

years and reevaluated for a mean of 6.5 years. Selenium therapy brought a 63 percent reduction in prostate cancer. In the selenium-treated group were 13 cases of prostate cancer, compared with 35 cases in the control group. Selenium provided no protection from skin cancer, which was the primary reason for the study.[8]

A study team at Brigham and Women's Hospital and other facilities in Boston found that men given 200 mcg/day of selenium for a mean of 4.5 years had a relative risk of 0.35 percent for prostate cancer, compared to controls. While selenium did not protect against skin cancer, it brought a reduced incidence of lung and colorectal cancer in those taking the supplement. The researchers added that selenium levels in the United Kingdom have been decreasing for several decades, largely because of a reduction in imported flour from North America in favor of selenium-poor flour from European countries. A recent survey found that the average intake of selenium in England is as low as 30 to 40 mcg/day. Consequently, there has been an increase in prostate cancer incidence and mortality.[9]

Researchers from China and the National Cancer Institute in Bethesda, Maryland, found that a combination of selenium (50 mcg), beta-carotene (15 mg), and vitamin E (60 IU) reduced the risk of dying from esophageal cancer and other diseases in Linxian, China, where there is little selenium in the soil. Of the almost 30,000 men and women studied ranging in age from 40 to 69, those who took the nutrients daily for five years had a 13 percent decline in cancer deaths and a 9 percent reduction in total death rates.[10]

Abram Hoffer, M.D., Ph.D., reported that L-selenomethionine can protect against skin cancer, both by retarding the number of lesions and by reducing the damage by UV radiation. He recommends 200 mcg/day of selenium and has given 600 mcg/day to patients for years without any toxic effects. Vitamin C (3,000 mg), vitamin E (800 IU), and selenium (200 mcg) daily help to protect against excessive UV radiation.[11]

At Kings College in London, a 24-hour dietary survey of 901 volunteers found the average intake for selenium was 50 mcg for women and 59 mcg for men. Selenium from cereals had fallen from 50 to 18 percent of total intake, but meat sources had increased from 28 to 39 percent in 1992, the last year tabulated. Those eating vegetarian and vegan diets might be most at risk for low selenium intakes, and intakes were found to be lower in vegans than in vegetarians. Some vegetarians received selenium from tuna: 100 g of tuna has about the same selenium content as four or five Brazil nuts.[12]

In evaluating 40 surgical patients at the London Health Science Center, Ontario, Canada, researchers reported that the patients had low levels of selenium and zinc. Surgical patients are at risk for deficiencies in the two minerals secondary to both increased needs and losses.[13]

A crossover study at Beijing Hospital, People's Republic of China, determined the effect of selenium for reducing the toxicity of cisplatin, a chemotherapy drug. Twenty-one patients were given 4,000 mcg/day of selenium versus another 21 who did not take the mineral. The patients were being treated for cancers of the lung, breast, stomach, esophagus, and colon. Selenium was given four days before and four days after chemotherapy treatments. On day 14 following chemotherapy, white blood cell counts were significantly higher in the selenium-treated patients versus the controls. Since there was no toxicity related to the selenium supplement, the researchers suggested that the mineral can reduce nephrotoxicity and bone marrow suppression brought on by the chemotherapy drug.[14]

Researchers in Bratislava, Slovakia, evaluated 16 patients with Down's syndrome and found they had lower levels of zinc and selenium than matched controls. The patients had elevated copper levels, but there was no difference in magnesium stores.[15]

In a French study involving 24 hospitalized women between the ages of 76 and 99, it was found that they had low selenium and zinc levels. Copper levels were adequate. The low levels of selenium and zinc could compromise the women's immune systems.[16]

A selenium deficiency is frequently found in sick preterm infants, according to researchers in Japan. The study involved 57 healthy term infants and 23 preterm children who had a history of respiratory problems.[17]

It has been estimated that infertility among married couples in Western countries is as high as 15 percent. Factors blamed on infertility in males include chemicals with an estrogenic effect that may have migrated from the food chain; phytoestrogens in plants, such as soybeans; and chemotherapeutic agents. To determine whether a decline in selenium intake might be related to infertility, researchers at the Glasgow Royal Infirmary in Scotland and other facilities gave 69 volunteers from an infertility clinic 100 mcg of selenium; 1 mg of vitamin A, 10 mg of vitamin C, and 15 mg of vitamin E; or a placebo daily for three months.[18] After taking semen samples, the researchers determined that sperm motility increased in the selenium-treated men, but there was a slight decline in the control group. Five men (11 percent) in the treatment group achieved paternity in contrast to none in the placebo group. "In the light of the recent report of early miscarriage in women with a low selenium status in Wales, it is possible that a higher pregnancy rate would have been achieved if both parents had been taking supplements," the researchers said.

A variety of selenium supplements are available over the counter. The recommended dietary allowance (RDA) is 70 mcg/day for most males and 55 mcg/day for most females. For pregnant women, the RDA is 65 mcg/day, and for breast-feeding women it is 75 mcg/day. Brazil nuts are the richest food source of selenium. Other food sources include wheat germ, brewer's yeast, fish, lobster, blackstrap molasses, beer, clams, crab, eggs, lamb, mushrooms, oysters, pork, Swiss chard, turnips, whole grains, spices, and nuts.

References

1. Ensminger, A., et al., *Foods and Nutrition Encyclopedia* (Clovis, Calif.: Pegus Press, 1983), 1976ff.

2. Foster, Harold D., "Selenium and Cancer: A Geographical Perspective," *Journal of Orthomolecular Medicine* 13(1): 8–10, 1998.

3. Clark, Larry C., "Effects of Selenium Supplementation for Cancer Prevention in Patients with Carcinoma of the Skin: A Randomized Control Trial," *Journal of the American Medical Association* 276(24): 1957–63, 1996.

4. Taylor, Ethan Will, "Selenium and Viral Diseases: Facts and Hypothesis," *Journal of Orthomolecular Medicine* 12(4): 227–39, 1997.

5. Johnson, Mary Ann, and Kimberly H. Porter, "Micronutrient Supplementation and Infection in Institutionalized Elders," *Nutrition Reviews* 58(11): 400–04, 1998.

6. Charnow, Jody A., "Selenium Supplements Reportedly Lower the Risk of Some Cancers in Humans," *Medical Tribune*, Jan. 23, 1997, 1.

7. Yoshizawa, Kazuko, et al., "Study of Prediagnostic Selenium Level in Toenails and Risk of Advanced Prostate Cancer," *Journal of the National Cancer Institute* 90(16): 1219–24, Aug. 19, 1998.

8. Clark, L. C., "Decreased Incidence of Prostate Cancer with Selenium Supplementation: Results of a Double-Blind Cancer Prevention Trial," *British Journal of Urology* 81: 730–34, 1998.

9. Giovannucci, E., "Selenium and the Risk of Prostate Cancer," *The Lancet* 352: 755–56, Sept. 5, 1998.

10. Li, Jun-Yao, et al., "Nutrition Intervention Trials in Linxian, China: Multiple Vitamin/Mineral Supplementation, Cancer Incidence, Disease-Specific Mortality Among Adults with Esophageal Dysplasia," *Journal of the National Cancer Institute* 85(18): 1492–98, 1993.

11. Hoffer, Abram, "Protection Against Ultraviolet Radiation," *Canadian Medical Association Journal* 147(6): 839–40, Sept. 15, 1992.

12. Judd, Patricia A., et al., "Vegetarians and Vegans May Be Most at Risk from Low Selenium Intakes," *British Medical Journal* 314: 1834, June 21, 1997.

13. Alfieri, M. A., et al., "Selenium and Zinc Levels in Surgical Patients Receiving Total Parenteral Nutrition," *Biological Trace Element Research* 61: 33–39, 1998.

14. Hu, Ya-Jun, et al., "The Protective Role of Selenium on the Toxicity of Cisplatin-Contained Chemotherapy Regimen in

Cancer Patients," *Biological Trace Element Research* 56: 331–41, 1997.

15. Kadrabova, Jana, et al., "Changed Serum Trace Element Profile in Down's Syndrome," *Biological Trace Element Research* 54: 201–6, 1996.

16. Schmuck, Anne, et al., "Analyzed Dietary Intakes, Plasma Concentrations of Zinc, Copper and Selenium, and Related Antioxidant Enzyme Activities in Hospitalized Elderly Women," *Journal of the American College of Nutrition* 15(5): 462–68, 1996.

17. Tsukahara, Hirokazu, et al., "Urinary Selenium Excretion in Infancy: Comparison Between Term and Preterm Infants," *Biology of the Neonate* 70: 35–40, 1996.

18. Scott, R., et al., "The Effect of Oral Selenium Supplementation on Human Sperm Motility," *British Journal of Urology* 82: 76–80, 1998.

83

Shark Cartilage and Shark Liver Oil

Environmentalists have expressed concern over the diminishing shark population, particularly in the Gulf of Mexico, where unregulated killing of the animals takes place. The sharks are hunted for their fins or sport by fishermen who consider it the "poor man's marlin." Sharks have a low reproductive capability and long reproductive cycles, and they are slow in reaching sexual maturity. A diminished shark population could have major ecological effects, since the animals maintain an important relationship with the ocean environment by controlling fish overpopulation and ridding the ocean of diseased fish. At one time shark cartilage was used as a component of artificial skin for burn victims, and it was a source of vitamin A until the vitamin was synthesized in 1940. Shark oil is used in supplements and in hemorrhoid remedies.[1] Producers

of shark cartilage and shark liver oil products maintain that they do not have to kill more sharks, since they use parts from sharks that have already been killed.

A February 1993 installment of the newsmagazine *60 Minutes* focused on Cuban researchers who used shark cartilage enemas to treat 29 breast and prostate cancer patients during a 16-week trial. X rays showed a shrinkage of the tumors. Two U.S. doctors who reviewed the records reported that the results were favorable. At the time, however, the National Institutes of Health said that it did not recommend shark cartilage.[2]

Julian Whitaker, M.D., reported that a survey of users of shark cartilage yielded interesting results. Although anecdotal, the results are encouraging: 106 cancer patients (78.3 percent) reported fair, good, or excellent results; 140 of 158 arthritis patients

(88.6 percent) reported fair, good, or excellent results; and 25 of 30 patients with psoriasis (83.3 percent) reported fair, good, or excellent results. He noted that the National Cancer Institute had planned to research shark cartilage in 1992 with studies on Kaposi's sarcoma in rats, but the institute later told Dr. William Lane, the developer of the product, that it had decided not to do the study, since it didn't want to appear to endorse the product.[3]

Some of the components in shark cartilage may escape digestion, enter the bloodstream, and find their way to a cancer site, according to C. Brian Blackadar, M.D., of the University of Guelp in Canada. By this mechanism, an orally ingested protein could exert a biological effect on a tumor outside the gastrointestinal tract. Whether shark cartilage exerts a biological effect on tumors by this route of administration remains to be seen. Skepticism is certainly warranted on any new cancer therapy, but we should not be too quick to dismiss anyone's work, Blackadar said.[4] "The skeptics correctly recalled that oral administration of insulin was virtually ineffective in the treatment of diabetes," he added. "The conclusion that the oral administration of shark cartilage on the treatment of cancer will also be futile is not so simple because of recent advances in our understanding of the digestion and assimilation of proteins."

The Journal of Naturopathic Medicine reported that seven out of eight cancer patients (87 percent) responded in a highly significant way to shark cartilage treatment. Shark fin soup, popular in China, is used for a variety of ailments, including inflammation and arthritis pain. For cancer, the mechanism of action for stopping tumor growth and bringing tumor necrosis is an inhibition of angiogenesis by a large protein molecule found in shark cartilage. Angiogenesis is the formation and differentiation of blood vessels.[5]

In the study, eight terminal cancer patients were started on shark cartilaginous material (91 percent protein) at a dose of 30 g/day. Seven women were given 15 g rectally as a retention enema, and 15 g/day as an aqueous suspension placed into the vaginal body cavity. One man was given two 15-g retention enemas. The enemas were retained for 30 minutes before being expelled. Of the eight patients, two had cervical cancer; one had a uterine adenocarcinoma; one had a bone metastasis from a primary cervical cancer; one had a soft tissue sarcoma; one had a large hemangioma of the vagina; one had peritoneal carcinoma from a primary colon cancer; and one had breast cancer that invaded the chest cavity. No toxic effects had been reported with shark cartilage given up to 30 g/day.

In his book, *Cancer Prevention and Nutritional Therapies,* Richard A. Passwater, Ph.D., interviewed William Lane, Ph.D. Lane discussed his first study in Mexico, in which cancer patients were given the equivalent of 60 g/day of shark cartilage based on a body weight of under 140 pounds. In advanced cases, researchers used as much as 120 g/day.[6] "An average of 60 to 80 g/day is generally used," Lane said, "and the success rate with solid tumors has been higher than 80 percent. The supplement is administered orally in juice or buttermilk at the rate of 15 to 20 grams each time, spread throughout the day and taken between meals. In some advanced cases, as in a Cuban study, the supplement is administered rectally at the rate of 15 to 20 grams in four ounces of body-temperature water. The enemas are given four times daily. When the patient becomes tumor free, a preventive dose of 10 to 15 g/day of shark cartilage should probably be used for an extended period."

Unlike animals, sharks have no bones, and their cartilaginous skeleton is the same today as it was when the fish evolved more than 400 million years ago. Shark cartilage is gristle made of long strands of tough, elastic tissue that the animals' immunity protects against carcinogens, mutagens, and pollutants. In addition, a substance in shark cartilage inhibits the growth of new blood vessels toward tumors in humans, thereby starving cancer cells and shutting down tumor growth. Other studies show that shark cartilage blocks angiogenesis.[7]

An oral dose of 9 g/day of shark cartilage, equally divided before meals, was given to a 49-year-old woman with chronic pain, degenerative joint disease, and low back syndrome. This brought a 50 percent reduction in pain scores after two weeks and an additional 50 percent reduction in six weeks, reported Lane. Positive results were also obtained when six osteoarthritic and degenerative joint disease patients were given 9 g/day of shark cartilage orally. Lane suggests that shark cartilage can be used in conjunction with other therapies in treating a variety of health conditions.[8]

Shark cartilage was effective in treating osteoarthritis in dogs, according to Melvyn Werbach, M.D. In an open trial, six patients with osteoarthritis who were unable to benefit from NSAIDs said that joint inflammation decreased, pain was reduced, and they were able to walk more easily. For this application, Werbach recommends four 740-mg capsules four times daily. Noticeable results usually manifest at the end of three weeks of therapy.[9]

"Shark liver oil is richer in alkylglycerols than any substance in our bodies outside of bone marrow and breast milk," Werbach continued. "When alkylglycerols are given prior to, during, and after radiation therapy for the treatment of uterine cancer, radiation injuries have been reduced by as much as two-thirds. And when they are given prior to radiation therapy for uterine cancer, alkylglycerols have been shown to enhance the success of the treatments."

Werbach recommends a shark liver oil concentrate (85 percent free alkylglycerols) in 200-mg supplements three times daily. Take the supplement a week prior to radiation therapy and continue during therapy and for one to three months afterward, he said.

Scientists have discovered that sharks found near Greenland and Iceland seem to have some of the most potent healing compounds, wrote Neil Solomon, M.D., Ph.D. The shark's liver contains alkylglycerols (AKGs), initially discovered in 1922 by M. Tsujimoto and Y. Toyama, two Japanese researchers. Studies have suggested that although shark liver oil may not cure a specific disease, it can boost the immune system.[10]

Solomon said that Ingemar Joelsson, M.D., Ph.D., a Swedish physician, and Drs. Sven and Astrid Brohults have published some interesting results on the use of shark liver oil and cancer. Many of the cancer patients they studied were undergoing radiation and/or chemotherapy from 1955 to 1990, and there was a significant decrease in mortality rates in the patients who were consuming shark liver oil.

Henry Brem, M.D., of Johns Hopkins University in Baltimore has found that squalamine, a chemical extracted from shark liver, slows angiogenesis and inhibits the growth of cancer in laboratory animals.[11] "Our results suggest that squalamine may be well suited for humans in the treatment of brain tumors and other diseases characterized by and dependent on new blood-vessel growth," Brem said. Squalene, a constituent of shark liver oil, is used in natural cosmetics, but it is usually processed from olives rather than animal sources.

Shark cartilage supplements are available commercially in a number of formulations, including capsules and powder.

Shark liver oil is available over the counter in a number of products, such as softgel capsules, which contain 50 and 100 mg, respectively, of alkylglycerols.

References

1. Mathews, James, "Shark Endangerment Concerns Researchers," *Journal of the National Cancer Institute* 84(3): 1001, July 1, 1992.

2. McKeown, L. A., "Shark Cartilage Data Skimpy: NIH Office Denies Recommending Study as Television Report Claimed," *Medical Tribune,* March 25, 1993, 10.

3. Whitaker, Julian, *Dr. Whitaker's Guide to Natural Healing* (Rocklin, Calif.: Prima Publishing, 1995), 334–35, 341–42.

4. Blackadar, C. Brian, "Skeptics of Oral Administration of Shark Cartilage," *Journal of the National Cancer Institute* 85(23): 1961–62, Dec. 1, 1993.

5. Lane, L. W., and E. Contreras, Jr., "High Rate of Bioactivity (Reduction in Gross Tumor Size) Observed in Advanced Cancer Patients Treated with Shark Cartilage Material," *Journal of Naturopathic Medicine* 3(1): 86–88, 1992.

6. Passwater, Richard A., *Cancer Prevention and Nutritional Therapies* (New Canaan, Conn.: Keats Publishing, 1993), 54ff.

7. Walters, Richard, *Options: The Alternative Cancer Therapy Book* (Garden City, N.Y.: Avery Publishing Group, 1993), 186–87.

8. Lane, William, "Shark Cartilage: Its Potential Medical Application," *Journal of the Advance of Medicine* 4(4): 263–71, Winter 1991.

9. Werbach, Melvyn, *Healing with Food* (New York: HarperPerennial), 1993, 54, 287.

10. Solomon, Neil, "The Promise of Shark Liver Oil," *Let's Live,* Aug. 1997, 55–56.

11. Christensen, Damaris, "Shark Liver Substance May Block Angiogenesis," *Medical Tribune,* Sept. 3, 1998, 22.

84

St. John's Wort

St. John's Wort *(Hypericum perfora-tum L.)* has been used as an herbal remedy since Greek and Roman times to treat wounds, ulcers, diabetes mellitus, the common cold, gastrointestinal disorders, jaundice, and liver disorders. In medieval Europe, it was used to ward off witches. More recently, hypericin and pseudohypericin, two constituents in the herb, have been shown to have antiviral properties for treating HIV and AIDS. Based on recent clinical studies, researchers in Turkey have found extracts from St. John's Wort to be effective for the treatment of mild and moderate depression.[1]

The favored therapy for depression in Germany, St. John's Wort was named for St. John the Baptist, whose birthday is June 24, about the time the plant's yellow blossoms begin to appear. *Wort* is an Old English name for plant. Because a month's supply of the herb costs only about $10, compared to $80 for Prozac, it has become popular in the United States for treating mild depression. Compared to Prozac, however, St. John's Wort produces less distressing side effects.[2]

In 1994, German physicians prescribed almost 66 million doses of preparations containing hypericum. Hypericin was recognized as a monoamine oxidase inhibitor in 1984 and was allowed for medicinal purposes in an average daily dose of 2 to 4 g/day for psychogenic disturbances, depressive states, anxiety, and nervous tension. While this therapy continues to be investigated, no serious drug interactions or toxicity have been reported by German physicians.[3]

Researchers at Ludwig-Maximilians University in Munich evaluated the efficacy of St. John's Wort in 23 randomized trials involving 1,757 patients with mild to moderately severe depression. Fifteen of the studies were placebo controlled, and eight compared hypericum with another drug treatment. The hypericum extracts were far superior to placebo and were also effective as standard medications for depression. Side effects were recorded for 19.8 percent of the patients on hypericum, compared with 52.8 percent of the patients given standard antidepressants. The daily dose of St. John's Wort extract and the dose of total extracts varied from 0.4 and 2.7 mg to 300 and 1,000 mg, respectively.[4]

Writing in the *Journal of Women's Health*, Shari Lieberman, Ph.D., C.N.S., reported that hypericum has a long history as a natural sedative, an anti-inflammatory, an astringent, and an anxiety reliever. A typical dose ranges from 900 to 1,800 mg/day. She analyzed 25 studies utilizing St. John's Wort and found it a safe and effective alternative to tricyclic antidepressants for the treatment of various forms of mild to moderate depression. German and European researchers consider hypericum as a first-line treatment for disturbances such as restlessness, anxiety, and irritability. The herb is also used to treat seasonal affective disorder, the so-called winter blues.[5]

Hypericum is a well-tolerated alternative to synthetic drugs for the treatment of mild to moderate depression, especially in patients who are intolerant of standard antidepressants, according to David Wheatley, M.D., of the Charter Chelsea Clinic in London. In 14 double-blind, placebo-controlled trials, of the patients given hypericum, 55.1 percent were said to be responders, compared to 22.3 percent getting a placebo. A responder was defined as showing a 50 percent reduction in severity of depression since beginning the study. Hypericum was found to produce less dry mouth and drowsiness than the antidepressant amitriptyline.[6]

Researchers in Germany evaluated 607 people aged 17 and older who suffered from depressive mood disorder. They were given one or two capsules of hypericum extract at dosages of 425 to 850 mg/day for six weeks. Following the trial, both the Hamilton Depression Scale and the von Zerssen Depression Scale readings improved by 60 percent. Disturbances in well-being—dejection, loss of interest, and so forth—and generalized physical complaints diminished during the therapy. Tolerance of the herbal therapy was rated as very good or good in 89.4 percent of the patients. After three weeks of therapy, dosage for 128 patients (21.1 percent) was reduced to one capsule daily.[7]

In Darmstadt, Germany, 1,800 mg/day of St. John's Wort extract and 150 mg/day of imipramine were administered to 209 severely depressed patients selected from 20 treatment centers. While both therapies were very effective by the end of the six-week study, the herbal remedy produced fewer side effects. The researchers concluded that the hypericum extract may be a treatment alternative for the majority of patients with severe depression.[8]

St. John's Wort is said to be remarkably safe as an antidepressant with a unique mode of action, according to researchers at the National Institute of Mental Health in Bethesda, Maryland. While the current mechanism of the herb remains unclear, it appears to affect multiple neurotransmitters without easily fitting into known antidepressant categories. St. John's Wort inhibits not only serotonin, but also norepinephrine and dopamine if the concentration is kept at a high level. Side effects are usually mild and include gastrointestinal complaints, fatigue, and photosensitization (from the sun) in fair-skinned people.[9]

Hypericum may be an effective treatment for patients with seasonal affective disorder. A study involved 20 patients between 29 and 63 years of age who were randomly assigned to get either 900 mg/day of hypericum or less than 300 lux phototherapy. When the patients took 900 mg/day of St. John's Wort, there was a significant reduction in their scores on the Hamilton Depression Scale. There was little difference when the volunteers received bright-light therapy combined with hypericum.[10]

St. John's Wort supplements are available in a variety of formulations. Capsules should contain a standardized formula of 0.3 percent hypericin. Tinctures, fluid extracts, powdered extracts, and other products are also available. Follow the directions on the label or ask your health care provider.

References

1. Ozturk, Y., et al., "Effects of *Hypericum perforatum* L. and *Hypericum calycinum* L. Extracts on the Central Nervous System in Mice," *Phytomedicine* III(2): 139–46, 1996.

2. Brody, Jane E., "Personal Health," *New York Times,* Sept. 10, 1997, C10.

3. De Smet, Peter A. G. M., and William A. Nolen, "St. John's Wort as an Antidepressant," *British Medical Journal* 313: 241–42, 1996.

4. Linde, Klaus, et al., "St. John's Wort for Depression—An Overview and Meta-Analysis of Randomized Clinical Trials," *British Medical Journal* 313:253–58, 1996.

5. Lieberman, Shari, "Nutraceutical Review of St. John's Wort *(Hypericum perforatum)* for the Treatment of Depression," *Journal of Women's Health* 7(2): 177–82, 1998.

6. Wheatley, David, "Hypericum Extract: Potential in the Treatment of Depression," *CNS Drugs* 9(6): 431–40, June 1998.

7. Mueller, Barbara M., "St. John's Wort for Depressive Disorders: Results of an Outpatient Study with Hypericum Preparation HYP 811," *Advances in Natural Therapy,* 109–16, 1998.

8. Vorbach, E. U., et al., "Efficacy and Tolerability of St. John's Wort Extract LI 160 versus Imipramine in Patients with

Severe Depressive Episodes According to ICD-10," *Pharmacopsychiatry* 30: 81–85, 1997.

9. Cott, J. M., and A. Fugh-Berman, "Is St. John's Wort *(Hypericum perforatum)* an Effective Antidepressant?" *Journal of* *Nervous and Mental Disease* 186(8): 500–01, 1998.

10. Kasper, Siegfried, "Treatment of Seasonal Affective Disorder (SAD) with Hypericum Extract," *Pharmacopsychiatry* 30: 89–93, 1997.

85

Tea Tree Oil

When Captain James Cook, the English navigator and explorer, arrived in New South Wales, Australia, in 1770, some of his sailors went ashore and made a tea from the leaves of a tree growing in the swampy lowlands. That tree, *Melaleuca alternifolia,* eventually became known as the tea tree. The natives had long used the leaves as a local antiseptic, and so settlers also began using the leaves and its volatile oil for treating cuts, abrasions, burns, insect bites, athlete's foot, and other conditions.[1]

Tea tree oil is unusual in that it is effective against all three varieties of infectious organisms; namely bacteria, fungi, and viruses. Its principal constituents include terpinen-4-ol (up to 30 percent), cineol, pinens, terpinenes, cymene, sesquiterpenes, and sesquiterpene alcohols.[2]

About 100 compounds in tea tree oil have antimicrobial activity, with the most prominent probably being terpinen-4-ol. Australian researchers tested eight different brands of tea tree oil and found that of 12 organisms tested, 11 were inhibited by all eight brands. In one study in which 5 percent tea tree oil and 5 percent benzoyl peroxide were tested in the treatment of acne, both substances were found to be beneficial, but tea tree oil had fewer side effects. The researchers theorize that there are other compounds in tea tree oil besides terpinen-4-ol that may be therapeutic.[3]

"Tea tree oil is the best treatment I know for fungal infections of the skin (athlete's foot, ringworm, jock itch)," said Andrew Weil, M.D. "It will also clear up fungal infections of the toenails or fingernails, a condition notoriously resistant to treatment, even by strong systemic antibiotics. You just paint the oil on affected areas two or three times a day."[4]

Weil went on to say that tea tree oil is nontoxic and nonirritating. Apply it full strength to boils and other localized infections. A 10 percent solution (about 1½ tablespoons to a cup of warm water) can be used to rinse and clean infected wounds with good results. The same solution makes an effective vaginal douche for treatment of both yeast and *Trichomonas* infections. *Trichomonas* are a variety of sexually transmitted disorders.

A study at the Queen Elizabeth II Medical Centre in Nedlands, Western Australia, tested the effectiveness of tea tree oil against *Malassezia furfur*, a normal component of skin microflora implicated in seborrheic dermatitis, dandruff, and other conditions. Researchers concluded that while tea tree oil cannot be used as an alternative systemic treatment because of its oral toxicity, it may have applications as a topical agent where previous treatments have failed or where prophylaxis is required.[5]

Since tea tree oil has received a great deal of attention as a natural remedy for bacterial and fungal infections, researchers at Wilmington Hospital in Delaware conducted a test to determine the oil's activity against 58 clinical isolates, including *Candida albicans, Trichophyton rubrum, Trichophyton mentagrophytes, Trichophyron tonserans, Asperagillus niger, Penicillin* species, *Epidermophyton floccosum,* and *Microsporum gypsum.* Tea tree oil showed inhibitory activity against all the organisms except one strain of *E. floccosum*. It was concluded that tea tree oil may be useful in the treatment of yeast, fungal, mucosal, and skin infections.[6]

Researchers at King's College in London tested three constituents in tea tree oil for their effectiveness against three organisms. They found that tea tree oils are active against *Staphylococcus aureus, Staph. epidermidis,* and *Propionibacterium* acnes. Their study supports the use of tea tree oil in the treatment of acne, and that terpinen-4-ol may not be the sole active constituent in the oil.[7]

Onychomycosis (ringworm of the nails) is a superficial fungal infection that destroys the entire nail, for which there seems to be no satisfactory cure. A double-blind study at the University of California at San Francisco involved 60 outpatients ranging in age from 18 to 80 who had this toenail problem. The volunteers were divided into two groups, with the treatment group getting a cream containing 2 percent butenafine hydrochloride and 5 percent tea tree oil. The cream was rubbed on the nails. After 16 weeks, 80 percent of the patients using the medicated cream were cured, as opposed to none in the placebo group. Four treated patients experienced mild inflammation but continued to use the cream.[8]

Oral candidiasis (thrush) is the most common opportunistic infection found in patients with HIV/AIDS. About 80 to 90 percent of these patients will develop thrush, which is caused by *Candida albicans,* at some stage of their infection. In one study, 12 patients were given 15 ml of tea tree oil solution four times daily, which they swished in their mouths and then spit out, for two to four weeks. At a four-week evaluation, 8 out of 12 showed a response (2 cured, 6 improved); 4 did not respond. In the two- to four-week follow-up, there was no relapse in the two patients who were cured. The patients had not responded to fluconazole, an antifungal drug.[9]

Because of its antibacterial activity, tea tree oil may be a useful topical treatment for *Staphylococcus aureus* and *S. pyrogenes,* which cause the childhood infection impetigo, a highly contagious disorder.[10] In the United States, impetigo is often referred to as the seven-year itch. Its thick, yellowish crust often leaves scars. Allergic reactions to tea tree oil have been seen by Australian dermatologists. A patch test can confirm the diagnosis.[11]

Speaking at a seminar at Macquarie University in Sydney, L. R. Williams stated that a program is now under way in Australia to produce the highest amount of terpinen-4-ol in a new variety of tea trees. The trees will produce commercial quantities of the oil.[12]

Tea tree oil is available in a variety of over-the-counter products, including pure tea tree oil, shampoos, conditioners, hand and body lotions, antiseptic creams, liquid soaps, vegetable soaps, toothpastes, mouthwashes, suppositories, and other products. It can be used as a germicide in the bathroom; as an antiseptic and cleanser in other parts of the home; as a diaper cleanser; for insect bites; to kill fleas on dogs; and as a treatment for head lice, among other uses. If tea tree oil is used full strength on sensitive parts of the body, it should be diluted with water or a carrier oil first.

References

1. Foster, Steven, and Varro E. Tyler, *Tyler's Honest Herbal* (New York: Haworth Herbal Press, 1999), 369–70.
2. Lawless, Julia, *The Encyclopedia of Essential Oils* (Shaftesbury, Dorset, England: Element Books, Ltd., 1992), 177–78.
3. Carson, Christine F., and Thomas V. Riley, "The Antimicrobial Activity of Tea Tree Oil," *Medical Journal of Australia* 160: 236, Feb. 21, 1994.
4. Weil, Andrew, *Natural Health, Natural Medicine* (Boston: Houghton Mifflin, 1990), 241–42.
5. Hammer, K. A., et al., "In Vitro Susceptibility of *Malassezia Furfur* to the Essential Oil of *Melaleuca alternifolia,*" *Journal of Medical and Veterinary Mycology* 35: 375–77, 1997.
6. "1998 William J. Stickel Bronze Award: Antifungal Activity of *Melaleuca alternifolia* (Tea Tree) Oil Against Various Pathogenic Organisms," *Journal of the American Podiatric Medical Association* 88: 489–92, Oct. 1998.
7. Raman, A., et al., "Antimicrobial Effects of Tea Tree Oil and Its Major Components on *Staphylococcus Aureus, Staph.*

Epidermidis, and *Propionibacteriaum* Acnes," *Letters in Applied Microbiology* 21: 242–45, Oct. 1995.

8. Syed, T. A., et al., "Treatment of Toenail Onychomycosis with 2 percent Butenafine and 5 percent *Melaleuca alternifolia* (Tea Tree) in Cream," *Tropical Medicine and International Health* 4: 284–87, April 1999.

9. Jandourek, Alena, et al., "Efficacy of *Melaleuca* Oral Solution for the Treatment of Flucorazole Refectory Oral Candidiasis in AIDS Patients," *AIDS* 12(9): 1033–37, 1998.

10. Carson, C. F., et al., "In Vitro Activity of the Essential Oil *Melaleuca alternifolia* Against *Streptococcus* spp.," *Journal of Antimicrobial Chemotherapy* 37: 1177–81, 1996.

11. Moss, Andrew, "Tea Tree Oil Poisoning," *Medical Journal of Australia* 160: 236, Feb. 21, 1994.

12. Williams, L. R., "Clonal Production of Tea Tree Oil High in Terpinen-4-ol for Use in Formulations for the Treatment of Thrush," *Complement. Their. Nurs. Midwifery* 4: 133–36, Oct. 1998.

86

Turmeric

Long used as a spice, turmeric *(Curcuma longa)*—often misspelled tumeric—lends its fragrance and flavor to Indian curries. It also has a variety of medicinal applications. As an example, an extract of turmeric is used in India as an eyewash for conjunctivitis. Chinese and Ayurvedic practitioners combine turmeric with other herbs to relieve gas, liver problems, toothaches, and sores. There is evidence that the active compound in turmeric—curcumin—protects the liver by increasing bile secretion, which is instrumental in digesting fats.[1]

Curcumin, taken from the rhizome of *Curcuma longa,* is a potent anti-inflammatory agent that has been studied for its ability to scavenge reactive oxygen radicals implicated in inflammation, reported researchers at the College of Pharmaceutical Sciences in Manipal, India. At high concentrations, it is a potent scavenger of hydroxyl radical. It is also a potent scavenger of superoxide radical, which may be the reason for its excellent anti-inflammatory activity.[2]

An anti-inflammatory agent on a par with cortisone, curcumin has reduced inflammation in animals and symptoms of rheumatoid arthritis in humans. It has been reported that 1,200 mg of curcumin are equivalent to 300 mg of phenylbutazone, an anti-inflammatory drug.[3]

Turmeric can easily be added to food. However, it is more potent when taken as a supplement in doses of 400 to 600 mg three times daily. Retail stores carry turmeric combined with bromelain, an enzyme found in pineapple, which enhances curcumin's absorption rate and has anti-inflammatory effects as well.[4]

Curcumin inhibits the synthesis of prostaglandins in the body that are involved in pain, such as those found in gout. The mechanism is similar to the pain-relieving properties of aspirin and ibuprofen, only weaker. In high doses, though, curcumin stimulates the adrenal glands to release the body's cortisone, a potent reliever of inflammation.[5]

A study at the All-India Institute of Medical Sciences in New Delhi, using laboratory animals, found that *Curcuma longa* appears to possess significant anti-inflammatory properties in animal testing. It is also effective in delayed hypersensitivity as judged by adjuvant arthritis methods. Adjuvant arthritis results in an immunologic process similar to that which underlines rheumatic and arthritic symptoms in humans. There were no toxic effects from the turmeric extract.[6]

At the Gandhi Medical College in Bhopal, India, researchers treated arthritic rats with oral doses of turmeric and cortisone acetate injections. Arthritic swelling on day 13 was significantly less in the animals treated with turmeric and cortisone, compared to controls. The protective effect of turmeric is attributed to its antihistamine properties.[7]

Since curcumin is known to act as an antioxidant, antimutagen, and anticarcinogen in experimental animals, researchers at the National Institute of Nutrition in Hyderabad, India, decided to test turmeric's antimutagenic effects on 16 chronic smokers. The volunteers were given 1.5 g/day of turmeric for 30 days, which significantly reduced the urinary excretion of mutagens in the smokers. The researchers said that turmeric is an effective antimutagen and that it may also be important in chemoprevention.[8]

Researchers have determined that turmeric oil and turmeric oleoresins are excellent scavengers of free radicals in lab glassware. Patients suffering from submucous fibrosis (cancer) benefited from turmeric oil and turmeric extract, as well as turmeric oleoresin, which contains turmeric oil, curcumin, and other resinous materials. Turmeric oil and turmeric oleoresin apparently act synergistically in protecting against DNA damage.[9]

At Northwestern University in Chicago, Curcumin I was found to inhibit benzo-pyrene-induced stomach tumors in female Swiss mice, and Curcumin III inhibited dimethylbenzathracene (DMBA), which induced skin tumors in bald Swiss mice. Both curcumins are the yellow phenolic compounds in turmeric. Also, Curcumin I inhibited DMBA-initiated skin tumors in female Swiss mice. It appears that the curcumins exert their anticarcinogenic activity by altering the activation and/or detoxification process of cancer-causing metabolism. Both curcumins also inhibited in vitro cytotoxicity of a human form of leukemia. The curcumins apparently exert an anticarcinogenic effect by inhibiting the reproduction of fully developed neoplastic cells.[10]

In a bacteriological study, Haridra eye-drops (derived from turmeric) were shown to help protect against *E. coli*, St. Aureus, *Klebsiella,* and *Pseudomonas*. Based on 50 cases of conjunctivitis, researchers reported that the eyedrops play an active role in treating conjunctivitis.[11]

At Tohoku University in Sendai, Japan, a turmeric extract exhibited intense preventive activity against carbon tetrachloride–induced liver damage in both humans and lab glassware. Carbon tetrachloride, a toxic chemical with an odor similar to that of chloroform, is used as a solvent and refrigerant.[12]

Although anecdotal, John S. James reported in *AIDS Treatment News* that in Trinidad, about 40 percent of the population is of Indian descent and regularly use curry in their diets. Another 40 percent is of African descent and seldom use curry. A study of AIDS patients in Trinidad found that those of African descent were more than 10 times likely to have AIDS as were curry-eating people of Indian descent.[13]

In another anecdotal story James wrote that an AIDS patient began taking turmeric extract with a concentration of curcumin of about 100 times the concentration of ordinary turmeric. The product, in capsules, contained 300 mg of turmeric extract concentrated and standardized for a minimum of preferred 95 percent curcumin. The patient took three capsules, or about 2.5 g of curcumin. The product was bought at a health food store. A week after beginning the therapy, the patient's regularly scheduled blood tests showed a substantial drop in p24 antigen, a typical measure of viral activity.

While much of the research on turmeric has been performed on animals and in vitro (lab glassware), there are sufficient human studies to suggest that this herb has considerable promise in dealing with inflammation, cancer, and other health problems. Ask your doctor for guidelines, and add this familiar spice to your kitchen and medicine cabinets.

References

1. Guinness, Alma E., ed., *Family Guide to Natural Medicine* (Pleasantville, N.Y.: Reader's Digest Association, 1993), 324.

2. Kunchandy, Elizabeth, and M. N. A. Rao, "Oxygen Radical Scavenging Activity of Curcumin," *International Journal of Pharmaceutics* 58: 237–40, 1990.

3. Loes, Michael, et al., *Arthritis: The Doctors' Cure* (New Canaan, Conn.: Keats Publishing, 1998), 173.

4. Weil, Andrew, *Spontaneous Healing* (New York: Alfred A. Knopf), 1995, 256.

5. Duke, James A., *The Green Pharmacy* (Emmaus, Pa.: Rodale Press, 1996), 223.

6. Arora, R. B., et al., "Anti-Inflammatory Studies on Curcuma Longa (Turmeric)," *Indian Journal of Medical Research* 59(8): 1289–95, Aug. 1971.

7. Chandra, Dinesh, and S. S. Goupta, "Anti-inflammatory and Antiarthritic Activity of Volatile Oil of *Curcuma Longa* (Haldi)," *Indian Journal of Medical Research* 60(1): 138–42, Jan. 1972.

8. Polasa, Kalpagam, et al., "Effect of Turmeric on Urinary Mutagens in Smokers," *Mutagenesis* 7(2): 107–9, 1992.

9. Hastak, K., et al., "Effect of Turmeric Oil and Turmeric Oleoresin on Cytogenetic Damage in Patients Suffering from Oral Submucous Fibrosis," *Cancer Letters* 116: 265–69, 1997.

10. Nagabhushan, M., and S. V. Bhide, "Curcumin as an Inhibitor of Cancer," *Journal of the American College of Nutrition* 11(2): 192–98, 1992.

11. Srinivas, C., and K. V. S. Prabhakaran, "Haridra (*Curcuma Longa*) and Its Effect on Abhisayanda (Conjunctivitis)," *Ancient Science of Life* VIII(3–4): 279–83, Jan.–April 1989.

12. Kiso, Yoshinobu, et al., "Antihepato-toxic Principles of *Curcuma Longa* Rhizomes," *Planta Medica* 49: 185–87, 1983.

13. James, John S., "Curcumin Update: Could Food Spice Be Low-Cost Antiviral?" *AIDS Treatment News* 176: 1, June 4, 1993.

87

Vanadium

First identified in 1831 by a Swedish researcher, vanadium was named after the Norse goddess of beauty, Vanadis. It was not obtained in pure form, however, until 1927. In 1970, Klaus Schwarz, Ph.D., demonstrated that this trace mineral is needed by both animals and humans. Vanadium-deficient diets resulted in retarded growth, impaired reproduction, and other complications in animals.[1]

Rodney J. French and Peter J. Jones of the University of British Columbia, Vancouver, Canada, reviewed the metabolism, essentiality, and dietary contentions concerning vanadium. The mineral, they said, is a transitional metal that has biochemical attributes similar to chromium, molybdenum, manganese, and iron. Because of the mineral's increasing use in industrial applications, atmospheric concentrations of vanadium are being absorbed through the lungs. It may substitute for other minerals, such as phosphorus, in the development of teeth and bones.[2]

French and Jones went on to say that pharmacological doses of the mineral have been implicated as a stimulatory agent in glucose metabolism, vanadate-dependent NADPH oxidation reactions, lipoprotein lipase activity, growth of red blood cells, and transport of amino acids. In the early 1900s, French researchers used vanadium to treat diabetes, anemia, chronic rheumatism, and tuberculosis.

In clinical trials, the authors wrote, vanadium therapy reduces blood glucose levels and maintains normal glycemic states for at least three months after treatment has stopped. Dietary requirements have not been established but are probably about 10 mcg/day. The typical Western diet provides between 15 and 30 mcg/day of the mineral. Food sources include mushrooms, parsley, dill, and black pepper.

An intake of 10 to 100 mcg/day of vanadium should be safe for humans. Toxicity can be prevented by using EDTA, a chelating agent, which is said to inhibit the absorption of the mineral. Toxicity can also be eliminated with vitamin C, chromium, protein, iron, chloride, and aluminum hydroxide. Vanadium intake in five regions of the United States ranged from 30.9 mcg/day in the Southeast to 50.5 mcg/kg dry weight in the West.[3]

Animal studies suggest that vanadium might be involved in lipid and catecholamine (neurotransmitter) metabolism, building bones and teeth, formation of erythrocytes (red blood cells), and thyroid function. Recent studies have found that in higher amounts, the mineral has anticarcinogenic activity and helps manage diabetes as well as stimulate cell division.[4]

The supplement has become popular with bodybuilders and power athletes, since vanadium seems to function in glucose metabolism, plays a role as an insulin cofactor, and mimics the action of insulin. Vanadium is claimed to be an anabolic-steroid alternative that increases protein synthesis and reduces fat. Studies have suggested that vanadium is needed for cellular metabolism, among other things.[5]

Insulin, a hormone, is a primary substance involved in fat storage, so it is reasonable to presume that foods and nutrients that make insulin more effective and that mimic insulin's actions in the body might aid in controlling appetite and weight gain. Among the nutrients that seem to perform these functions are vanadium, chromium, and *Gymnema sylvestre* (an Ayurvedic herb), as well as bay leaves, allspice, cinnamon, cloves, and turmeric.[6]

Although the various functions of vanadium are unclear, high doses seem to have a pharmacologic action, according to Sheldon Saul Hendler, M.D., Ph.D. As an example, vanadium has been known to have an insulin-mimicking effect on laboratory animals. Artificially induced diabetes in rats can actually be reversed with a form of vanadium called vanadate.[7] "If and how vanadium affects glucose tolerance and fat and cholesterol levels in humans is entirely unclear," Hendler continued. "Epidemiologic studies have indicated that low vanadium intake may be associated with human cardiovascular disease. Given the fact that vanadium, in pharmacologic doses, does have insulinlike activity in rats, it is conceivable that some form of vanadium could be developed to regulate glucose and lipid metabolism in humans."

At the University of Massachusetts at Amherst, researchers observed that vanadium and chromium seem to enhance insulin's action in diabetes. Sodium vanadate at 125 mg/day has been shown to lower insulin requirements in insulin-dependent diabetics, as well as lower the cholesterol amounts in their blood. Niacinamide (B$_3$) in doses up to 3,000 mg/day may help to prevent or delay the onset of Type 1 diabetes, since it is involved in DNA damage/repair and in providing protection against free radical damage. Vitamin E at 100 IU/day and vitamin C at 250 to 600 mg/day may also help diabetics.[8]

Writing in *Natural Prescriptions,* Robert M. Giller, M.D., emphasized that vanadium is a natural element that has been beneficial to many diabetics. It's available in buffered form, and its insulinlike properties increase the uptake of glucose and protein by the muscles and liver.[9]

Using laboratory animals, researchers in Brussels, Belgium, determined that vanadium compounds can mimic actions of insulin through alternative signaling pathways. Animals given vanadyl acetylacetonate exhibited the highest levels of plasma or tissue vanadium, probably due to a greater intestinal absorption. Organic vanadium compounds, especially vanadyl acetylacetonate, correct the hyperglycemia and impaired kidney glycolysis of diabetic rats more safely and potently than vanadyl sulfate. This is not particularly due to improved intestinal absorption, but indicates more potent insulinlike properties. Hyperglycemia indicates an abnormally high concentration of glucose in circulating blood, especially in diabetics.[10] Researchers in Reus, Spain, using young and old Sprague-Dawley rats, reported that their findings agree with a higher kidney concentration of vanadium in the group of adult rats treated with vanadate/vanadium than in the untreated vanadate group.[11]

Because of vanadium's potent insulin-mimicking ability, long-term vanadium therapy causes marked and sustained decreases in plasma glucose, triglycerides, and cholesterol. Since they counter insulin resistance, vanadium compounds also provide protection against high blood pressure. Vanadium has provided positive effects in recent clinical trials.[12]

Researchers in France studied 68 wine samples from different regions of France and California to determine their vanadium content. Levels ranged from 7.0 to 90.0 mcg/L in red wine and from 6.6 to 43.9 mcg/L in white wine. The vanadium content of 12 grape samples was also studied, and it was found that the vanadium content varied from 2 to 17 mcg/kg for white wine and from 5 to 11 mcg/kg for red varieties. The longer the wine is stored, the more vanadium it contains. It was concluded that the daily individual dietary intake of the French population was estimated to be 11 mcg/day.[13]

With diabetes, obesity, and cardiovascular disease among the leading causes of ill health in the United States, it would seem that vanadium is a much-neglected mineral. Vanadium is available over the counter in a variety of formulations, such as vanadyl sulfate.

References

1. Ensminger, A., et al., *Foods and Nutrition Encyclopedia* (Clovis, Calif.: Pegus Press, 1983), 2145.

2. French, Rodney J., and Peter J. Jones, "Role of Vanadium in Nutrition Metabolism, Essentiality and Dietary Considerations," *Life Sciences* 52(4): 339–46, 1993.

3. Hartland, Barbara F., and B. A. Harden-Williams, "Is Vanadium of Human Nutritional Importance Yet?" *Journal of the American Dietetic Association* 94(8): 891–95, Aug. 1994.

4. Garrison, Robert, Jr., and Elizabeth Somer, *The Nutrition Desk Reference* (New Canaan, Conn.: Keats Publishing, 1995), 227.

5. Gastelu, Daniel, and Fred Hatfield, *Dynamic Nutrition for Maximum Performance* (Garden City, N.Y.: Avery Publishing Group, 1997), 97–98.

6. Clouatre, Dallas, *Anti-Fat Nutrients* (San Francisco: Pax Publishing, 1993), 20ff.

7. Hendler, Sheldon Saul, *The Doctors' Vitamin and Mineral Encyclopedia* (New York: Simon & Schuster, 1990), 194–95.

8. Cunningham, J. J., "Micronutrients as Nutraceutical Intervention in Diabetes Mellitus," *Journal of the American College of Nutrition* 17(1): 7–10, 1998.

9. Giller, Robert M., and Kathy Matthews, *Natural Prescriptions* (New York: Ballantine Books, 1994), 116.

10. Reul, B. A., et al., "Effects of Vanadium Complexes with Organic Ligands on Glucose Metabolism: A Comparison Study in Diabetic Rats," *British Journal of Pharmacology* 126: 467–77, January 1999.

11. de la Torre, A., et al., "Effect of Age on Vanadium Nephrotoxicity in Rats," *Toxicology Letters* 105: 75–82, March 8, 1999.

12. Verma, Sudodh, et al., "Nutritional Factors That Can Favorably Influence the Glucose/Insulin System: Vanadium," *Journal of the American College of Nutrition* 17(1): 11–18, 1998.

13. Teiss'edre, P. L., et al., "Vanadium Levels in French and California Wines: Influence on Vanadium Dietary Intake," *Food Additives and Contaminants* 15: 585–91, July 1998.

88

Vitamin A

Also known as retinol (pre-formed vitamin A), vitamin A was discovered in 1912 by Elmer V. McCollum and Marguerite Davis at the University of Wisconsin at Madison. It was isolated when McCollum and Davis determined that something in butterfat and egg yolk made the difference between moderate success in the nutrition of young rats on certain diets. Their discovery was confirmed several months later by Thomas Burr Osborne and Lafayette Benedict at Yale University in New Haven, Connecticut.[1]

Vitamin A is found in such animal sources as milk, butter, eggs, liver, and fish liver oils, and it can be formed in the liver from carotenes, which come from green and yellow vegetables. Carotene is often referred to as pro-vitamin A, but carotene is not utilized as effectively as vitamin A. Vitamin A is essential for the health of eyes,

skin, teeth, gums, and mucous membranes. If you have difficulty seeing at night or when you enter a darkened theater, or if the glare from sunlight or car headlights at night bothers you, you may have a vitamin A deficiency. The retina of the eye contains a pigment (visual purple) composed of vitamin A and protein. When visual purple is converted to visual yellow and then to visual white when exposed to light, vitamin A is lost in the conversion. But visual purple is regenerated if a fresh supply of the vitamin is available. Without this regeneration, night blindness can occur.

A deficiency in vitamin A injures the epithelial tissues throughout the body, including cells in the outer layer of the skin; the mucous membranes that line the mouth; and the digestive, respiratory, and genitourinary tracts. When vitamin A is lacking, epithelial cells dry, flatten, and slough off, becoming hard and dry, like the scales of dry skin. Like vitamins D, E, and K, vitamin A is fat soluble.

The World Health Organization has stated that vitamin A deficiency is a public health problem in more than 60 countries, and puts at risk the lives and eyesight of about 250 million preschool-aged children. Patients with xerophthalmia (a serious eye disorder) need an oral dose of 200,000 IU of vitamin A immediately, again on the following day, and a third dose a week later. For children under one year of age, the dose is half that amount. Children six months of age and younger should receive one-quarter that amount. Periodic oral supplementation with a megadose of vitamin A in children at high risk has reduced mortality.[2]

After reviewing data collected between 1985 and 1987 as part of the National Institute of Child Health and Human Development Neural Tube Defects Study, researchers at the National Institutes of Health, headed by James L. Mills, M.D., reported no increase in risk for women taking daily doses of between 8,000 and 10,000 IU of vitamin A around the time of conception. This is about triple the Recommended Dietary Allowance for the vitamin (2,670 IU). Mills said that this amount does not result in malformations in general or neural tube defects.[3]

Researchers from Berman-Gund Laboratory, Harvard Medical School, and Massachusetts Eye and Ear Infirmary in Boston reported that large daily doses of vitamin A, in this case 15,000 IU, can impede the slide toward blindness for patients with retinitis pigmentosa, saving many years of eyesight for those prone to this inherited disease. A patient who began taking vitamin A supplements at age 32 could retain vision until age 70, rather than lose his sight at age 63. The study evaluated 601 patients ranging in age from 18 to 49. Ninety-five percent of the volunteers completed the study, and all were suffering from retinitis pigmentosa. Vitamin E in this study was not beneficial.[4]

Vitamin A supplements are currently being used to treat retinitis pigmentosa and some forms of cancer. The daily need for the vitamin is estimated to be 2,667 IU for adult women and 3,300 IU/day for adult men. Since vitamin A is fat soluble and stored in the liver, potential toxicity has been widely publicized. However, a study found that people 18 to 54 years of age with retinitis pigmentosa could ingest prolonged amounts of 25,000 IU/day of vitamin A without any problems.[5]

UNICEF reported that vitamin A supplements saved the lives of about 300,000 children in developing countries in 1997. Deaths from diarrhea, which kills about 2.2 million children annually, were reduced by 35 to 50 percent with the vitamin; measles kills almost one million children each year, and vitamin A supplements reduced these deaths by one-half; malaria, which kills some 600,000 children annually, caused one-third fewer deaths in New Guinea with vitamin A supplements.[6]

Researchers in Canada evaluated 138 men between the ages of 40 and 75 in a study that began in 1986. Those who had the highest intake of vitamin A had a 54 percent lower risk of duodenal ulcer than those with the lowest intake of the vitamin. Also, the men with the highest intake of dietary fiber had a 45 percent lower risk of duodenal ulcer. Duodenal ulcers were 33 percent less likely to develop in those who had seven or more servings of fruit and vegetables daily than in the men who had fewer than three servings per day. A reduced risk was also found in those who ate vitamin A–rich foods such as apples, yams, and liver. An increased risk was tabulated for those who ate bacon, hot dogs, and cold cereal.[7]

When Chinese researchers evaluated 58 volunteers with lung cancer and 22 people with stomach cancer, compared with controls, they found that lung cancer patients had significantly lower serum levels of vitamin A, beta-carotene, and vitamin E. Lower levels of the three vitamins were associated with an increase in lung cancer, and lower levels of vitamin A and beta-carotene were associated with a higher risk of stomach cancer.[8]

The role of vitamin A deficiency in infectious disease morbidity and mortality has been known for hundreds of years. For example, vitamin A supplementation in hospitals reduced child mortality by 20 to 30 percent. The use of vitamin A supplements is one of the most cost-effective interventions for improving health and is as important as vaccination and rehydration therapy in public health. Vitamin A and related retinoids have a therapeutic potential as immune modulators in dealing with health of hair and nails, health of mucous membranes, formation of blood and blood cells, white blood cell function, natural killer cell function, Langerhans cell function, T lymphocyte function, immunoglobulin production, interleukin production, tumor necrosis factor production, and other attributes.[9]

In a study in Brazil, improvement in lung function tests was observed after volunteers were given vitamin A supplements. This supports the assumption of a local vitamin A deficiency in patients with chronic obstructive pulmonary disease.[10]

Researchers at Johns Hopkins Hospital in Baltimore reported that at least a dozen trials show that vitamin A supplementation brings a reduction in severe morbidity and mortality from infectious diseases among children who have acute measles or who are from areas where vitamin A deficiency is pronounced. A deficiency in the vitamin is characterized by alterations in immunity, changes in mucosal surfaces, impaired antibody responses, altered T and B cell function, and other complications. Since vitamin A costs only about two cents per capsule, it is one of the most cost-effective means of reducing childhood mortality.[11]

A study at the National Cancer Institute in Bethesda, Maryland, evaluated 2,440 men aged 50 and older who were tracked for 10 years. It was reported that 84 of the men developed prostate cancer, and that the mean serum vitamin A levels were significantly lower in the prostate cancer patients than in those without the disease. The inverse relationship between blood levels of vitamin A and prostate cancer was independent of age and other variables. This was reportedly the first prospective study of a large number of participants to equate low blood levels of the vitamin and prostate cancer.[12]

At the New York City Department of Health and Memorial Miller Children's Hospital in Long Beach, California, studies showed that young children in the United States, like those in less developed countries, would benefit from increased intake of vitamin A. In 1990, there were 27,000 cases of childhood measles in the United States and almost 50 percent of the afflicted children were less than five years old. Measles incidence rose 137 percent from 1989 in children less than one year of age, and of the 6,247 evaluated, 89 died from complications of the disease.[13]

Researchers at the Harvard School of Public Health found that vitamin A supplements brought a 49 percent reduction in mortality risk in HIV-infected children in Tanzania. Beginning in April 1993, the researchers conducted a double-blind study involving 687 children aged six months to five years who were hospitalized with pneumonia. In addition to the usual therapy, the children received 400,000 IU of vitamin A (half that for infants). The same therapy was given four and eight months after the children were discharged. Low-cost vitamin A supplements reduced mortality in HIV-infected children, many of them living where vitamin A deficiency is common.[14]

Milk in plastic jugs exposes vitamin A and riboflavin (B_2) to light, thereby reducing the amount of the vitamins. This can also produce an "off" flavor. A translucent plastic jug of skim milk in a lighted dairy case for one day can lose up to 70 percent of vitamins A and B_2. Milk that comes in a cardboard carton loses only 2 percent of B_2 and 15 percent of vitamin A.[15]

Various vitamin A supplements are available at your nearest health food store. If you are not eating vitamin A–rich foods on a regular basis, you may want to investigate taking a vitamin A supplement. Pregnant women should consult their health care providers.

References

1. McCollum, Ernestine B., and Elmer V. McCollum, "Vitamins A, D, E, K," *Food—The Yearbook of Agriculture* (Washington, D.C.: U.S. Department of Agriculture, 1959), 130ff.

2. Potter, Andrew R., "Reducing Vitamin A Deficiency Could Save the Eyesight and Lives of Countless Children," *British Medical Journal* 314: 317–18, Feb. 1, 1997.

3. Mills, James L., "Vitamin A and Birth Defects," *American Journal of Obstetrics and Gynecology* 177: 31–36, 1997.

4. Berson, Eliot L., et al., "A Randomized Trial of Vitamin A and Vitamin E Supplementation for Retinitis Pigmentosa," *Archives of Ophthalmology* 111: 761–72, 1993.

5. Sibulesky, Lena, et al., "Safety of 7,500 RE (25,000 IU) Vitamin A Daily in Adults with Retinitis Pigmentosa," *American Journal of Clinical Nutrition* 69: 656–63, 1999.

6. Runestad, Todd, "Vitamin A Saved 300,000 Children's Lives in 1997," *Nutrition Science News* 3(3): 99, March 1998.

7. Charnow, Jody A., "Vitamin A and Fiber May Cut Risk of Duodenal Ulcer," *Medical Tribune,* Feb. 6, 1997, 15.

8. Kumagai, Y., et al., "Serum Antioxidant Vitamins and Risk of Lung and Stomach Cancer in Shenyang, China," *Cancer Letters* 129: 145–49, 1998.

9. Semba, R. D., "The Role of Vitamin A and Related Retinoids in Immune Function," *Nutrition Reviews* 56: S38–S48, 1998.

10. Paiva, Sergio, A. R., et al., "Assessment of Vitamin A Status in Chronic Obstructive Pulmonary Disease Patients and Healthy Smokers," *American Journal of Clinical Nutrition* 64: 928–34, 1996.

11. Semba, R. D., "Vitamin A, Immunity, and Infection," *Clinical Infectious Diseases* 19: 489–99, 1994.

12. Reichman, Marsha E., et al., "Serum Vitamin A and Subsequent Development of Prostate Cancer in the First National Health and Nutrition Examination Survey Epidemiologic Follow-Up Study," *Cancer Research* 50: 2311–15, April 15, 1990.

13. Frieden, T., et al., "Vitamin A Levels and Severity of Measles," *American Journal of Clinical Nutrition* 146: 182–86, 1992. Also, A. Arrieta, et al., "Vitamin A Levels in American Children with Measles," *Clinical Research* 40: A131, 1992.

14. Fawsi, W. W., et al., "A Randomized Trial of Vitamin A Supplements in Relation to Mortality Among Human Immunodeficiency Virus-Infected and Uninfected Children in Tanzania," *Pediatric Infectious Disease Journal* 18: 127–33, Feb. 1999.

15. "Milk and Light Exposure," *Nutrition Week* 26(38): 7, Oct. 4, 1995.

89

Vitamin B$_1$ (Thiamine)

In 1911, while working at the Lister Institute in London, Polish scientist Casimir Funk, M.D., isolated a substance from rice polishings that prevented beriberi. The substance turned out to be vitamin B$_1$, the first vitamin to be identified. At the time, beriberi was decimating large groups of people in the Far East who favored white rice over brown rice. Funk was convinced that there was something in food that prevented beriberi, scurvy, and pellagra and that this something was important to life. His rice polishings preparation, which was effective in curing beriberi in birds, was an amine compound, from which he coined the name *vitamine*. In 1919, the *e* was dropped when it became obvious that there were any number of unknown essential factors that might not have the amine structure. Funk also conducted pioneering research on vitamin B$_3$, and later did work in the United States.[1]

Among other things, vitamin B$_1$ serves as a coenzyme in the metabolism of carbohydrates and amino acids, the building blocks of protein. Those in the initial stages of a B$_1$ deficiency or marginal deficiency may experience vague symptoms of loss of appetite, weight loss, apathy, decrease in short-term memory, confusion, and irritability, according to the Vitamin Nutrition Information Service. Research in Canada and the Republic of Ireland has shown that marginal deficiencies of B$_1$ are fairly common among the elderly. For those who have borderline deficiencies, B$_1$ supplements often improve well-being, increase appetite, and decrease fatigue in the elderly. A survey by the USDA in 1997 found that 74.6 percent of men and 60.9 percent of women aged 70 and over were meeting the RDA for B$_1$.[2]

Beriberi is considered a rather uncommon disorder, but Ruth Ryan, M.D., and colleagues found that three women between the ages of 36 and 44 complained of symptoms associated with beriberi, including sleep disturbances, posttraumatic stress disorder, panic attacks, depression, leg cramps, constant fatigue, visual disturbances, unsteady gait, abdominal cramps, and hair loss. The women were relieved of their symptoms after being given 100 mg of B_1 intramuscularly as well as oral supplements of the entire B-complex of vitamins. Since the B vitamins work synergistically, nutritionists prefer to prescribe the whole complex of eight vitamins, rather than a single B vitamin. Ryan suggested that a B_1 deficiency should be evaluated in psychiatric patients who are difficult to manage.[3]

Researchers at Ainslie Hospital in Edinburgh reported that thiamine deficiency may have played a role in brain damage in a group of patients with head injuries who either were alcoholics or had Wernicke-Korsakoff syndrome. This syndrome is caused by a deficiency of B_1 and other B vitamins and is usually related to malnutrition due to alcohol abuse.[4] There has been a significant reduction in patients with Wernicke-Korsakoff syndrome in Australia following the enrichment of bread flour with B_1.[5]

Unless high doses of B_1 are given, patients with Wernicke-Korsakoff syndrome risk irreversible brain damage, according to researchers in England. In fact, B vitamin deficiencies directly affect the brain and are common in alcohol misuse. Vitamins B_1,

B_2, B_3, and B_6 serve as coenzymes and are necessary for glucose, lipid, and amino acid metabolism. The therapeutic dose in this instance is thought to be 500 mg once or twice a day and up to 1 g for 3 to 5 days for B_1.[6]

One's need for vitamin B_1 is highest when carbohydrates are the main source of energy. Doctors at Hospital Universitari Val d'Hebron in Barcelona recommend a multivitamin treatment for all patients with a history of alcoholism so as to rule out polyneuropathy caused by a vitamin deficiency. Their recommendation came after studying a 43-year-old male who had been drinking 150 mg/day of alcohol for a year before admission. There was progressive weakness in his hands and legs, and he was diagnosed as having a classic case of beriberi. Progressive improvement was observed after he was given 200 mg/day of B_1 intravenously.[7]

At the University of South Florida College of Medicine at Tampa, researchers reported that giving Alzheimer's patients 3 to 5 g/day (3,000 to 5,000 mg) of B_1 is often beneficial. A significant number of patients with senile dementia of the Alzheimer's type were found to have a thiamine deficiency, which may impact on cognitive function.[8]

Researchers in Turkey found that giving 250 mg of B_6 and 250 mg of B_1 twice daily for four weeks over a six-month period was useful in alleviating leg cramps in 25 pregnant women. Ten of the patients were relieved of all of their symptoms, and

14 reported significant improvement. Only one patient failed to respond to the therapy. The two vitamins are depleted during pregnancy, since the fetus apparently takes what it needs. The authors said that magnesium is a reliable therapy for leg cramps, but that the mineral is not available in supplement form in their country.[9]

Vitamin B_1 may be the best therapy for women with painful menstrual cramping, according to a study reported in the *Indian Journal of Medical Research*. For example, 556 females ranging in age from 12 to 21, with moderate to severe dysmenorrhea, were given 100 mg/day of B_1 or a placebo for 90 days. For those getting the vitamin, 87 percent said they no longer had the problem; 8 percent reported a significant improvement; and 5 percent reported no effect. The women getting the B_1 therapy had no complaints for two months after the study, even though they were no longer taking the vitamin.[10]

A thiamine deficiency may be related to congestive heart failure, which affects about four million Americans. An estimated 200,000 patients die from this disease, according to researchers at the University of Michigan at Ann Arbor. They theorize that a deficiency in the vitamin may be related to long-term use of diuretics, which are routinely given to treat the edema (swelling) associated with congestive heart failure.[11]

In their study, the researchers investigated the B_1 status of 38 consecutively treated patients with ischemic or nonis-chemic heart disease after they were admitted to a cardiology clinic at the university. Eight (21 percent) of the 38 patients had a thiamine deficiency; 7 were labeled severe; and 1 had a marginal reading. The remaining patients did not have a B_1 deficiency. In addition to overusing diuretics, a thiamine deficiency is related to inadequate amounts of the vitamin in diet and supplements.

A study at Sheba Medical Center, Tel-Hashomer, Israel, found that thiamine supplements are beneficial in the treatment of some patients with moderate to severe heart failure who have been given long-term therapy with furosemide. Furosemide is prescribed for high blood pressure. While hospitalized, the patients received 200 mg/day of B_1 by injection or a placebo. Upon discharge, all 30 patients were given oral doses of 200 mg/day of B_1 as outpatients for six weeks. B_1 therapy is simple, cheap, and safe, and may improve elements of left ventricular systolic dysfunction and decreased functional capacity, which are related to both heart disease and an unsuspected B_1 deficiency.[12]

A report published in the *Journal of the American Medical Association* stated that since November 1996, there has been a nationwide shortage of intravenous multivitamins used in the United States, and that patients given total parenteral nutrition without multivitamins are at risk for thiamine deficiency. Physicians giving patients intravenous feedings were warned to be on the lookout for B_1 deficiencies and lactic acidosis.[13]

The best food sources of B_1 include wheat germ, brewer's yeast, beans and peas, whole-grain breads and cereals, rice bran, lean pork, ham, soybean flour, nuts, eggs, fish, plums, prunes, broccoli, asparagus, cauliflower, corn, endive, dandelion greens, kale, and Brussels sprouts. The RDA of thiamine ranges from 1 to 1.8 mg/day. For adults 51 years of age and older, the RDAs are 1.2 mg/day for men and 1.1 mg/day for women.

References

1. Murray, Frank, *Program Your Heart for Health* (New York: Larchmont Books, 1977), 291.

2. *Back-Grounder,* Vitamin Nutrition Information Service, Parsippany, N.J.: April 1999.

3. Ryan, Ruth, et al., "Beriberi Unexpected," *Psychosomatics* 38(3): 291–94, June 1997.

4. Ferguson, R. K., et al., "Thiamine Deficiency in Head Injury: A Missed Insult?" *Alcohol and Alcoholism* 32(4): 493–500, 1997.

5. Harper, Clive G., et al., "Prevalence of Wernicke-Korsakoff Syndrome in Australia: Has Thiamine Fortification Made a Difference?" *Medical Journal of Australia* 168: 542–45, June 1, 1998.

6. Cook, Christopher C. H., and Allan D. Thomson, "B Complex Vitamins in the Prophylaxis and Treatment of Wernicke-Korsakoff Syndrome," *British Journal of Clinical Practice* 57(9): 461–65, 1997.

7. Comabella, M., et al., "High Istrogenic Fulminant Beriberi," *The Lancet* 346: 182–83, July 15, 1995.

8. Gold, Michael, et al., "Plasma and Red Blood Cell Thiamine Deficiency in Patients with Dementia of the Alzheimer's Type," *Archives of Neurology* 52: 1081–85, Nov. 1995.

9. Avsar, A. Filiz, et al., "Vitamin B₁ and B₆ Substitution in Pregnancy for Leg Cramps," *American Journal of Obstetrics and Gynecology* 175(1): 233–34, July 1996.

10. Gokhale, L. B., "Curative Treatment of Primary (Spasmodic) Dysmenorrhea," *Indian Journal of Medical Research* 103: 227–31, 1996.

11. Brady, Jennifer, et al., "Thiamin Status, Diuretic Medications, and the Management of Congestive Heart Failure," *Journal of the American Dietetic Association* 95: 541–44, May 1995.

12. Shimon, Ilan, et al., "Improved Left Ventricular Function After Thiamine Supplementation in Patients with Congestive Heart Failure Receiving Long-Term Furosemide Therapy," *American Journal of Medicine* 98: 485–90, May 1995.

13. "Lactic Acidosis Traced to Thiamine Deficiency Related to Nationwide Shortage of Multivitamins for Total Parenteral Nutrition—United States, 1997," *Journal of the American Medical Association* 278(2): 109–11, July 9, 1997.

90

Vitamin B$_2$ (Riboflavin)

Formerly known as vitamin G, vitamin B$_2$ is a yellow, water-soluble pigment. Research began in 1879, but the function and importance of this vitamin were not completely understood until the 1930s. In 1932, Otto Warburg and W. Christian of Germany studied a yellow enzyme in yeast and split it into a protein and a pigment (flavin). B$_2$ was later determined to be an important human nutrient that is merged with protein in the body to form various key enzymes. These flavoproteins function in the respiration of tissue and serve closely with enzymes containing vitamin B$_3$.[1]

Some flavoproteins are called oxidases, since they catalyze the oxidation of various chemical substances. The association of riboflavin- and niacin-containing enzymes explains the similarity of certain findings related to deficiencies of the vitamins B$_2$ and B$_3$. A deficiency of either creates soreness and redness of the tongue and lips; atrophy of papillae on the surface of the tongue; and cracks at the corners of the mouth. In B$_2$ deficiency, dermatitis often involves the scrotum, face, and ears.

A low-cost treatment for migraine headaches seems to be 400 mg/day of riboflavin. In a double-blind study in Belgium, 55 patients with migraine were given a megadose of B$_2$ for three months. The vitamin brought relief to 59 percent of the volunteers, compared to 15 percent of the controls who were free of pain.[2]

Vitamin B$_2$ and magnesium are also effective in treating migraine headaches, reported Alexander Mauskop, M.D., of State University of New York/Downstate Medical Center in Brooklyn. He added that a magnesium deficiency has been suspected in between 30 and 50 percent of migraine sufferers. This deficiency causes blood vessel spasm and blocks pain messages from being sent and received along the nervous system. While the mechanism by which the two nutrients relieves migraines is not well understood, Mauskop recommends 400 mg/day each of B$_2$ and magnesium.[3]

Elderly people may have a B$_2$ deficiency, even though they may seem to be getting sufficient amounts from their diets, according to researchers at the University of Ulster in Northern Ireland. The same was said for vitamin B$_6$. The study involved 83 elderly volunteers aged 65 and older who were living at home.[4]

"The lower supplementation level (1.6 mg/day), shown to be effective in up to one-half of the apparently healthy elderly people in this study, could reasonably be achieved through normal dietary means; i.e., increased consumption of riboflavin-rich foods such as milk and dairy products, and riboflavin-fortified foods such as breakfast cereals," said lead researcher Sharon M. Madigan. "Our findings suggest that older people have an increased requirement for riboflavin and, on this basis, we conclude that current U.K. and U.S. dietary recommendations for riboflavin are likely to be insufficient for elderly people."

In *Clinical Pearls with The Experts Speak,* Kirk Hamilton interviewed Bruno M. Lesourd, M.D., Ph.D., of Faculte de Medecine Pitie-Salpetriere in Paris, who participated in the European Euronut/Seneca study to determine the nutritional status of the elderly. Lesourd reported low intakes for

vitamin B$_1$ (0 to 64 percent); B$_2$ (0 to 33 percent); B$_6$ (0 to 29 percent); C (0 to 14 percent); A (0 to 94 percent); and folic acid (2 to 11 percent).[5]

Researchers at Wageningen Agricultural University in The Netherlands surveyed 40 nursing home residents, 21 people recently admitted to a nursing home, and 186 individuals living at home. They found that diet intakes for a number of vitamins were below the minimum requirement in half of the nursing home residents. Nutrients in short supply were B$_1$, B$_2$, B$_6$, and vitamin C.[6] Of 102 patients in intensive care facilities, those who died within a week of discharge had vitamin B$_2$ deficiencies, compared to the patients who survived.[7]

In evaluating 62 male and female cancer patients, researchers at Virginia Polytechnic Institute and State University at Blacksburg reported that the patients had substantial dietary deficiencies and might need dietary counseling and/or supplements. The patients were deficient in 10 vitamins and minerals; namely, A, C, D, E, B$_1$, B$_2$, B$_3$, B$_6$, B$_{12}$, and zinc.[8]

At the University of Colorado Health Sciences Center in Denver, a 46-year-old woman with AIDS, who had been on triple-drug therapy for four months, was admitted to the hospital with lactic acidosis, fatty liver, and other complications. She was discharged in good condition after getting B$_2$ therapy.[9]

Researchers at the Royal Masonic Hospital in London said that in mental patients, deficiencies of B$_2$, B$_6$, and folic acid are linked to depression, and that a B_1 deficiency is associated with schizophrenia. Deficiencies of B_2 and B_6 are thought to be due to insufficient amounts in the food of the mentally ill patient. In addition, psychotropic drugs, anticonvulsants, oral contraceptives, antibiotics, and other drugs deplete vitamin stores. While classic B vitamin deficiencies are not common, subclinical deficiencies of B_1, B_2, B_6, B_{12}, and folic acid are rather common. These deficiencies are especially noticeable in depression and alcoholism.[10]

In *Pediatric Neurology,* researchers in Milan recorded the history of a child who had normal development until age 3, at which time he developed leukodystrophy, a degenerative disease of white matter in the brain. The child had unusually high levels of glutaric acid, dicarboxylic acid, and glycine derivatives in his urine. After being given 50 mg/day of riboflavin, there was a rapid improvement in his case.[11]

Between 1991 and 1993, an epidemic of optic and peripheral neuropathy affected more than 50,000 people in Cuba. The nerve and eye damage was related to deficiencies in B_2, B_3, B_{12}, and the amino acid methionine, plus excess tobacco use. One of the reasons for the deficiencies was a severe storm that restricted the availability of many foods, especially animal products, according to the Centers for Disease Control and Prevention in Atlanta.[12]

Plastic jugs expose vitamins A and B_2 in milk to light, reducing their potency. Light can also trigger an "off" flavor. Translucent plastic jugs of skim milk in a lighted dairy case can lose up to 70 percent of their vitamin A and B_2 in only one day. In a cardboard carton, milk loses only 2 percent of its riboflavin and 15 percent of its vitamin A.[13]

Food sources of B_2 include milk, meat, whole-grain breads and cereals, brewer's yeast, wheat germ, rice bran, cheese, eggs, nuts, corn, beans, asparagus, broccoli, endive, kale, dandelion greens, soybeans, beet greens, Brussels sprouts, chicory, peas, turnip greens, kohlrabi, parsley, and spinach. The recommended daily intake of B_2 ranges from 1.1 to 1.8 mg/day.

References

1. *Food, the Yearbook of Agriculture* (Washington, D.C.: U.S. Department of Agriculture, 1959), 141–42.

2. Schoenen, Jean, et al., "Effectiveness of High-Dose Riboflavin in Migraine Prophylaxis: A Randomized Controlled Trial," *Neurology* 50: 466–70, 1998.

3. Johnson, Kate, "Neurologist Urges Use of Dietary Supplements to Treat Migraine," *Medical Tribune* 40(11): 17, June 10, 1999.

4. Madigan, S. M., et al., "Riboflavin and Vitamin B_6 Intakes and Status and Biochemical Response to Riboflavin Supplementation in Free-Living Elderly People," *American Journal of Clinical Nutrition* 66: 389–95, 1998.

5. Hamilton, Kirk, "Elderly, Immune System, and Nutrition," *Clinical Pearls with The Experts Speak,* Sacramento, Calif., 1997,

301. Also, Bruno M. Lesourd, "Nutrition and Immunity in the Elderly: Modification of Immune Responses with Nutritional Treatments," *American Journal of Clinical Nutrition* 66: 478S–84S, 1997.

6. van der Wielen, Reggy P. J., "Dietary Intakes of Energy and Water-Soluble Vitamins in Different Categories of Aging," *Journal of Gerontology: Biological Sciences* 51A(1): B100–B07, 1996.

7. Shenkin, S. D., et al., "Subclinical Riboflavin Deficiency Associated with Outcome of Seriously Ill Patients," *Clinical Nutrition* 8: 269–71, 1989.

8. Bass, Faye B., et al., "The Need for Dietary Counseling of Cancer Patients as Indicated by Nutrient and Supplement Intake," *Journal of the American Dietetic Association* 1319–21, 1995.

9. Fouty, B., et al., "Riboflavin to Treat Nucleoside Analogue–Induced Lactic Acidosis," *The Lancet* 352: 291–92, July 25, 1998.

10. Carney, M. P., "Vitamins and Mental Health," *British Journal of Hospital Medicine* 48(8), Oct. 21–Nov. 3, 1992.

11. Uziel, Graziella, et al., "Riboflavin-Responsive Glutaric Aciduria Type II Presented as a Leukodystrophy," *Pediatric Neurology* 13(4): 333–35, 1995.

12. Philen, Roseanne M., et al., "Epidemic Optic Neuropathy in Cuba—Clinical Characterizations and Risk Factors," *New England Journal of Medicine* 333(18): 1176–82, Nov. 2, 1995.

13. "Milk and Light Exposure," *Nutrition Week* 26(38): 7, Oct. 4, 1996.

Vitamin B₃ (Niacin)

Niacin, a member of the B complex of vitamins, is a combination that includes nicotinic acid, nicotinamide, and niacinamide. These often serve with two other B vitamins, thiamine and riboflavin, in producing energy in cells. Niacin's role in nutrition was first described by Spanish physician Gaspar Casal in 1730, soon after corn was introduced into Europe. Corn is deficient in niacin and thus caused a disease called pellagra to spread throughout the world. It reached epidemic proportions in the southern United States after the Civil War, when thousands of poor succumbed. Today, pellagra is rarely found in the United States, although orthomolecular physicians often refer to subclinical pellagra, in which deficiencies of B₃ are related to a number of illnesses.[1]

Niacin is found in body tissues as part of two coenzymes, nicotinamide adenine dinucleotide (NAD) and nicotinamide adenine dinucleotide phosphate (NADP). As a water-soluble vitamin, little of it is stored in the body. Major food sources include liver, kidney, lean meat, rabbit, poultry, fish, mushrooms, nuts, milk, cheese, eggs, and enriched cereals.

Psychiatrist Abram Hoffer, M.D., Ph.D., has successfully treated thousands of patients with schizophrenia and other mental illnesses. He has found that 90 percent of these patients, treated with orthomolecular therapy for at least two years, will recover. He has trained more than 50 physicians in this new approach to schizophrenia. Although vitamin B₃ is the backbone of his therapy, he also uses other nutrients:

- vitamin B₃ (niacin or niacinamide): 500 mg three times daily after meals, ranging up to 2 g three times daily

When using niacin, more is often needed. Inositol hexaniacinate has the beneficial properties of niacin and rarely has side effects.

- vitamin C: 1 to 2 g three times daily after meals
- pyridoxine (B_6): 250 to 500 mg/day
- zinc: any form, equivalent to 50 mg/day
- any combination of any B complex preparation
- essential fatty acids such as flaxseed oil, 2 to 4 tablespoons daily
- These nutrients are combined with any necessary antidepressant, tranquilizer, or any other medication indicated, but the aim is to reduce drug medications as soon as possible, consistent with continuing improvement.[2]

A research team at the University of Massachusetts at Amherst reported that niacinamide can help prevent or delay the onset of Type 1 diabetes mellitus. Doses up to 3,000 mg/day are considered non-toxic. The role of the B vitamin may be involved in DNA repair/damage processes or in protecting against free radical damage. Vitamin C, vitamin E, chromium, and vanadium may also be helpful. For example, 125 mg/day of vanadium can lower insulin requirements in insulin-dependent diabetics and can lower blood levels of cholesterol.[3]

Nicotinamide and vitamin E have been shown to have similar effects in protecting residual beta cell function in patients with recent onset insulin-dependent diabetes mellitus. The two vitamins have minimal adverse effects and may prove beneficial in future intervention trials of insulin-dependent diabetes mellitus in those who have recently been diagnosed with the disease.[4]

One study evaluated 108 individuals with cholesterol levels greater than or equal to 200 mg/dl; serum triglycerides greater than or equal to 200 and less than or equal to 800 mg/dl; as well as apoliprotein-B of greater than or equal to 110 mg/dl. The volunteers received either 10 mg/day of atorvastatin (Lipitor), a cholesterol-lowering drug, or 1 g three times daily of timed-release niacin for 12 months. The drug lowered LDL cholesterol by 30 percent and total cholesterol by 26 percent, while increasing HDL cholesterol by 4 percent. Total triglycerides went down by 17 percent. Niacin reduced LDL cholesterol by 2 percent, and total cholesterol by 7 percent; increased HDL cholesterol by 25 percent; and lowered triglycerides by 29 percent.[5]

Aggressive lipid reduction can prevent both primary and secondary coronary episodes and reduce mortality rates. Lipoprotein-a, which is made up of an LDL particle linked by a disulfide bridge to apoprotein-a, can become oxidized and contribute to fatty deposits in the arteries. Further, elevated levels of lipoprotein-a, more than 25 to 30 mg/dl, are a significant risk for cardiovascular disease, according to Antonio Gotto Jr., M.D.[6]

In gram doses, nicotinic acid, or niacin, can significantly increase low HDL cholesterol and reduce elevated LDL cholesterol, triglycerides, and lipoprotein-a, Gotto said. Niacin, the most cost-effective hypolipidemic medication available, was the first nutrient shown to reduce coronary events. In the Coronary Drug Project in the 1970s, long-term treatment with niacin resulted in a 27 percent reduction in recurrent myocardial infarction in men. After 15 years of follow-up, there was a significant 11 percent drop in mortality in the niacin-treated group. New formulations of niacin, such as an extended-release formulation, have improved tolerance as a lipid-modifying therapy, Gotto added.

A study at Texas Southwestern Medical Center in Dallas involved 44 men with HDL-cholesterol levels of less than 40 mg/dl. The trial included three phases: first, a 30 percent–fat diet; second, the volunteers were given 1.5 g/day of niacin; third, they were given 3 g/day of niacin. In the 1.5 g/day treatment group, B_3 brought an average 20 percent increase in HDL cholesterol as well as significantly lower triglyceride levels.[7]

For alcoholics who refuse to stop drinking, the low cost of nicotinamide and the absence of side effects at doses twice as high as those used in the study (1.25 g/day with meals) might make it a cost-effective intervention strategy It also has a wide margin of safety in preventing liver disease, according to Italian researchers.[8]

Using laboratory mice, topical nicotinamide reduced skin tumors from 75 percent to 42.5 percent in animals who had been exposed to UV radiation.[9]

In The Netherlands, seven patients with bullous pemphigoid (blistering skin lesions) were given a daily regimen of 2 g of tetracycline and 2 g of nicotinamide. Total remission was achieved in six to eight weeks, at which time the dose was gradually reduced.[10]

A pilot study at the National Institutes of Health, Bethesda, Maryland, involved 72 patients with osteoarthritis who received either 3,000 mg/day of niacinamide or a placebo for 12 weeks. Arthritis symptoms improved 29 percent with the niacin therapy and worsened by 10 percent in the control group. Although pain levels did not change, the vitamin B_3 group reduced their anti-inflammatory medications by 13 percent. The beneficial effect was noted between one and three months of therapy, with the maximum benefit reported in one to three years.[11]

Not many researchers are aware of the landmark work achieved by William Kaufman, M.D., a New York physician, in using niacinamide and other supplements to treat arthritis. Some of his patients needed almost 1,000 mg/day of B_3. It is unfortunate that his important work has not been duplicated, since he was able to relieve arthritis symptoms in many patients. His book, now out of print, was *The Common Form of Joint Dysfunction: Its Incidence and Treatment*, published in 1949.[12]

When some people take niacin, they will experience a vasodilation (niacin flush)—a dilation of the blood vessels—beginning in the forehead and extending downward, in which the skin may itch and turn red. This is probably due to a sudden release of histamine. The flush usually goes away in a few hours and often diminishes the longer the vitamin is taken. It is not harmful except for those who are highly susceptible to the flush. The intensity of the flush can be reduced by taking aspirin or antihistamine before or at the time the niacin is taken. Or, niacinamide can be used instead. Niacinamide usually does not cause a flush.[13]

Various forms of vitamin B_3 are available over the counter. If you are suffering from schizophrenia, Type 1 diabetes, high cholesterol levels, or arthritis, for example, ask your health care provider about this unique vitamin.

References

1. Ensminger, A., et al., *Foods and Nutrition Encyclopedia* (Clovis, Calif: Pegus Press, 1983), 1589ff.

2. Hoffer, Abram, "Orthomolecular Treatment for Schizophrenia," *Natural Medicine Journal* 2(3): 12–13, March 1999.

3. Cunningham, J. J., "Micronutrients as Nutraceutical Interventions in Diabetes Mellitus," *Journal of the American College of Nutrition* 17(1): 7–10, 1998.

4. Pozzilli, Paolo, et al., "Vitamin E and Nicotinamide Have Similar Effects in Maintaining Residual Beta Cell Function in Recent Onset Insulin-Dependent Diabetes (the IMDIAB IV Study)," *European Journal of Endocrinology* 137: 234–39, 1997.

5. McKenney, James M., et al., "A Randomized Trial of the Effects of Atorvastatin and Niacin in Patients with Combined Hyperlipidemia or Isolated Hypertriglyceridemia," *American Journal of Medicine* 104: 137–43, 1998.

6. Gotto, Antonio M., Jr., "The New Cholesterol Education Imperative and Some Comments on Niacin," *American Journal of Cardiology* 81: 492–94, Feb. 15, 1998.

7. Martin-Jadraque, Raquel, et al., "Effectiveness of Low-Dose Crystalline Nicotinic Acid in Men with Low High-Density Lipoprotein Cholesterol Levels," *Archives of Internal Medicine* 156: 1081–88, 1996.

8. Volpi, Elena, et al., "Nicotinamide Counteracts Alcohol-Induced Impairment of Hepatic Protein Metabolism in Humans," *Journal of Nutrition* 127: 2199–2204, 1997.

9. Gensler, Helen L., "Prevention of Photoimmunosuppression and Photocarcinogenesis by Topical Nicotinamide," *Nutrition and Cancer* 29(2): 157–62, 1997.

10. Kolbach, D. N., et al., "Bullous Pemphigoid Successfully Controlled by Tetracycline and Nicotinamide," *British Journal of Dermatology* 133: 88–90, 1995.

11. Jonas, W. B., et al., "The Effect of Niacinamide on Osteoarthritis: A Pilot Study," *Inflammation Research* 45: 330–34, 1996.

12. Adams, Ruth, and Frank Murray, *Arthritis* (New York: Larchmont Books, 1979), 89ff.

13. Hoffer, Abram, *Orthomolecular Medicine for Physicians* (New Canaan, Conn.: Keats Publishing, 1989), 36, 151.

92

Vitamin B$_6$ (Pyridoxine)

When John M. Ellis, M.D., retired from his medical practice in Mount Pleasant, Texas, alternative medicine lost a great champion for vitamin B$_6$. Ellis had spent a lifetime researching and studying the vitamin. He and his sometime collaborator, Karl Folkers, Ph.D., of the University of Texas at Austin, were essentially protégés of the Hungarian-American scientist Paul Gyorgy, M.D., who discovered vitamin B$_6$ in 1934. They had frequently discussed their research with Gyorgy prior to his death. Gyorgy, who worked at the University of Pennsylvania School of Medicine at Philadelphia, also discovered two other B vitamins—biotin and riboflavin (B$_2$). It was Gyorgy who named B$_6$ pyridoxine. The vitamin consists of three closely related substances: pyridoxine, pyridoxal, and pyridoxamine.

One of Ellis and Folkers's more interesting experiments revealed that newborn infants in Austin had more vitamin B$_6$ circulating in their blood than did some of Ellis's patients with rheumatism/arthritis, carpal tunnel syndrome, premenstrual edema, toxemia of pregnancy, and other health problems.

In his book, *Free of Pain,* which mentions many of the nutritional pioneers of the twentieth century, Ellis lists the signs and symptoms of a vitamin B$_6$ deficiency: paresthesia of the hands (numbness and tingling); impaired sensation in the fingers; impaired finger flexion in the joints; fluctuating edema in hands; morning stiffness of finger joints; pain in the hands; impaired coordination in finger function; weakness of pinch (pressure between thumb and index finger); dropping of objects; tenderness over the carpal tunnel with Tinel's and

Phalen's signs; painful shoulders; painful movement of the thumb at the knuckle (the metacarpophalangeal joint); painful elbows; and sleep paralysis.[1]

The following conditions, which give rise to the above symptoms, will respond to vitamin B$_6$ therapy: idiopathic carpal tunnel syndrome; acute, subacute, and chronic noninflammatory tenosynovitis; acute, subacute, and chronic noninflammatory tendinitis; de Quervain's disease (synovitis of thumb tendons); diabetic neuropathy as related to carpal tunnel syndrome; periarticular synovitis around multiple joints; shoulder-hand syndrome; premenstrual edema; menopausal arthritis; edema of pregnancy; toxemia of pregnancy; use of birth control pills; arterial subendothelia proliferation; and hardening of the arteries.

"After five years of study and collaboration, Karl Folkers and I had blood data that showed B$_6$ deficiency in 33 patients with idiopathic carpal tunnel syndrome, all of whom were treated with pyridoxine and only two underwent surgery of the carpal tunnel," Ellis said. "The balance of 31 were cured of their complaint by being cured of their B$_6$ deficiency through taking 100 milligrams of B$_6$ daily."

He added, "I further state without reservation that all pregnant women should have at least 50 mg/day of B$_6$ as a supplement throughout their pregnancies, and many will require a larger dose. All pregnant women should also receive at least 500 mg/day of magnesium. Vitamin and mineral supplements prevent many complications of pregnancy."

From 1962 to 1972, Ellis gave B$_6$ in varying amounts to more than 200 pregnant women, the dosage determined by the degree of edema (swelling) in their hands and feet. Twenty-five of the women exhibited symptoms identical with carpal tunnel syndrome, and every one responded to treatment with 50 to 300 mg/day of B$_6$.

Carpal tunnel syndrome, a painful condition of the wrist, begins with a major nerve that carries signals between the hand and the brain. Traveling through the wrist, the nerve passes through a tunnel formed by the wrist bones (the carpals) and a tough membrane on the underside of the wrist that binds the bones together. Since the tunnel is rigid, swollen tissues press on and pinch the nerve, causing excruciating pain. The problem affects computer operators, post office employees, pianists, and others who constantly flex their wrists.

More than 200,000 carpal tunnel syndrome operations are performed every year in the United States, at an annual estimated cost of more than $1 billion.[2] Carpal tunnel syndrome may be reversed using special exercises, better hand posture, inexpensive hand splints worn at night, or nonsteroidal anti-inflammatories. Surgery—sometimes unnecessary—on the median nerve can cost anywhere from $3,000 to $10,000.[3]

Writing in *Physician Management* in 1994, Paul C. Gerber explained that therapies given by Alan R. Gaby, M.D., could possibly save up to 20 percent of the health care dollar, including the use of vitamin B_6 for carpal tunnel syndrome. B_6 costs about $5 for a three-month supply versus conventional surgical treatment.[4]

According to the *Journal of the American College of Nutrition*, 100 to 200 mg/day of B_6 has been shown to relieve the symptoms of carpal tunnel syndrome in 12 weeks. The dosage is well below the 500 mg/day dosage that has been suggested as the upper range to avoid toxicity.[5]

A study at Kaiser Permanente Medical Center in Hayward, California, evaluated 20 patients between the ages of 27 and 63 who were diagnosed with carpal tunnel syndrome. They had been taking 200 mg/day of B_6 for three months. Pain scores dramatically improved during the course of the study, and 200 mg/day of B_6 did not produce any toxicity.[6]

Researchers at the Portland Hand Surgery and Rehabilitation Center in Oregon recruited 441 adult volunteers and reported that B_6 is beneficial to some people with carpal tunnel syndrome. The vitamin apparently may act as a diuretic, reducing fluid accumulation and possibly helping the carpal tunnel syndrome as well. Dosages range from 100 to 200 mg/day of B_6, and the treatment period is usually 12 weeks.[7]

Kilmer S. McCully, M.D., was perhaps the first researcher to detail how elevated levels of homocysteine, the amino acid, damage intimal cells that lead to heart attacks and strokes. Deficiencies of B_6 and folic acid, which aid in the formation of homocysteine, are related to insufficient intakes of the two B vitamins in foods, as well as losses of the nutrients due to processing, preservation, and the marketing of foods such as white flour, white rice, sugar, fats, and oils. McCully recommends daily supplements of 3 mg of B_6 and 400 mcg of folic acid to reduce the risk of hardening of the arteries and other problems, assuming these amounts are not being provided by the diet.[8]

At the Queen's University of Belfast in Ireland, researchers determined that B vitamins and antioxidants are an effective way of reducing homocysteine levels, reducing LDL-cholesterol oxidation, and therefore lowering the risk of cardiovascular disease. The study involved 101 men who completed an eight-week intervention program. The B vitamins consisted of 1 mg/day of folic acid; 7.2 mg/day of B_6; and 0.02 mg/day of B_{12}, which reduced homocysteine levels by 27.9 percent. The antioxidants were 150 mg/day of vitamin C; 100 mg/day of vitamin E; and 9 mg/day of beta-carotene, which brought homocysteine levels up by an insignificant 5.1 percent. But the antioxidants significantly increased resistance to LDL oxidation.[9]

In 18 consecutive studies on autism between 1965 and 1996, almost half of the children in the study benefited from vitamin B_6 therapy. The average amount of the vitamin that proved to be beneficial was 8 mg per body weight per day. B_6, combined with 4 mg/day per body weight of magnesium, often results in improvement within several days. For adults, the B_6 recommendation is 1,000 mg/day for a 120-pound person, and up to 400 mg/day of magnesium. Also beneficial for autistic children is dimethylglycine (DMG), which usually comes in 125-mg tablets. A five-year-old boy needed to take 16 DMG tablets daily to bring results. Folic acid (250 mcg per pound of body weight) and vitamin C (8,000 mg/day) have also brought results in autistic individuals.[10]

Doses of vitamin B_6 up to 100 mg/day are likely to be of benefit in treating premenstrual symptoms and premenstrual depression. PMS symptoms include bloating, weight gain, abdominal pain, lack of energy, and headache.[11]

In a placebo-controlled study involving 342 pregnant women, 30 mg/day of B_6 significantly reduced the severity of nausea and the number of vomiting bouts daily in the treated women. This amount of B_6 apparently did not affect the fetus.[12]

Turkish researchers studied 25 pregnant women who were given 250 mg of B_6 and 250 mg of B_1 orally twice daily for four weeks over a six-week period to study the effect on leg cramps. The women were healthy and revealed no nutritional deficiencies. In 10 of the patients, the vitamin therapy completely relieved their cramps, and 14 showed significant improvements. One patient did not respond to the therapy. Normally, B_6 and B_1 levels are reduced during pregnancy, probably because the fetus gets first dibs on the nutrients.[13]

Analysis of food intake surveys, using previous RDAs, indicates that 10 to 25 percent of men and 25 to 50 percent of women 51 years of age and older have vitamin B_6 intakes below the newly established Estimated Average Requirement (EAR). In the Boston Nutritional Status Survey of the Elderly, researchers found that even in seemingly well-nourished populations, B_6 intakes were often below the EAR.[14]

Since B_6 acts as a coenzyme in the metabolism of amino acids and carbohydrates, B_6 intakes in the elderly are essential because the vitamin plays an active role in homocysteine metabolism and because a B_6 deficiency can impair immune function. The vitamin is also necessary for the maintenance of glucose tolerance and normal cognitive function in the elderly. B_6 requirements are higher for older adults than for younger people, and they are higher for men than for women. The new RDAs for those aged 51 and older are 1.7 mg/day for men and 1.5 mg/day for women. For younger men and women, the RDA is 1.3 and 1.2 mg/day, respectively.

Supplementation with multivitamins and minerals is appropriate therapy for patients with rheumatoid arthritis. In evaluating 41 patients with rheumatoid arthritis, researchers found that both men and women were getting less than the RDA for vitamin B_6, magnesium, and zinc. Folic acid and copper levels were deficient when compared to typical American diet intakes.[15]

In Munich, researchers reported that vitamin B_6 is beneficial for B_6-dependent epilepsy patients to avoid mental retardation. Doses range from 10 to 90 mg/kg body weight daily.[16]

Researchers at the Beltsville Human Nutrition Research Center in Maryland studied 15 adult bronchial asthma patients whose B_6 levels were considerably lower than the controls. Although 50 mg of B_6 twice daily did not elevate B_6 levels in the treatment group, these patients did experience a decrease in severity of their wheezing and asthma attacks.[17]

It has been known for 40 years that a deficiency in B_6 causes seizures in infants. The preventive dosage ranges from 200 to 300 mg/day to 0.2 to 30 mg/kg of body weight per day. Most children can be protected with 50 mg/day of B_6. In small children, this translates to 5 mg/kg of body weight daily.[18]

At the University Hospital of Louis Pasteur in Kosice, Slovakia, a vitamin B_6 deficiency was often found in chronic kidney failure patients. The deficiency is due to decreased amounts of the vitamin in the diet, losses during dialysis, and other reasons. For patients without erythropoietin treatment, the B_6 dosage is 5 mg/day. For those with erythropoietin treatment, the recommendation is 20 mg/day. Erythropoietin is a hormonal substance formed in the kidneys that stimulates red blood cell formation. In addition, 50 mg/day of B_6 stimulates the immune system in hemodialysis patients.[19]

In a study at Dalhouse University in Halifax, Nova Scotia, Canada, B_6 and vitamin E restored the health of a 74-year-old woman with a long-standing history of schizophrenia. Upon admission, she was experiencing auditory and visual hallucinations and paranoid delusions. Among the several drugs she had been taking was risperidone, an antipsychotic drug used for treating schizophrenia. She was diagnosed as having neuroleptic malignant syndrome, possibly related to the risperidone. The drugs were eventually discontinued and she was given 1,600 IU/day of vitamin E and 200 mg/day of B_6. After two weeks of vitamin therapy, her abnormal involuntary movement scores decreased from 39 to 19, her psychiatric rating scale also went down from 74 to 45, and she fully recovered.[20]

Pancreatic cancer ranks eleventh for cancer incidence and fifth among cancer deaths in the United States. Finland has a relatively high mortality rate for the disease. There are few risk factors for pancreatic cancer, but cigarette smoking and age have been implicated.[21] At the National Cancer Institute in Bethesda, Maryland, and other facilities in the United States and Finland, researchers conducted a case-control study within the Alpha-Tocopherol, Beta-Carotene Cancer Prevention Study of 29,133 male Finnish smokers ranging in age from 50 to 69. The results support the hypothesis that maintaining adequate folic acid and vitamin B_6 status—especially in a diet rich in fruits and vegetables—may reduce the risk of pancreatic cancer and confirm the risk associated with cigarette smoking.

"The level of folic acid grain fortification in the U.S. has been estimated to reduce the risk of neural tube defects by 22 to 26 percent in women with marginal folate status, and, in view of our study, could conceivably have an impact on pancreatic cancer in those with marginal folic acid status," the research team said.

Since B$_6$ is found in a variety of foods, there should be no reason why people are deficient in the vitamin, but as we have seen, that is not the case. Some of the best food sources are liver, wheat germ, brewer's yeast, brown rice, fish, eggs, nuts, soybeans, peas, whole-grain cereals, bananas, pears, grapes, cabbage, carrots, kale, tomatoes, spinach, cauliflower, and turnips. To get larger amounts, B$_6$ supplements are probably needed by most people.

References

1. Ellis, John Marion, *Free of Pain* (Dallas: Southwest Publishing Co., 1983), 29–144.

2. Franzblau, Alfred, and Robert A. Werner, "What Is Carpal Tunnel Syndrome?" *Journal of the American Medical Association* 282(2): 186–87, July 14, 1999.

3. "Repetitive-Motion Ills Worsened by Quick Ergonomic Fixes in Workplace," *Medical Tribune,* July 23, 1992, 12.

4. Gerber, Paul C., "Alternative Medicine: All Eyes on NIH's Office of Alternative Medicine," press release, March 1994, 30–42.

5. Reynolds, Robert, "Vitamin Supplements: Current Controversies," *Journal of the American College of Nutrition* 13(2): 118–26, 1994.

6. Bernstein, Allan L., and Jamie S. Dinesen, "Brief Communication: Effect of Pharmacologic Doses of Vitamin B$_6$ on Carpal Tunnel Syndrome, Electroencephalographic Results, and Pain," *Journal of the American College of Nutrition* 12(1) 73–76, 1993.

7. Keniston, Richard C., et al., "Vitamin B$_6$, Vitamin C, and Carpal Tunnel Syndrome: A Cross-Sectional Study of 441 Adults," *Journal of Occupational and Environmental Medicine* 39(10): 949–59, Oct. 1997.

8. McCully, Kilmer S., "Homocysteine, Folate, Vitamin B$_6$, and Cardiovascular Disease," *Journal of the American Medical Association* 279(5): 392–93, Feb. 4, 1998.

9. Woodside, J., et al., "The Effects of Vitamin Supplementation on Cardiovascular Risk," *Journal of Inheritable and Metabolic Disease* 19(Suppl. 1): 26, 1996.

10. Rimland, Bernard, "What Is the Right 'Dosage' for Vitamin B$_6$, DMG, and Other Nutrients Useful in Autism?" *Autism Research Review International* 11(4): 3, 1997.

11. Wyatt, Katrina M., et al., "Efficacy of Vitamin B$_6$ in the Treatment of Premenstrual Syndrome: Systematic Review," *British Medical Journal* 318: 1375–81, May 22, 1999.

12. Baker, Barbara, "Vitamin B$_6$ Can Ease Pregnancy-Related Nausea," *Family Practice News,* Sept. 1, 1997.

13. Avsar, A. Filiz, et al., "Vitamin B$_1$ and Vitamin B$_6$ Substitution in Pregnancy for Leg Cramps," *American Journal of Obstetrics and Gynecology* 175(1): 233–34, July 1996.

14. Rosenberg, Irwin H., "Vitamin Needs of Older Americans," *Vitamin Nutrition Information Service Back-Grounder* 7(1): 2–3, April 1999.

15. Kremer, Joel M., and Jean Bigaouette, "Nutrient Intake of Patients with Rheumatoid Arthritis Is Deficient in Pyridoxine, Zinc, Copper, and Magnesium," *Journal of Rheumatology* 23(6): 990–94, 1996.

16. Baumeister, F. A. M., and J. Egger, "Diagnosis and Therapy of Vitamin B$_6$–Dependent Epilepsy," *Monatsschr Kinderheilkd* 144: 534–36, 1996.

17. Reynolds, Robert D., and Clayton Natta, "Depressed Plasma Pyridoxal Phosphate Concentrations in Adult Asthmatics," *American Journal of Clinical Nutrition* 41: 684–88, April 1985.

18. Gospe, S. M., Jr., "Current Perspectives on Pyridoxine-Dependent Seizures," *Journal of Pediatrics* 132(6): 919–23, June 1998.

19. Mydlik, Miroslav, et al., "Metabolism of B$_6$ and Its Requirement in Chronic Renal Failure," *Kidney International* 52(Suppl. 62): S56–S59, 1997.

20. Dursun, S. M., et al., "High-Dose Vitamin E Plus Vitamin B$_6$ Treatment of Risperidone-Related Neuroleptic Malignant Syndrome," *Journal of Psychopharmacology* 12(2): 220–21, 1998.

21. Stolzenberg-Solomon, Rachael Z., et al., "Pancreatic Cancer Risk and Nutrition-Related Methyl-Group Availability Indicators in Male Smokers," *Journal of the National Cancer Institute* 91(6): 535–41, March 17, 1999.

93

Vitamin B$_{12}$

In *New Scientist* in 1964, E. Lester Smith, Ph.D., wrote that May 5 is still celebrated in his laboratory as "red crystal day." It was on that date in 1948 that the first microscopic crystals of vitamin B$_{12}$ appeared, isolated from liver. B$_{12}$ is also variously called cobalamine and cyanocobalamin. Containing probably the most complex chemical formula of any vitamin, the water-soluble B$_{12}$ is the only vitamin to contain a metal—cobalt—as well as phosphorus. Since B$_{12}$ cannot be duplicated in the laboratory, it is the most potent of vitamins. B$_{12}$ does not have to be extracted from natural sources such as liver, but it can be synthesized from fermentation procedures similar to those used in making penicillin and other antibiotics.[1]

Pernicious anemia is a disease of the blood cells that can be deadly if left untreated. B$_{12}$ is a curative agent. A sub-stance called intrinsic factor, present in the human stomach, allows a healthy person to absorb B$_{12}$ from food. When this substance is lacking, the individual cannot absorb the vitamin and may well develop pernicious anemia. B$_{12}$ injections are usually given to alleviate the problem; however, large doses given orally can apparently be properly absorbed for those who do not have intrinsic factor.

The late Roger J. Williams, Ph.D., of the University of Texas at Austin, said that B$_{12}$ is definitely a link in the nutritional chain that protects against mental illness. But in pernicious anemia, the mental symptoms are not necessarily uniform and can range from difficulty in concentrating or remembering to stuporous depression, severe agitation, hallucinations, and even manic or paranoid behavior. Like the symptoms of pellagra (caused by a B$_3$ deficiency), those caused by B_{12} deficiency may be similar to those observed in schizophrenia.

Homocysteine, a breakdown product of the amino acid methionine, can reach elevated levels and become a risk factor for heart attacks and strokes. These levels can be reduced with 0.65 to 10 mg/day of folic acid, 250 mg/day of vitamin B_6, and 1 mg/day of B_{12} given by injection. Ingestion of multivitamins may also lower homocysteine levels.[2]

At the Siebens-Drake/Roberts Research Institute in London, Ontario, Canada, vitamin therapy reduced homocysteine levels and hardening of the arteries among 38 men and women who were observed for 4.4 years. The supplement regimen consisted of 5 mg/day of folic acid beginning in 1994, and in 1996, 2.5 mg/day of folic acid, 25 mg/day of B_6, and 250 mcg/day of B_{12}.[3]

Vitamin therapy can reduce damage to the lining of the arteries, even for patients who have had a stroke. Researchers evaluated 29 men and 21 women who had strokes, all 50 years of age or older. The 27 patients in the treatment group received 5 mg of folic acid, 100 mg of B_6, and 1 mg of B_{12} daily, which brought a 27 percent reduction in homocysteine in the treatment group.[4]

Researchers at the University of Colorado Health Sciences Center at Denver stated that a B_{12} deficiency is present in up to 15 percent of the elderly. Many of the seniors have elevated homocysteine levels with an undiagnosed B_{12} deficiency. However, they should not be given folic acid supplements until their B_{12} stores have been evaluated. The researchers suggested 100 to 1,000 mcg/day of B_{12} to raise B_{12} concentrations and lower methylmalonic acid levels. The latter acid is an intermediate in fatty acid metabolism and is often elevated when there is a B_{12} deficiency. Since B_{12} and folic acid are so intimately intertwined, it is important that B_{12} status be monitored in the elderly because of the increasing fortification of foods with folic acid.[5]

Patients undergoing high-flux hemodialysis often have a drop in levels of B_{12}. In one study, 22 patients whose levels of B_{12} dropped considerably had to be given supplements. A B_{12} deficiency is related not only to losses during dialysis, but also to low amounts of the vitamin in the patients' food.[6]

An expert panel suggested that B_{12} should probably be added to any supplement containing folic acid to avoid masking a B_{12} deficiency. While homocysteine levels are an indicator of folate, B_{12}, and B_6 deficiency, an excess of methylmalonic acid may be an even more reliable indicator of a B_{12} deficiency.[7]

Researchers at West Virginia University at Charleston have stated that high risk groups for B_{12} deficiency include the elderly, those taking ulcer medications for long periods, AIDS patients, vegetarians, those who have had stomach or bowel surgery, and patients with dementia. The recommendation is 1,000 mcg of B_{12} injections given weekly and then monthly, or the same amount given orally. Intranasal doses of 500 mcg can be given once a week.[8]

In *Medical Hypotheses,* John V. Dommisse, M.D., wrote that the psychiatric conditions most associated with B_{12} deficiency include organic brain syndrome, paranoia, violence, and depression. Oral doses of 1,000 to 5,000 mcg/day of B_{12} have been used for patients with pernicious anemia. But oral doses between 1,000 and 2,600 mcg/day after breakfast and supper seem to be the best way to maintain high levels of the vitamin.[9]

Patients with HIV-positive infections who experience chronic diarrhea should be screened for B_{12} deficiency, since the water-soluble vitamin is lost during the day in urine and feces. Of 36 patients tested, 39 percent had low levels of the vitamin.[10]

Of six patients with Alzheimer's disease in another study, four had low levels of B_{12}. Since many elderly have low B_{12} stores in their blood, this was not a surprising finding.[11]

Sulfites, often used in salad bars and in the processing and storage of foods and beverages, can cause asthma in susceptible people. In an Italian study, B_{12} was able to block a sulfite-induced bronchospasm in four of five asthmatic children.[12]

In 10 of 12 patients with asthma, researchers reported good results by giving them 30 mg/day of B_{12} for 15 to 20 days. One patient reported weight gain and improvement in constipation, while another experienced an improvement in dyspepsia due to hyperacidity.[13]

At the Karolinska Institute in Huddinge, Sweden, 16 patients with multiple sclerosis (MS) were evaluated. Blood levels of B_{12} in these patients were lower than in the healthy controls. MS patients often have elevated levels of homocysteine and a B_{12} deficiency. The researchers recommended B_6 and B_{12} therapy.[14]

In studying 61 patients who had gastric surgery for peptic ulcer, and 107 controls, researchers discovered that 48 percent of the patients versus 21 percent of the controls had low blood levels of B_{12}. They also found that 80 percent of 19 B_{12}-deficient postsurgery patients had elevated blood levels of methylmalonic acid, and 63 percent had raised levels of both methylmalonic acid and homocysteine. The levels went down following B_{12} supplementation.[15]

It is estimated that 28 million Americans have hearing impairments, and this number is expected to increase as the population ages. Five to 15 percent of the elderly may be deficient in B_{12}, and between two and 20 percent may be lacking in folic acid. High homocysteine concentrations, accompanied by low levels of B_{12} and folic acid, may be related to hearing loss, since deficiencies in the vitamins may adversely affect blood flow to the cochlea of the inner ear, where much of the hearing loss occurs.[16]

A study at the University of Athens in Greece evaluated a 55-year-old man who had been dieting for 10 years. Unable to lose weight, he opted for an operation to treat his obesity, but the dieting and the operation depleted his B_{12} stores and he almost lost his eyesight. B_{12} therapy did not restore his vision. In four other cases, however, B_{12} supplements resulted in an improvement in vision.[17]

Researchers studied 38 men, all heavy smokers, who had bronchial squamous metaplasia. In the treatment group of 21, who received 10 to 20 mg/day of folic acid and 750 mg/day of B_{12} for one year, there was a significant decrease in lesions, compared to the controls.[18]

At University Hospital in Uppsala, Sweden, vitamin B_{12} and folic acid were used to treat patients with vitiligo, a skin disorder characterized by smooth white spots on various parts of the body. In the study, 33 males and 67 females aged 9 to 75 were given 1 mg of B_{12} and 5 mg of folic acid twice daily. They were encouraged to expose their skin to the sun in summer and UVB radiation in winter to cause a slight reddening of the white areas. The treatment lasted from three to six months. Repigmentation was noticeable in 52 patients, including 37 who sunned themselves in the summer and six who used UVB lamps in the winter. Following therapy, the spread of vitiligo had stopped in 64 percent of the treatment group. Supplementing with the two B vitamins, combined with sun exposure, can induce repigmentation better than either of the vitamins or sun exposure alone. Therapy should continue as long as the white areas continue to repigment.[19]

In studying 21 strict vegans compared to 21 omnivorous controls, a lower concentration of B_{12} was found in the blood of vegans, compared to the controls, according to researchers in Finland. In following nine vegans, there was a deterioration of B_{12} levels over a two-year period. While some seaweeds they consumed in large amounts might have provided enough bioavailable B_{12}, the average use of seaweed and fermented foods did not provide enough of the vitamin to maintain B_{12} status.[20]

G. P. Oakley Jr. believes that foods fortified with folic acid should also contain added B_{12}. Older people often do not absorb B_{12} as readily as young people because of a reduction in gastric acidity. Another concern is that those with severe B_{12} deficiency may have a delay in diagnosis and treatment if they don't exhibit pernicious anemia.[21]

B_{12} is not widely available in foods. Some of the best sources include beef kidney, beef liver, sole, ham, and powdered milk. The recommended daily amount is about 2 mcg/day for most adults. Pregnant women need 2.2 mcg/day, while breastfeeding women should get 2.6 mcg/day.

References

1. Adams, Ruth, and Frank Murray, *Body, Mind, and the B Vitamins* (New York: Larchmont Books, 1981), 176ff.
2. Malinow, M. R., et al., "Plasma Homocysteine: A Risk Factor for Arterial Occlusive Diseases," *Journal of Nutrition* 126:1238S–43S, 1996.
3. Peterson, John C., and J. David Spence, "Vitamins and Progression of Atheroscle-

rosis in Hyper-Homocysteinemia," *The Lancet* 351: 263, Jan. 24, 1998.

4. Peck, Peggy, "Homocysteine Response Seen with B Vitamins," *Family Practice News,* April 1, 1998, 32.

5. Stabler, Sally P., et al., "Vitamin B$_{12}$ Deficiency in the Elderly: Current Dilemmas," *American Journal of Clinical Nutrition* 66: 741–49, 1997.

6. Chandna, Shahid M., et al., "Low Serum Vitamin B$_{12}$ Levels in Chronic High-Flux Hemodialysis Patients," *Nephron* 75: 259–63, 1997.

7. Rowe, Paul M., "Institute of Medicine Examines Folate, B$_{12}$, and Choline Needs," *The Lancet* 349: 780, March 15, 1997.

8. Swain, Randall, "An Update on Vitamin B$_{12}$ Metabolism and Deficiency States," *Journal of Family Practice* 41(6): 595–600, Dec. 1995.

9. Dommisse, J., "Subtle Vitamin B$_{12}$ Deficiency and Psychiatry: A Largely Unnoticed But Devastating Relationship?" *Medical Hypotheses* 34: 131–40, 1991.

10. Ehrenpreis, E., et al., "Malabsorption and Deficiency of Vitamin B$_{12}$ and HIV-Infected Patients with Chronic Diarrhea," *Digestive Diseases and Sciences* 39(10): 2159–62, Oct. 1994.

11. McCaddon, A., and C. Kelly, "Familial Alzheimer's Disease and Vitamin B$_{12}$ Deficiency," *Age and Ageing* 23: 334–37, July 1994.

12. Peroni, D. G., and A. L. Boner, "Sulfite Sensitivity," *Clinical and Experimental Allergy* 25: 680–81, 1995.

13. Caruselli, M., "Vitamin B$_{12}$ in Asthma," *Riforma Medica* 66: 841–64, Aug. 2, 1952.

14. Baig, Shadid M., and G. A. Qureshi, "Homocysteine and Vitamin B$_{12}$ in Multiple Sclerosis," *Biogenic Amines* 11(6): 479–85, 1995.

15. Kapadia, Cyrus R., "Vitamin B$_{12}$ Deficiency After Gastric Surgery: Its Early Indication," *Gastroenterology* 11(4): 1151–55, 1996.

16. Houston, Denise K., et al., "Age-Related Hearing Loss, Vitamin B$_{12}$, and Folate in Elderly Women," *American Journal of Clinical Nutrition* 69: 564–71, 1999.

17. Moschos, Michael, "A Man Who Lost Weight and His Sight," *The Lancet,* 351–1174, April 15, 1998.

18. Saito, M., et al., "Chemoprevention Effects on Bronchial Squamous Metaplasia by Folate and Vitamin B$_{12}$ in Heavy Smokers," *Chest* 106: 496–99, Aug. 1994.

19. Juhlin, Lennart, and Mats J. Olsson, "Improvement of Vitiligo After Oral Treatment with Vitamin B$_{12}$ and Folic Acid and the Importance of Sun Exposure," *Acta Dermatologica Venerologica* (Stockholm) 77: 460–62, 1997.

20. Rauma, Anna-Lisa, et al., "Vitamin B$_{12}$ Status of Long-Term Adherents of a Strict Uncooked Vegan Diet (Living Food Diet) Is Compromised," *Journal of Nutrition* 125: 2511–15, 1995.

21. Oakley, Godfrey P., Jr., "Let's Increase Folic Acid Fortification and Include Vitamin B$_{12}$," *American Journal of Clinical Nutrition* 65: 1889–90, 1997.

94

Vitamin C

In 1974, Emil Ginter, M.D., of the Institute of Human Nutrition Research in Bratislava, Czechoslovakia (now Slovakia), explained to me that if infants were given ascorbic acid and tracked throughout their lives, he was convinced they would never develop heart disease, because the vitamin C would keep cholesterol deposits at bay. In one study, 1,000 mg/day of vitamin C lowered cholesterol by about 10 percent during a 47-day trial. In another study, Ginter gave adults 300 mg/day of the vitamin for 47 days and found that in 13 of the adults, cholesterol deposits dropped by an average of 33 mg/200 ml. In still another trial, 1,000 mg/day brought a decrease in triglycerides from an average of 230 mg/100 ml to an average of 126. For the vitamin C, Ginter used a novel pink wafer that fizzed when it was placed in a glass of water.[1]

Numerous researchers have concurred with Ginter's findings. Constance Spittle, M.D., reported that 1,000 mg/day of vitamin C decreased cholesterol levels. Irwin Stone, Ph.D., said that, based on more than 40 years of research, he found that 3,000 to 5,000 mg/day of vitamin C in spaced doses may be sufficient to prevent the high incidence of heart disease and strokes. H. L. Loh, M.D., of the University of Dublin in Ireland also supported the use of vitamin C in lowering cholesterol levels. Omer Pelletier, Ph.D., of Ottawa University in Canada, said that for people who smoke 20 or more cigarettes a day, there is a 40 percent reduction in vitamin C in the blood, which could lead to health problems. More recently, scores of researchers have echoed these sentiments, such as Ishwarlal Jialal, M.D., of the University of Texas/Southwestern Medical Center at Dallas.

Anitra C. Carr and Balz Erei of the Linus Pauling Institute, Oregon State University at Corvallis, noted that the recommended dietary allowance (RDA) for vitamin C for nonsmoking adults is 60 mg/day, based on a mean requirement of 46 mg/day to prevent scurvy (the RDA for smokers is 100 mg/day). However, recent scientific evidence suggests that an increased intake of vitamin C is associated with a reduced risk of chronic diseases such as cancer, cardiovascular disease, and cataract. It is likely that the amount of the vitamin needed to prevent scurvy is not sufficient to protect against these diseases.[2]

With this in mind, Carr and Erei reviewed the biochemical, clinical, and epidemiologic evidence to date concerning vitamin C and chronic disease. The data suggest that an intake of 90 to 100 mg/day of vitamin C is necessary for optimum reduction of chronic disease risk in nonsmoking men and women. They suggest that a new RDA for vitamin C should be 120 mg/day.

The great apes, which are as large or larger than adult Americans depending on species and sex, consume from 2,000 to 6,000 mg/day or more of vitamin C. This contrasts with the recommended vitamin C allowance for the average American of 60 mg/day. Like humans, apes are unable to synthesize vitamin C and must obtain it from their diets. Many wild primates ingest higher amounts of many minerals, vitamins, essential fatty acids, dietary fiber, and other necessary nutrients than most human beings, and the increasingly strong recommendation for humans to consume more fresh fruits and vegetables seems to be well supported when examining wild primate diets.[3]

Speaking at an international conference on nutrition and cancer, Mark Levine, M.D., of the National Institute of Diabetes and Digestive and Kidney Diseases said that the RDA for vitamin C should be raised from 60 to 200 mg/day. The vitamin is very safe, he continued, but there can be an elevation of oxalate and uric excretion at daily doses of 1,000 mg/day and higher in susceptible people. A daily serving of five fruits and vegetables provides 210 to 280 mg of the vitamin, but less than one in 10 Americans follows this recommendation.[4]

Researchers at the San Francisco VA Medical Center in California evaluated 6,624 men and women enrolled in the Second National Health and Nutrition Examination Survey (NHANES II). They found that blood levels of vitamin C were associated with the prevalence of coronary heart disease and stroke. For example, a 0.5 mg/dl increase in serum vitamin C brought an 11 percent reduction in coronary heart disease and stroke. Compared with people with low to marginally low vitamin C levels, there was a 27 percent decreased risk of coronary heart disease and 26 percent decreased prevalence of stroke among those with higher blood levels of the vitamin. When results from the NHANES I Follow-Up Study data were published, it was reported that the highest intakes of vitamin C had a 25 to 50 percent reduction in deaths from cardiovascular disease.[5]

British researchers have found that homocysteine damages the vascular endothelium, which could promote a heart attack or stroke. Methionine, an amino acid, is the metabolic precursor of homocysteine, and when volunteers were given 1,000 mg/day of vitamin C for a week before being given oral methionine, oxidative damage was prevented with the vitamin therapy.[6]

Elderly people with relatively low intakes of vitamin C may be at increased risk of illness and death, according to Irwin H. Rosenberg, M.D., of Tufts University School of Medicine in Boston. A study of supposedly well-nourished seniors in Massachusetts showed that those with the lowest vitamin C intakes (less than 91 mg/day) had significantly higher all-cause and coronary heart disease mortality rates than those with higher vitamin C intakes. A British study reported higher death rates from stroke in those with low blood levels of vitamin C or low dietary intakes of the vitamin.[7]

Rosenberg went on to say that several studies revealed a positive association between vitamin C intake and bone density. Vitamin C is essential for the normal synthesis of collagen, a crucial bone protein. Epidemiologic trials have shown an inverse relationship between vitamin C intake and the risk of cataract. While none of the volunteers in the studies had classic scurvy, differences in vitamin C intake within the "normal" range may have important health consequences for elders.

Researchers studied 633 seniors living in East Boston, none of whom had Alzheimer's disease. In a 4.3-years follow-up, 91 of the volunteers developed the disease; however, none had taken vitamins C and E. Of the 27 users of vitamin E supplements and 23 who took vitamin C supplements, none developed the disease. The data suggest that higher doses of vitamins C and E may lower the risk of Alzheimer's disease.[8]

In a study at the University of California at San Francisco, women with high blood levels of vitamin C were half as likely to develop gallbladder problems as people with lower levels of the vitamin. The data, involving medical records of more than 9,000 men and women, suggest that the vitamin may also help to prevent gallstones by assisting in the transformation of cholesterol, one of the main components in most gallstones, into bile acids.[9]

Researchers at Tufts University and other Boston-area facilities evaluated 247 women ranging in age from 56 to 71 who were recruited from the Nurses' Health Study, using those with both high and low intakes of vitamin C. Those who took vitamin C supplements for more than 10 years had a 77 percent lower incidence of cataracts than those who did not take the vitamin. In this study at least, 1,000 mg/day of vitamin C is needed to ward off lens opacity. It seems that larger amounts are needed to keep the lens supplied with vitamin C. Many of the women took at least 500 mg/day of vitamin C in addition to what was ingested from food and multivitamin sources.[10]

The dietary intake of vitamins A, C, and E and lung cancer incidence were evaluated among 3,968 men and 6,100 women between the ages of 25 and 74 (NHANES I Study). After 19 years of follow-up, 248 of the people had developed lung cancer. Those consuming the highest dietary amounts of vitamin C, beta-carotene, and other carotenoids, and vitamin E from foods, had the lowest risk of developing lung cancer.[11]

In general, most people in Western countries are getting sufficient vitamin C from diet and supplements. Researchers at Arizona State University at Tempe, however, were surprised to find a high rate of vitamin C deficiency and depletion among generally healthy, middle-class patients using a health care facility for routine health, gynecological, and pregnancy exams. Six percent of the volunteers had plasma vitamin C levels suggesting a vitamin C deficiency, and 30.4 percent had depleted levels. Vitamin C deficiency is frequently reported in critically ill patients admitted to hospital, suggesting that the condition has created increased utilization and metabolism of the vitamin. A person who does not have full-blown scurvy may still experience generalized weakness and fatigue.[12]

In three controlled trials at the University of Helsinki in Finland, each trial found a considerably lower incidence of pneumonia in the group given between 0.05 g and 2 g/day of vitamin C.[13]

There may be a correlation between deficiencies in antioxidants—especially vitamin C—and asthma. Children of those who smoke have a higher rate of asthma. Cigarette smoke is known to deplete vitamin C stores. Eleven studies, dating from 1973, investigated the relationship between vitamin C supplements and asthma. In 7 of the 11 studies, there was considerable improvement in respiratory function and asthma symptoms when patients were given 1,000 to 2,000 mg/day of vitamin C.[14]

Researchers at the University of Texas Medical Branch at Galveston evaluated the amount of lead in the blood of 75 males between the ages of 20 and 35. The volunteers were given either no vitamin C, 200 mg/day, or 1,000 mg/day of vitamin C for one month. There was no change in the men getting no vitamin C or 200 mg, but for those given 1,000 mg/day, lead levels dropped 81 percent.[15]

The intake of vitamin C in a man's diet can protect his sperm from genetic damage that can cause inherited diseases or cancer in his children, according to Bruce N. Ames, Ph.D., of the University of California at Berkeley. In men who reduced their dietary intake of vitamin C from 250 mg/day to 5 mg/day, a form of DNA damage in their sperm nearly doubled. When the men consumed 60 or 250 mg/day of the vitamin, DNA damage ceased.[16]

According to researchers in Finland, large, therapeutic doses of vitamin C early in the course of a common cold significantly decreases the severity of symptoms. The vitamin may increase the production of T lymphocyte cells and interferon. While some people may experience diarrhea and other gastrointestinal complaints while taking 4 g/day, others may ingest 30 g/day without complications, apparently because the vitamin is being used up to fight the infection. The Finnish study is a rebuttal to the trial by Thomas Chalmers in 1975, who suggested that the vitamin was of no benefit in fighting the common cold.[17]

Studies have suggested that free radicals assist in the proliferation of the HIV virus and diminish the immune response. In a three-month trial, 49 HIV-infected patients received 1,000 mg/day of vitamin C, 800 IU/day of vitamin E, or a placebo. The vitamins greatly reduced free radical activity and slightly reduced concentrations of the virus.[18]

Ultraviolet radiation is responsible for such acute problems as sunburn, suppression of immune function, and photosensitivity reactions, as well as long-term effects such as aging and skin cancer. In a study involving 20 healthy volunteers, researchers compared the protective effects of 2,000 mg/day of vitamin C, 1,000 IU/day of vitamin E, or a placebo against sunburn. The combined use of antioxidants reduced the sunburn reaction, which might suggest a subsequent risk for later skin damage.[19]

The old saw that vitamin C causes kidney stones has been continuously rebutted, yet still turns up in the literature. In fact, vitamin C can prevent kidney stones. In the Harvard Prospective Health Professional Follow-Up Study, volunteers with the highest intakes of vitamin C (around 1,500 mg/day) had a lower risk of kidney stones than those getting lesser amounts of the vitamin. Dosages as high as 10 g/day have not produced any stones. Of course, those on hemodialysis or who have a history of kidney stones, severe kidney disease, or gout should consult their health care professionals.[20]

Numerous ascorbic acid supplements are available in stores. Food sources include citrus fruits, acerola cherries, strawberries, pineapple, black currants, guava, cabbage, turnip greens, broccoli, tomatoes, kale, corn, parsley, cantaloupe, green peppers, papaya, peaches, collards, mustard greens, blueberries, and blackberries.

References

1. Murray, Frank, *Program Your Heart for Health* (New York: Larchmont Books, 1977), 303ff.

2. Carr, Anitra C., and Balz Frei, "Toward a New Recommended Dietary Allowance for Vitamin C Based on Antioxidant and Health Effects in Humans," *American Journal of Clinical Nutrition* 69: 1086–1107, 1999.

3. Milton, Katharine, "Nutritional Characteristics of Wild Primate Foods: Do the Diets of Our Closest Living Relatives Have Lessons for Us?" *Nutrition* 15(6): 488–98, 1999.

4. Jancin, Bruce, "Expert Says Vitamin C RDA Should Be Raised to 200 Mg,"

Family Practice News, Nov. 1, 1997, 21.

5. Simon, Joel A., et al., "Serum Ascorbic Acid and Cardiovascular Disease Prevalence in U.S. Adults," *Epidemiology* 9: 316–21, 1998.

6. Chambers, J. C., et al., "Demonstration of Rapid Onset Vascular Endothelial Dysfunction After Hyperhomocysteinemia: An Effect Reversible with Vitamin C Therapy," *Circulation* 99: 1156–60, March 9, 1999.

7. Rosenberg, Irwin H., "Vitamin Needs of Older Americans," *VNIS Backgrounder* 7(1), April 1999.

8. Morris, M. C., et al., "Vitamin E and Vitamin C Supplement Use and Risk of Incident Alzheimer Disease," *Alzheimer Disease and Associated Disorders* 12: 121–26, 1998.

9. Carroll, Linda, "Vitamin C Helps Prevent Gallstones in Women," *Medical Tribune,* Sept. 17, 1998, 25.

10. Jacques, Paul F., et al., "Long-Term Vitamin C Supplement Use and Prevalence of Early Age-Related Lens Opacities," *American Journal of Clinical Nutrition* 66: 911–16, 1997.

11. Yong, L. C., et al., "Intake of Vitamins E, C, and A and Risk of Lung Cancer: The NHANES I Epidemiologic Follow-Up Study," *American Journal of Epidemiology* 146: 231–43, 1997.

12. Johnston, Carol S., and Lori L. Thompson, "Vitamin C Status of an Outpatient Population," *Journal of the American College of Nutrition* 17(4): 366–70, 1998.

13. Hemila, Harri, "Vitamin C Intake and Susceptibility to Pneumonia," *Pediatric Infectious Disease Journal* 16(9): 836–37, 1997.

14. Hatch, Gary E., et al., "Asthma, Inhaled Oxidants, and Dietary Antioxidants," *American Journal of Clinical Nutrition* 61: 625S–30S, 1995.

15. Dawson, E. B., et al., "Effect of Ascorbic Acid Supplementation on Blood Lead Levels," *Journal of the American College of Nutrition* 16(5): 480/Abstract 42, 1997.

16. "Daily Vitamin C Protects Sperm from Genetic Damage," *Medical Tribune,* Jan. 16, 1992, 23.

17. Hemila, Harri, et al., "Vitamin C and the Common Cold: A Retrospective Analysis of Chalmers's Review," *Journal of the American College of Nutrition* 14(2): 116–23, 1995.

18. Allard, J. P., et al., "Effects of Vitamin E and C Supplementation on Oxidative Stress and Viral Load in HIV-Infected Subjects," *AIDS* 12: 1653–59, 1998.

19. Eberlein-Konig, B., et al., "Protective Effect Against Sunburn of Combined Systemic Ascorbic Acid (Vitamin C) and D-Alpha Tocopherol (Vitamin E)," *Journal of the American Academy of Dermatology* 38: 45–48, 1998.

20. Gerster, H., "No Contribution of Ascorbic Acid to Renal Calcium Oxalate Stones," *Annals of Nutrition Metabolism* 41: 269–82, 1997.

95

Vitamin D

Vitamin D, which is both a vitamin and a hormone, promotes calcium absorption from the intestines, calcium resorption from the bone, and calcium deposition into bone tissue. Since vitamin D came to fame as a treatment for rickets, it is called the antirachitic vitamin. But 10 different compounds have antirachitic characteristics, and they are called D_1, D_2, D_3, and so on. The best known of these is D_2 (ergocalciferol from plant sources) and D_3 (cholecalciferol from animal sources). D_3 is the form of vitamin D found in fish oils and eggs, and produced in human skin. When calcium in the blood declines, parathyroid hormone stimulates the synthesis of D_3 in the kidneys. The two hormones increase absorption of calcium from the intestines and increase resorption from bone. When blood levels of calcium increase, parathyroid hormone

no longer stimulates its synthesis and D_3 production declines.[1]

Vitamin D can be obtained from the sun through the conversion of 7-dehydrocholesterol to previtamin D, which is spontaneously converted to vitamin D. The vitamin obtained from food or from the skin is then converted to 25-hydroxyvitamin D in the liver and 1,25-dihydroxyvitamin D—the active hormone—in the kidneys. A vitamin D deficiency is associated with increased parathyroid hormone secretion, increased bone turnover, osteoporosis, and mild osteomalacia, as well as increased risk of hip and other fractures, according to the Food and Nutrition Board of the Institute of Medicine. The board added that as much attention should be given to increasing vitamin D intake as has been publicized in increasing calcium intake in older people. For example, adults probably need 800 to

1,000 IU/day of vitamin D. The board further suggested that adult intake of supplemental multivitamins (containing vitamin D) or calcium supplements should be increased substantially.[2]

For adults, the recommendation of 200 IU of vitamin D per day may prevent osteomalacia in the absence of sunlight, but more of the vitamin is needed to help prevent osteoporosis and secondary hyperparathyroidism, reported Reinhold Vieth of the University of Toronto and Mount Sinai Hospital in Canada. Vitamin D supplements are also beneficial in the prevention of some cancers, and the progression of osteoarthritis, multiple sclerosis, and high blood pressure.[3] "If vitamin D is similar to a drug, then dose-finding studies are needed to use it properly, especially if nonclassical benefits are potentially relevant," Vieth said. "Alternatively, if by analogy with other nutrients, vitamin D supplementation is intended to make up for what some people may not be getting from its natural source, in this case the sun, then the current adult daily reference intake of 200 IU/day is woefully inadequate."

A study involving 290 men and 469 women aged 67 to 95 found that data from a population-based sample of elderly people suggest that low levels of vitamin D are an important public health problem that could readily be addressed by adequate vitamin D intake or sunlight exposure. The study confirms earlier studies that elderly people who took a vitamin supplement or drank two or three glasses of milk per day

had sufficient vitamin D levels in their blood. But 75 percent of women and 80 percent of men in this study did not regularly take vitamin D supplements, and among this group, 68 percent of women and 64 percent of men consumed less than 8 ounces of milk daily.[4]

If older Americans consumed extra vitamin D and calcium, this might substantially reduce the enormous cost—$13.8 billion in 1995—of treating broken bones in the elderly. That was the conclusion of a three-year study of 389 men and women over the age of 65. The group that took calcium and vitamin D supplements daily had less than half as many broken bones during the study as the control group: 11 fractures versus 26. The supplements contained 500 mg of calcium and 700 IU of vitamin D.[5]

The study participants consumed a little more than 700 mg of calcium daily from their diets. By adding the supplements, they averaged about 1,200 mg, which is now the recommended amount for those aged 51 and over. To get that amount from food, a person would have to consume a well-balanced diet, including three daily sources of dairy products.

At Massachusetts General Hospital, Boston, researchers found that serum 25-hydroxyvitamin D levels were below normal in many of the patients studied. Sixty-six percent consumed less than the recommended dietary allowance for vitamin D, and 37 percent of those with intakes above the RDA were also deficient in the vitamin. Reasons for the deficiency included inadequate vitamin D in the diet, the winter season, and housebound patients. In a subgroup of 77 patients less than 65 years of age without any known risk factors for hypovitaminosis D, the prevalence of vitamin D deficiency was 42 percent. Ironically, vitamin D deficiency sometimes surfaces in those who are taking more than the RDA.[6]

"Maintaining vitamin D intake at the level of the current recommended daily amount or using multivitamins/minerals may not be sufficient to ensure adequate vitamin D stores," said Melissa K. Thomas, M.D., Ph.D. "Because of the potential adverse effects of vitamin D deficiency on the skeleton and other organ systems, widespread screening for vitamin D deficiency or routine vitamin D supplementation should be considered."

Women begin to lose bone rapidly during the first five or so years following menopause. Megadoses of calcium can modestly reduce cortical loss from long bones but have little effect on the spine. However, vitamin D can boost the effectiveness of calcium. For postmenopausal women, 1,000 to 1,500 mg of calcium and 400 to 800 IU of vitamin D daily can reduce bone loss.[7]

African-American women living in northern latitudes apparently don't manufacture enough vitamin D during the summer to carry them through winter months, and they need to increase their vitamin D intake. Researchers found that African-American women had about half as much 25-hydroxyvitamin D circulating in their blood during the year as white women. In studying 51 African-American women and 39 white women living in the Boston area, the researchers said that in winter, when vitamin D levels are lowest, parathyroid hormone was raised only in the African-American women. The hormone signals when blood calcium is low, and it can stimulate loss of calcium from the bones.[8]

Vitamin D deficiency among the elderly is more prevalent than once believed, according to Cass Ryan, Ph.D., R.D., and colleagues at Louisiana Tech University at Ruston. The deficiency is related to insufficient time in the sun, wearing too much clothing when outdoors, and a decreased kidney mass, which decreases the production of D_3. The elderly are also less likely to get enough vitamin D from their diets. The major dietary source for the vitamin is fortified dairy products, which many elderly forego because of lactase deficiency. Lactase is an enzyme needed to digest the lactose (milk sugar) in milk. They also avoid dairy products to limit their intake of calories and saturated fat.[9]

A variety of drugs interfere with the metabolism, absorption, and utilization of vitamin D, the researchers continued. Laxatives, especially mineral oil, also interfere. Cholestyramine, a cholesterol-lowering drug, may bind vitamin D in the gut and interfere with its absorption. Anticonvulsive drugs, such as carbamazepine, phenytoin, and phenobarbital, also interfere with vitamin D metabolism.

"The requirement for vitamin D is known to be dependent on the concentration of calcium and phosphorous in the diet, the physiological state of development, age, sex, degree of exposure to the sun, and the amount of skin pigmentation," the researchers said. "Very dark skin can prevent up to 95 percent of ultraviolet rays from the sun from reaching the layers of the skin where the conversion of 7-dehydrocholesterol to the active form of vitamin D occurs."

Researchers from the Minerva Foundation Institute for Medical Research in Helsinki, Finland, evaluated vegetarians, lacto-ovo-vegetarians, and lacto-vegetarians. It was found that strict vegetarians were especially low in vitamin D. These vegetarians were noticeably vulnerable in Finland because of the northern latitude in the winter months, when sunlight is at a minimum.[10]

Human skin contains a sterol called cholesterol that is transformed into vitamin D_3 when exposed to ultraviolet light. Clouds, fog, and dust in the atmosphere absorb UV rays, so that sunlight in cities is inferior to sunlight in open country. Since window glass absorbs UV rays, the light that passes through ordinary glass has practically no activity to prevent against bone disorders.[11]

Does sunscreen inhibit the production of vitamin D? It is believed that exposure to sunlight two or three times weekly provides considerable amounts of the vitamin. In an Australian population, those staying longer in the sun were urged to use an SPF 15 sunscreen. Those who applied SPF 17 to head, neck, forearm, and hands did not inhibit vitamin D levels.[12]

An estimated 20 to 34 percent of Asian toddlers in Britain are deficient in vitamin D and may have low levels of iron as well. This puts many of the children at risk of developing rickets and iron deficiency anemia. It was suggested that all pregnant women and children up to the age of five should get a vitamin D supplement, unless they are getting sufficient amounts from sun and diet.[13]

In a study of 11 patients with amyotrophic lateral sclerosis (ALS), commonly known as Lou Gehrig's disease, blood levels of 25-hydroxyvitamin D were significantly lower than in the controls. Doctors ruled that two patients had deficient levels of the vitamin, while the other nine had insufficient amounts. Dietary vitamin D intake was below 100 IU in 10 patients. Ten lived in sunlight-poor areas. The researchers added that there is a disturbance in calcium metabolism in a significant portion of patients with ALS.[14]

At the UCLA School of Medicine, researchers evaluated 173 patients at high and moderate risk for coronary artery disease. It was determined that 1,25-vitamin D levels were inversely related to the extent of vascular calcification and the possible development of hardening of the arteries. Since vitamin D is associated with bone mineralization, this may explain the relationship between osteoporosis and vascular calcification, which occurs in over 90 percent of the patients with coronary heart disease.[15]

In a study of 142 Dutch diabetics aged 70 to 88, 39 percent had low levels of vitamin D. Total insulin concentration during the oral glucose tolerance test was also inversely associated with the concentration of 25-hydroxyvitamin D, suggesting that low levels of vitamin D may be a significant risk factor for glucose intolerance.[16]

Researchers in New York studied 181 cases of prostate cancer, involving 90 black patients and 91 white patients, and found that those with elevated risks of prostate cancer had the lowest summer blood levels of 1,25-hydroxyvitamin D. The researchers theorized that the conversion of 25-hydroxyvitamin D to 1,25-dihydroxyvitamin D contributes to the risk of prostate cancer.[17]

At the Veterans Affairs Medical Center, Bronx, New York, 50 patients with spinal cord injury and 50 controls were evaluated. About one-third of the spinal cord injury patients were deficient in vitamin D. It was recommended that these patients be treated with adequate amounts of vitamin D and calcium supplements. Some of the patients exhibited mild, secondary hyperparathyroidism and abnormally low levels of calcium circulating in the blood.[18]

A study at Mount Sinai Medical Center in New York City reported that two female patients with frequent migraine headaches and premenstrual syndrome (PMS) complaints got relief with vitamin D and cal-cium. One patient with low vitamin D levels was given 1,600 IU of vitamin D and 1,200 mg of calcium daily. Within two months, her migraine and PMS symptoms significantly eased. The second patient, although not deficient in either nutrient, was given 1,200 IU of vitamin D and 1,200 mg of calcium daily for three months. Again, there were significant improvements in both migraine and PMS symptoms. Additional migraine attacks were halted when she chewed the equivalent of 1,200 to 1,600 mg of calcium.[19]

Based on the research, vitamin D is a very neglected nutrient. One of the reasons for its deficiency is that it is not readily available in foods. Good sources include eggs, liver, milk, fatty fish, fish liver oils, and certain vitamin D–fortified foods. Sunlight provides considerable amounts, assuming you do not cover your skin with too much clothing.

References

1. Garrison, Robert Jr., and Elizabeth Somer, *The Nutrition Desk Reference* (New Canaan, Conn.: Keats Publishing, 1995), 78–82.

2. Utiger, Robert D., "The Need for More Vitamin D," *New England Journal of Medicine* 338(12): 828–29, March 19, 1998.

3. Vieth, Reinhold, "Vitamin D Supplementation, 25-Hydroxyvitamin D Concentrations, and Safety," *American Journal of Clinical Nutrition* 69: 842–56, 1999.

4. Jacques, Paul F., et al., "Plasma 25-hydroxyvitamin D and Its Determinants in an Elderly Population Sample," *American Journal of Clinical Nutrition* 66: 929–36, 1997.

5. McBride, Judy, "Rate of Broken Bones Could Fall," *USDA Food and Nutrition Research Briefs*, Oct. 1997, 1.

6. Thomas, Melissa, et al., "Hydro-Vitaminosis D in Medical Inpatients," *New England Journal of Medicine* 338(12): 777–83, March 19, 1998.

7. Dawson-Hughes, Bess, "Calcium and Vitamin D Nutritional Needs of Elderly Women," *Journal of Nutrition* 126: 1165S–67S, 1996.

8. McBride, Judy, "More Vitamin D May Benefit Black Women," *USDA Food and Nutrition Research Briefs*, Oct. 1998, 3–4.

9. Ryan, Cass, et al., "Vitamin D in the Elderly," *Nutrition Today* 30(6): 228–33, Nov./Dec. 1995.

10. Karkkainen, M., et al., "Low Serum Vitamin D Concentrations and Secondary Hyperparathyroidism in Middle-Aged, Caucasian Strict Vegetarians," *Challenges of Modern Medicine* 7: 342–44, 1995.

11. *Food: The Yearbook of Agriculture* (Washington, D.C.: U.S. Department of Agriculture, 1959), 133–36.

12. Holick, Michael F., "Regular Use of Sunscreen on Vitamin D Levels," *Archives of Dermatology* 131: 1337–38, Nov. 1995.

13. Wharton, B. A., "Low Plasma Vitamin D in Asian Toddlers in Britain," *British Medical Journal* 318: 2–3, Jan. 2, 1999.

14. Sato, Yoshihiro, et al., "Hypovitaminosis D and Decreased Bone Mineral Density in Amyotrophic Lateral Sclerosis," *European Neurology* 37: 225–29, 1997.

15. Watson, Karol E., et al., "Active Serum Vitamin D Levels Are Inversely Correlated with Coronary Calcification," *Circulation* 96: 1755–60, 1997.

16. Baynes, K. C. R., et al., "Vitamin D Glucose Tolerance and Insulinemia in Elderly Men," *Diabetologia* 40: 344–47, 1997.

17. Corder, Elizabeth H., et al., "Seasonal Variation in Vitamin D–Binding Protein and Dehydroepiandrosterone: Risk of Prostate Cancer in Black and White Men," *Cancer Epidemiology, Biomarkers, and Prevention* 4: 655–59, 1995.

18. Bauman, William A., "Vitamin D Deficiency in Veterans with Chronic Spinal Cord Injury," *Metabolism* 44(12): 1612–16, Dec. 1995.

19. Thys-Jacobs, Susan, "Vitamin D and Calcium in Menstrual Migraine," *Headache* 34(9): 544–46, Oct. 1994.

96

Vitamin E

When Ruth Adams and I were editing *Better Nutrition* magazine in the 1960s and early 1970s, it was almost impossible to find doctors or other professionals who would go on record recommending vitamin and mineral supplementation. Many of these professionals eventually became avid supporters of supplements, but at the time they preferred to remain on the sidelines. The notable exceptions were Evan Shute, M.D., and Wilfrid Shute, M.D., brothers who operated the Shute Clinic in London, Ontario, Canada. Ruth and I always looked forward to their periodic newsletter, which reported exciting research on the use of vitamin E to treat heart disease, intermittent claudication, varicose veins, gangrene, severe burns, and other conditions. Their provocative before-and-after color photos were enough to convince the most diehard skeptics as to the power of vitamin E, but the American Medical Association always refused to allow them to show their slides at AMA meetings. Fortunately, times have changed since, and although many doctors may not be bold enough to recommend vitamin E to their patients, the majority readily admit taking vitamin E themselves to possibly prevent a heart attack. Apparently the skeptics are not reading the literature.

Cardiovascular disease continues to be the number one cause of death in the United States, resulting in more than 954,000 deaths annually and accounting for nearly 42 percent of all deaths, according to Eric B. Rimm, Sc.D. In addition, more than 58 million Americans have one or more types of cardiovascular disease. Of these, about 13 million have had heart attacks or angina, and there are some 1.5

million new heart attack patients each year. The annual cost of heart disease in the United States in 1998 was estimated to be $274.2 billion. Antioxidants such as vitamins C and E and the carotenoids are believed to be important in disease prevention because they counteract the damaging effect of free radicals and other highly reactive chemical compounds produced by oxidation.[1]

Vitamin E is a collective name for two groups of compounds—the tocopherols and the tocotrienols—which share the same biological activity but to different degrees, Rimm said. There are four tocopherols (alpha, beta, gamma, and delta), which differ in the number and position of methyl groups on the ring. The tocotrienols are different in that their side chain is unsaturated.

The most active form of vitamin E is alpha-tocopherol. The naturally occurring form found in foods and in natural-source vitamin E is d-alpha-tocopherol. Synthetic vitamin E consists of a mixture of eight stereoisomers and is designated as dl-alpha-tocopherol. It has long been suggested that the bioavailability of d-alpha-tocopherol is about 35 percent higher than that of dl-alpha-tocopherol.

In studying data from the Third National Health and Nutrition Examination Survey (NHANES III), which tabulated the nutritional status of 16,295 adults aged 18 and older, researchers at the Centers for Disease Control and Prevention in Atlanta found that about 27 percent of the U.S. population had low levels of vitamin E. Twenty-nine percent of men, 28 percent of women, 26 percent of whites, 41 percent of African Americans, 28 percent of Mexican Americans, and 32 percent of other volunteers had low concentrations of the vitamin.[2]

An initial step in the development of cardiovascular disease is the oxidation of LDL cholesterol. In a study using healthy, nonsmoking men, 400, 800, or 1,200 IU of vitamin E was administered daily for eight weeks. The researchers found that 1,200 IU/day was far more effective than 400 IU/day in reducing LDL oxidation.[3]

In 1996 in *The Lancet*, researchers in England published the findings of the largest clinical trial of natural vitamin E in preventing coronary heart disease. They reported that 400 and 800 IU/day of vitamin E reduced the incidence of nonfatal heart attacks by 77 percent. More recently, researchers using that data in the CHAOS trial calculated the financial impact of supplementation would reduce the cost of treatment by $578 for the typical American patient suffering a nonfatal heart attack and $181 for a similar Australian patient over a three-year period. Extrapolating these hospitalization savings to U.S. patients, vitamin E supplements would bring a potential savings of $578 million.[4]

A Canadian study found that vitamin E reduced the risk of various health problems. Vitamin E intake from food and supplements was evaluated in 342 people who had had ischemic strokes and 501 people who were healthy. The volunteers consisted of a multiethnic group of elderly men and women. Ischemic strokes are the most common type of this disorder and are characterized by a narrowing of blood vessels in the brain, which inhibits the flow of blood. Those who took vitamin E supplements were 47 percent less likely to have an ischemic stroke, the second most common cause of cardiovascular-related deaths.[5]

In a two-year, randomized clinical trial funded by the National Institutes of Health, 2,000 IU/day of vitamin E, 10 mg/day of selegiline, or a combination of the two slowed the functional deterioration seen in moderately severe patients with Alzheimer's disease. Selegiline hydrochloride (Alzene, Deprenyl, or Eldepryl) is a monoamine oxidase inhibitor and anti-Parkinsonism drug. Of 341 patients, those taking either or both of the substances experienced a delay in reaching severe dementia, institutionalization, loss of the ability to perform basic activities of living, or death, compared to the control group. Doses of up to 2,000 IU/day of vitamin E resulted in no side effects in most cases. But oral intake of high amounts can exacerbate blood coagulation defects and is contraindicated in people with that problem.[6]

Robert N. Butler of *Geriatrics* magazine recommends that his patients take a multivitamin supplement with extra vitamin C and 200 IU/day of vitamin E. He adds that vitamin E supplements decrease the risk of heart attacks, slow the progression of Alzheimer's disease, and increase immunity in the elderly. The typical American diet does not provide sufficient vitamin E to achieve documented health benefits. Those who want to get 400 IU/day of vitamin E from their diets would have to eat 1,000 almonds, which would also provide 8,000 calories and roughly 1.5 pounds of fat.[7]

In assessing the cognitive function of almost 1,800 middle-aged and elderly men and women, Austrian researchers found that those with the poorest cognitive scores had the lowest blood levels of vitamin E and beta-carotene. Subsequent analysis showed that high levels of vitamin E were strongly associated with normal cognitive function. It is believed that adequate lifelong intake of vitamin E from foods and supplements may help people to maintain normal brain function in middle and old age and possibly ward off Alzheimer's.[8]

Researchers at the University Medical Center at Stony Brook, New York, evaluated the dietary habits, vitamin supplement usage, and blood levels of vitamin E for 764 volunteers in the Lens Opacities Case-Control Study. Those who took vitamin E supplements had a 57 percent lower risk of developing cataracts, especially after five years of supplementation, compared to those who did not take the vitamin. Those with high blood levels of the vitamin had a 42 percent lower risk. Further, those who took multivitamins had a 31 percent lower risk of developing a cataract.[9]

Macular degeneration involves the degeneration of the part of the eye responsible for sharp central vision and can lead to blindness. A study evaluated the diets, blood levels of various nutrients, and visual health of 2,500 volunteers. After examining the ratio of vitamin E to cholesterol and other blood fats, the researchers reported that those with the greatest concentrations of vitamin E were 82 percent less likely to develop macular degeneration. Vitamin E helps to prevent the oxidation of fats, and those with higher levels of blood fats may be able to compensate by increasing their vitamin E intake.[10]

Finnish men who took 50 mg/day of vitamin E for five to eight years had a 32 percent lower rate of prostate cancer than those who did not supplement with the vitamin. The men who took the vitamin also had a 41 percent lower death rate from the disease. Vitamin E may help to prevent some forms of prostate cancer by attacking free radical formation as well as boosting the immune system.[11]

Various studies have reported that men who supplement their diets with vitamin E over the long haul reduce their risk of prostate cancer by one-third. To determine whether vitamin E had any effect on prostate cancer and a high-fat diet, researchers injected laboratory mice with prostate cancer cells, and fed them a high- and low-fat diet, with or without added vitamin E. Animals fed a high-fat diet and supplemented with vitamin E had significantly lower tumor growth, suggesting that the vitamin may offset the tumor-promoting effect of high-fat diets.[12]

In one study levels of isoprostane, thromboxane B_2, and glucose were measured in 85 diabetics and 85 healthy controls. Isoprostane is a by-product of free radical reactions, and increased levels indicate oxidative stress. Thromboxane B_2 promotes blood clots, and glucose is the standard marker for diabetes. The diabetics had higher levels of isoprostane and thromboxane B_2 compared to the controls.[13] Ten of the diabetics were given 600 IU/day of vitamin E for two weeks. The vitamin brought a 37 percent decline in isoprostane levels and a 43 percent reduction in thromboxane B_2 levels. Vitamin E supplements also reduced oxidative stress and curbed the blood-clotting effect of thromboxane B_2.

Another study involved 29 diabetics and 21 nondiabetic siblings. It was found that the diabetics had higher levels of lipid peroxides (free radical–damaged fats) and thromboxane B_2, which increased the risk of blood clotting. Among the diabetics given 100 IU/day of vitamin E, lipid peroxide levels went down by 30 percent and thromboxane B_2 decreased by 51 percent.[14]

Preeclampsia, characterized by high blood pressure, headache, and water retention, is a fairly common problem during pregnancy. It can be a prelude to eclampsia, which can result in convulsions and death if not properly treated. A research team measured levels of vitamin E and malondialdehyde in 18 preeclamptic, 15 eclamptic, and 25 healthy women. Malondialdehyde is a marker of lipid peroxidation or free radical damage to fats. The researchers reported that, compared to healthy women, women with preeclampsia and eclampsia had higher levels of malondialdehyde and lower levels of vitamin E.[15]

Researchers in England reported that supplementing 160 women at risk for preeclampsia with either 400 IU/day of vitamin E or 1,000 mg/day of vitamin C lowered the risk of this disorder by 76 percent, compared to women given a placebo. Supplements were started between 16 and 22 weeks of gestation.[16]

Another group of researchers studied the effect of dietary intake of antioxidant vitamins on the increased risk of hip fractures associated with smoking, using data from a study of 66,651 women between the ages of 40 and 76. Smoking is a significant risk factor for fractures due to osteoporosis. Smokers with a low intake of vitamins C or E had a threefold higher risk of hip fractures. Women with low intakes of both vitamins had a 4.9-fold higher risk of bone fractures. In addition, the risk of hip fractures increased by only 10 percent in smokers with high intakes of vitamin E and 40 percent in those with high intakes of vitamin C.[17]

The skin is exposed to ultraviolet radiation from sunlight and air pollutants containing free radicals and ionizing radiation, which can result in melanoma, the deadliest form of skin cancer. Using laboratory animals, researchers applied topical vitamin E to the skin 24 hours prior to exposing them to UV radiation. The vitamin reduced free radical levels in the animals and increased antioxidant defenses in the skin by bolstering the antioxidant network and recycling other antioxidants. The higher antioxidant levels may also protect the skin against aging.[18]

In giving vitamin E dosages, researchers often refer to International Units (IUs) and milligrams (mg). For the record, 1.49 IU of vitamin E is equivalent to 1 mg of d-alpha-tocopherol. Natural-source vitamin E (d-alpha-tocopherol) is isolated from vegetable oils, mostly soy. However, sunflower, corn, peanut, canola, cottonseed, and rice bran oils can also be used. Synthetic vitamin E (dl-alpha-tocopherol) is produced from petrochemicals.[19]

In addition to d-alpha-tocopherol, natural vitamin Es include d-alpha-tocopheryl acetate and d-alpha-tocopheryl acid succinate. Natural mixed tocopherols are d-alpha, d-beta, d-gamma, and d-delta tocopherol. In addition to dl-alpha-tocopherol, synthetic vitamin Es include dl-alpha-tocopheryl acetate and dl-alpha-tocopheryl acid succinate. To buy natural-source vitamin E, you will find dosages of 200, 400, 600, 800, 1,000, and 1,200 IU. Synthetic vitamin Es are generally sold in dosages of 100, 200, and 400 IU.

The recommended dietary allowance (RDA) for vitamin E is 15 IU/day for men and 12 IU/day for women. Major food sources of vitamin E include wheat germ oil, sunflower oil, safflower oil, peanut oil, mayonnaise, soft and hard margarine, wheat germ, sunflower seeds, almonds, peanuts, soybean oil, butter, brown rice, oatmeal, and peanut butter.

References

1. Rimm, Eric B., "Vitamin E and Cardiovascular Disease," *VNIS Backgrounder* 7(2); Feb. 1999.

2. Ford, E. S., and A. Sowell, "Serum A-Tocopherol Status in the United States Population: Findings from the Third National Health and Nutrition Examination Survey," *American Journal of Epidemiology* 150(3): 290–300, 1999.

3. Fuller, C. J., et al., "Effects of Increasing Doses of Alpha-Tocopherol in Providing Protection of Low-Density Lipoprotein from Oxidation," *American Journal of Cardiology* 81: 231–33, 1998.

4. Davey, J., et al., "Cost-Effectiveness of Vitamin E Therapy in the Treatment of Patients with Angiographically Proven Coronary Narrowing (CHAOS Trial)," *American Journal of Cardiology* 82: 414–17, 1998.

5. Benson, R. T., et al., "Vitamin E Intake: A Primary Preventive Measure in Stroke," paper presented at the American Academy of Neurology, 51st Annual Meeting, Toronto, Canada, April 20, 1999.

6. Sano, Mary, et al., "A Controlled Trial of Selegiline, Alpha-Tocopherol, or Both as Treatment for Alzheimer's Disease," *New England Journal of Medicine* 336: 1216–22, April 24, 1997.

7. Butler, R. N., "Vitamin E Supplements: Clinical Practice Is Changing with New Data on Preventive Care of Older Patients," *Geriatrics* 52: 7–8, July 1997.

8. Schmidt, R., et al., "Plasma Antioxidants and Cognitive Performance in Middle-Aged and Older Adults: Results of the Austrian Stroke Prevention Study," *Journal of the American Geriatrics Society* 46: 1407–10, 1998.

9. Leske, M. C., et al., "Antioxidant Vitamins and Nuclear Opacities," *Ophthalmology* 105: 831–36, 1998.

10. Delcourt, C., et al., "Age-Related Macular Degeneration and Antioxidant Status in the POLA Study," *Archives of Ophthalmology* 117: 1384–90, 1999.

11. Heinomen, O. P., et al., "Prostate Cancer and Supplementation with Alpha-Tocopherol and Beta-Carotene: Incidence and Mortality in a Controlled Trial," *Journal of the National Cancer Institute* 90: 440–46, 1998.

12. Fleshner, N., et al., "Vitamin E Inhibits the High-Fat Diet Promoted Growth of Established Human Prostate LNCaP Tumors in Nude Mice," *Journal of Urology* 161: 1651–54, 1999.

13. Davi, G., et al., "In Vivo Formation of 8-Iso-Prostaglandin F2 Alpha and Platelet Activation in Diabetes Mellitus," *Circulation* 99: 224–29, 1999.

14. Jain, S., et al., "Relationship of Blood Thromboxane B_2 (TxB_2) with Lipid Peroxides and Effect of Vitamin E Supplementation on TxB_2 and LP Levels in Type 1 Diabetic Patients," paper presented at American Diabetes Association meeting, Chicago, Illinois, June 1998.

15. Yanik, F. A., et al., "Preeclampsia and Eclampsia Associated with Increased

Lipid Peroxidation and Decreased Serum Vitamin E Levels," *International Journal of Gynecology and Obstetrics* 64: 27–33, 1999.

16. Chappell, L. C., et al., "Effect of Antioxidants on the Occurrence of Pre-Eclampsia in Women at Increased Risk: A Randomized Trial," *The Lancet* 354: 810–16, 1999.

17. Melhus, H., et al., "Smoking, Anti-oxidant Vitamins, and the Risk of Hip Fracture," *Journal of Bone and Mineral Research* 14: 129–35, 1999.

18. Lopez-Torres, M., et al., "Topical Application of Alpha-Tocopherol Modulates the Antioxidant Network and Diminishes Ultraviolet-Induced Oxidative Damage in Murine Skin," *British Journal of Dermatology* 138: 207–15, 1998.

19. "The Vitamin E Fact Book," Vitamin E Research and Information Service, La Grange, Illinois, 1989.

97

Vitamin K

Known as the antihemorrhagic vitamin, vitamin K is necessary for the synthesis of prothrombin and other blood-clotting factors in the liver. Two naturally occurring forms of the vitamin are K_1 (phylloquinone), found in green plants, and K_2 (menaquinone), synthesized by various microorganism, such as bacteria in the intestinal tract. Since the intestines of a newborn infant are sterile at birth, the supply of vitamin K is not sufficient until normal bacterial flora in the intestine develops, usually by the third or fourth day of life.[1]

For this reason, pediatricians often give newborns vitamin K by mouth or injection to prevent hemorrhaging, although the practice remains controversial. The practice began in the 1940s and 1950s, according to Jean Golding, Ph.D., of the Institute of Child Health in Bristol, England. By 1970, the proportion of newborns getting vitamin K injections had increased to 25 percent, compared to 5 percent in 1958. It seems that a small number of children may develop leukemia from the intramuscular injections of vitamin K. There is apparently no risk for those getting the vitamin by mouth; however, oral doses to prevent hemorrhaging are not as effective as the injections.[2]

Writing in *Pediatrics,* Gerald B. Merenstein, M.D., took exception with studies by Golding et al. suggesting that vitamin K injections increase the risk of childhood leukemia. The American Academy of Pediatrics has stated that there has not been a sharp increase in childhood leukemia since vitamin K injections began in earnest in 1961, and the academy recommends that all newborns be given a single intramuscular injection of 0.5 to 1 mg of vitamin K. If available, vitamin K should be given orally at 2 mg at birth, again at one to two weeks, and at four weeks of age for breast-fed infants. If a breast-fed infant develops diarrhea, the dosage should be repeated.[3]

Researchers at the University of Lund in Sweden evaluated one million infants getting vitamin K injections at birth, compared to 272,080 children given the vitamin by mouth. They found that the risk of cancer following intramuscular injection of vitamin K was not elevated, compared to oral administration. Based on their study, the alleged association between intramuscular vitamin K therapy and childhood cancer could not be verified.[4]

In a study in The Netherlands, physicians gave 16 pregnant women on anticonvulsive therapy 10 mg/day of vitamin K from the 36th week of pregnancy to term. It was concluded that the therapy reduces the frequency of vitamin K deficiency in newborns of mothers on anticonvulsive therapy.[5]

Researchers at Brigham and Women's Hospital and Harvard Medical School and other facilities evaluated the diets of 72,327 women aged 38 to 63. Those who ate 109 to 242 mcg of vitamin K daily had a 30 percent less chance of breaking a hip than the women who consumed less than 109 mcg daily. The women who ate lettuce, a reliable source of vitamin K, at least once a day were 45 percent less likely to have a hip fracture as those who ate the vegetable once a week or less, according to Diane Feskanich, R.D. In addition to its associa-

tion with proteins in bone, vitamin K may influence bone metabolism through its effect on urinary calcium excretion or by inhibiting the production of bone-resorbing agents such as prostaglandin E_2 and interleukin-6.[6]

"We found a lower risk of hip fractures in middle-aged and older women with moderate and high intakes of vitamin K than in those with a low intake," Feskanich said. "Our results support the suggestion that dietary vitamin K requirements should be based on bone health as well as on blood coagulation."

A subclinical deficiency in the vitamin may be more prevalent than previously thought, based on using coagulation times as a marker for vitamin K deficiency. Vitamin K acts as a cofactor with several proteins which seem to have a regulatory role in calcium metabolism, tissue mineralization, and bone turnover. Postmenopausal women are especially at risk for subclinical vitamin K deficiency. And patients undergoing anticoagulant therapy involving vitamin K antagonists, such as coumadin (to prevent blood clots), may be ripe for subclinical vitamin K deficiency. These drugs apparently inhibit the activity of vitamin K in bone proteins.[7]

At Maastricht University in The Netherlands, C. Vermeer et al. reported that those who do not regularly eat green vegetables will have a decreased vitamin K intake. This can decrease further if cheese and curd are not eaten regularly. In people 60 to 70 years of age, it has been estimated that the ingestion of vitamin K drops by about 50 percent. A number of studies in Japan have demonstrated a reduction in postmenopausal bone loss when the patients were given vitamin K supplements. In two studies involving 50 and 140 postmenopausal women, it was shown that daily doses of 1 to 10 mg of vitamin K resulted in a reduction in urinary calcium loss, among other things.[8]

Researchers at Tufts University in Boston have found that vitamin K activates at least three proteins involved in bone formation, and that many people may need more than the current recommended dietary allowance of 60 to 80 mcg/day to maintain strong, healthy bones. One of these proteins, osteocalcin, must be saturated with carboxyl groups, and the attachment of carboxyl groups requires vitamin K. While the role of osteocalcin is not completely understood, a French research team has found that older women with elevated levels of osteocalcin had lower bone density and a higher risk of hip fracture.[9]

Another study at Tufts University determined that about 50 percent of our daily vitamin K requirements are made from bacteria in our intestines. However, this will satisfy only about 10 to 15 percent of our needs for the vitamin. Our actual needs may be 400 mcg/day instead of the currently recommended 65 mcg for women and 80 mcg for men. One-half cup of collard greens provides 440 mcg of vitamin K.[10]

Reduced amounts of vitamin K–dependent clotting factors have been found in patients getting antibiotic therapy, and they may need vitamin K supplements, according to researchers at the University of Wisconsin at Madison.[11]

Vitamin K may improve the bone health of athletic women. Strenuous exercise often results in low estrogen levels and irregular menstrual cycles, which often result in bone loss. In those with low estrogen levels, 10 mg/day of vitamin K brought a 15 to 20 percent increase in bone formation and a 20 to 25 percent decrease in bone resorption. The therapy stabilized a balance between bone formation and resorption.[12]

Government experts recommend eating five to nine servings of fresh vegetables and fruits daily to help build our vitamin K stores. But rich sources of the vitamin—including kale, parsley, lettuce, collard greens, broccoli, spinach, and cabbage—are not at the top of everyone's favorite vegetable list.

References

1. Ensminger, Audrey, et al., *Food and Nutrition Encyclopedia* (Clovis, Calif.: Pegus Press, 1983), 2271ff.
2. "Vitamin K and Childhood Cancer," *British Medical Journal* 304: 1264–65, May 16, 1992.
3. Merenstein, Gerald B., "Controversies Concerning Vitamin K in the Newborn," *Pediatrics* 91(5): 1001–02, May 1993.
4. Ekelund, Hans, et al., "Administration of Vitamin K to Newborn Infants and

Childhood Cancer," *British Medical Journal* 307: 89–91, 1993.

5. Cornelissen, Marlies, et al., "Supplementation of Vitamin K in Pregnant Women Receiving Anticonvulsant Therapy Prevents Neonatal Vitamin K Deficiency," *American Journal of Obstetrics and Gynecology* 168 (3/Part I): 884–88, March 1993.

6. Feskanich, Diane, "Vitamin K Intake and Hip Fractures in Women: A Prospective Study," *American Journal of Clinical Nutrition* 69: 74–79, 1999.

7. Ferland, Guylaine, "Subclinical Vitamin K Deficiency: Recent Development," *Nutrition Report* 12(1): 1, 8, Jan. 1994.

8. Vermeer, Cees, et al., "Vitamin K and Metabolic Bone Disease," *Journal of Clinical Pathology* 51: 424–26, 1998.

9. Murray, Frank, "Vitamin K Helps to Improve Bone Health," *Let's Live,* May 1997, 18.

10. "Vitamin K Requirements," *Nutrition Week,* Aug. 22, 1997, 7.

11. Suttie, J. W., "Vitamin K and Human Nutrition," *Journal of the American Dietetic Association* 92(5): 585–90, May 1992.

12. Craciun, A. M., et al., "Improved Bone Metabolism in Female Elite Athletes After Vitamin K Supplementation," *International Journal of Sports Medicine* 19: 479–84, 1998.

98

Wheat

Wheat germ is a nutritious addition to the diet because it is the heart of the wheat kernel and the embryo from which a new plant will grow. One cup of wheat germ contains 245 calories, 17 g of protein, 7 g of fat, 34 g of carbohydrate, 57 mg of calcium, 5.5 mg of iron, 1.39 mg of vitamin B_1, 0.54 mg of vitamin B_2, and 3.1 mg of vitamin B_3. Both wheat germ and wheat bran are reliable sources of fiber.

At a symposium of the New York Academy of Sciences, evidence was presented to show that wheat bran products protect against cancers of the breast and colon. For example, a diet containing 20 to 40 g/day of wheat fiber is associated with lower levels of circulating estrogens. Dietary fiber, such as that from wheat, is required for the reabsorption of estrogen into the bloodstream. It was pointed out that diets supplemented with 15 to 30 g/day of wheat fiber have shown significant reductions in serum estrogens, compared to corn and oat bran supplementation. Therefore, only wheat fiber produces significant reductions in secondary bile acids and bacterial enzymes associated with colon cancer.[1]

Colon cancer, the second deadliest form of cancer in the United States, kills almost 55,000 Americans annually. Researchers at the University of California at Davis, after conducting a 6½-month study with lab animals, reported that wheat bran that has been heated slightly may be more protective against colon cancer than raw wheat bran. Animals given processed wheat had 33 percent fewer growths in their colons compared to those who ate raw wheat bran.[2]

At the Royal Brisbane Hospital in Australia, 411 patients with colorectal adenomas were placed on a 25 percent fat reduction diet and supplemented with 25 g of wheat bran daily, along with a capsule of 20 mg/day of beta-carotene. A statistically significant drop in risk of large adenomas was observed. Patients on the low-fat diet and added wheat bran had no large adenomas during two and four years of follow-up.[3]

Researchers at the Arizona Cancer Center at Tucson found that wheat bran as a dietary supplement decreased the growth of rectal adenomatous polyps in patients with familial polyposis. In the trial, 13.5 g/day of wheat bran was given for eight weeks after a previous month in which the volunteers were given 2 g/day. There was a 22 percent decrease in rectal polyps. The researchers concluded that wheat bran fiber supplements can inhibit DNA synthesis and rectal mucosal cell proliferation in high-risk patients.[4]

To keep the gastrointestinal tract healthy, K. H. Soergel, M.D., of the Medical College of Wisconsin at Milwaukee, recommends: "Eat wheat bran, not oat bran, because it is slowly fermented all along the colon. Unrefined, unprocessed wheat bran in a plastic bag is preferred, because it is very cheap. Metamucil and other psyllium products are fermented rapidly in the cecum. They are more expensive and may be less effective."[5]

Danilo Badiali, M.D., and colleagues in Italy conducted a double-blind crossover study for two four-week periods in which 24 patients received 20 g of wheat bran or a placebo to test its effectiveness against constipation. The bran therapy was more effective than the placebo in improving bowel frequency and fecal transit time. However, the researchers admitted that wheat bran is more beneficial for those with slow colonic transit time.[6]

On separate days, researchers in France gave six men a low-fiber test meal containing 70 g of fat and 756 mg of cholesterol, enriched or not with 10 g of oat bran, rice bran, or wheat bran or 4.2 g of wheat germ. All of the fibers reduced cholesterol levels. There were no changes in serum glucose or insulin responses, but serum triglyceride levels were lower with oat bran, wheat bran, and wheat germ.[7]

Researchers at Loma Linda University in California evaluated more than 31,000 non-Hispanic white Seventh-Day Adventists concerning coronary artery disease. Volunteers who consumed nuts more than four times a week had fewer fatal coronary heart disease events, and those who ate whole-wheat bread also experienced lower rates of nonmyocardial infarction and fatal coronary disease, when compared with those who ate white bread. The researchers believe that the fiber or the higher concentration of vitamin E from wheat germ in the whole-grain bread was responsible for the protection. The nuts contain a healthy form of fat.[8]

Wheat germ oil (octacosanol) is present in small amounts in wheat germ and other vegetable oils. A valuable nutrient, it teaches us a lesson about the power of nutritional substances, according to Robert C. Atkins, M.D. From the 1930s through the 1960s, wheat germ oil was extensively researched by Thomas Cureton, Ph.D., of the University of Illinois, who recommended it for stamina, reaction time, and cardiovascular disease. Later, Carlton Fredericks, Ph.D., began recommending it for patients with impaired brain function.[9]

Omega-3 oils, found in wheat germ, flax, walnut, and soy, can improve the skin from both the inside out and the outside in, according to Donald O. Rudin, M.D. For example, 10 percent of wheat germ oil is omega-3 fatty acids and 40 percent is omega-6 fatty acids.[10]

Wheat germ, wheat bran, wheat germ oil, wheat grass, and numerous other wheat products are available in the marketplace. While wheat is a beneficial substance, it is also one of the most common causes of food allergies, which can lead to a variety of health problems, such as irritable bowel syndrome, celiac disease, and gluten intolerance. Blood and skin tests and the elimination diet can determine if wheat is a problem for you. Many people with gluten intolerance suffer many complications because they are allergic to wheat, rye, oats, and barley. For many others, wheat is a very beneficial food and supplement.

References

1. Baute, Linda, "Evidence of Protective Effects of Wheat Fiber Grows," *Journal of the National Cancer Institute* 83(22): 1614–15, Nov. 20, 1991.

2. "Colon Cancer and Wheat Bran," *Nutrition Week,* Sept. 4, 1998, 8.

3. MacLennan, Robert, et al., "Randomized Trial of Intake of Fat, Fiber, and Beta-Carotene to Prevent Colorectal Adenomas," *Journal of the National Cancer Institute* 87(23): 1760–66, Dec. 6, 1995.

4. Alberts, D. S., et al., "Effects of Dietary Wheat Fiber on Rectal Epithelial Cell Proliferation in Patients with Resection from Colorectal Cancer," *Journal of the National Cancer Institute* 82(15): 1280–85, Aug. 1, 1990.

5. Hamilton, Kirk, "Colonic Fermentation and the Medical Consequences," *The Experts Speak* (Sacramento, Calif.: I.T. Services, 1996), 84–86. Also, K. H. Soergel, "Colonic Fermentation: Metabolic and Clinical Implications," *Clinical Investigation* 72: 742–48, 1994.

6. Badiali, Danilo, et al., "Effect of Wheat Bran in the Treatment of Chronic, Nonorganic Constipation: A Double-Blind Controlled Trial," *Digestive Diseases and Sciences* 40(2): 349–56, Feb. 1995.

7. Cara, Louis, et al., "Effects of Oat Bran, Rice Bran, Wheat Fiber, and Wheat Germ on Postprandial Lipemia in Healthy Adults," *American Journal of Clinical Nutrition* 55: 81–88, 1992.

8. Fraser, Gary E., et al., "A Possible Protective Effect of Nut Consumption on Risk of Coronary Heart Disease: The Adventist Health Study," *Archives of Internal Medicine* 152: 1416–24, July 1992.

9. Atkins, Robert C., *Dr. Atkins' Health Revolution* (Boston: Houghton Mifflin Co., 1988), 344–45.

10. Rudin, Donald O., and Clara Felix, *The Omega-3 Phenomenon* (New York: Rawson Associates, 1987), 23, 58.

99

Yohimbine

With the vast publicity surrounding Viagra, consumers have become aware that there are many prescription drugs and over-the-counter preparations for erectile dysfunction. Unfortunately, some of these medications have unpleasant side effects. In response, consumers are turning to natural remedies such as yohimbine, but alas, it is not necessarily benign.

Yohimbine, which comes from the bark of the yohimbe tree *(Pausinystalia johimbe)*, is said to be one of the few aphrodisiacs in nature, according to Sheldon Saul Hendler, M.D., Ph.D. He discussed a double-blind study in which 48 men were treated with yohimbine. Half of the volunteers were suffering from psychologic impotence, while the impotence of the remaining half had a physical basis. Some 62 percent who were given 6 mg/day of the herb for 10 weeks

reported notable improvements in sexual function, compared to 16 percent getting a placebo. Improvement was judged on the frequency and quality (rigidity and lasting power) of erections. Among those who were suffering from psychogenic problems, 46 percent reported positive responses to the herb. In another study, Hendler said that overweight Polish women lost 5.3 pounds per week after being given yohimbine.[1]

In *Natural Prescriptions,* Robert M. Giller, M.D., calls yohimbine a natural remedy for impotence. The herb dilates the surface blood vessels in the penis and stimulates the release of norepinephrine, a hormone released during physical stress. The usual dose is three 5.4-mg tablets daily, and there should be some response in two to three weeks. The herb can increase heart rate and raise blood pressure, so the dosage should be lowered if symptoms appear, then gradually increased to the prescribed dose.[2]

At Valparaiso University in Indiana, a double-blind trial was conducted in which 11 patients with erectile dysfunction were recruited from an outpatient clinic. Controls did not have any sexual problems. In the treatment group, the men were given 10 mg three times daily of yohimbine. The men without functional sexual problems experienced no effect when the herb was given, and mixed effects were found in the sexual function of those with erectile dysfunction. Three of the 11 men experienced strong positive effects, and five others reported partial results. With the yohimbine therapy, frequency of sexual activity increased along with self-assessed genital response to visual sexual stimulation. Diaries kept by the men reported increased sexual arousal and erectile response during masturbation, but not during intercourse. The herb brought a slight decrease in sexual interest in the controls. It was concluded that yohimbine may exert an enhancing effect on sexual desire and improve sexual performance. In this and other studies, the improved erection response with the herb is about 20 percent or higher.[3]

Contrary to some reports, yohimbine does not increase testosterone levels. However, the herb and its isolated alkaloid have some potent effects on sexual function. The herb not only increases blood flow to the penis, but also enhances libido. In one study, yohimbine used alone was successful in 34 to 43 percent of the cases.

Combined in a formula with testosterone and strychnine, its effectiveness is further enhanced. However, consumers wishing to use the herb should consult a professional, since there is skepticism about the potency of some over-the-counter preparations. The FDA has approved the product by prescription. Side effects include an increase in heart rate and blood pressure, dizziness, skin flushing, and headache.[4]

"For at least 10 years, I have maintained that if there is a real herbal erection enhancer, yohimbe is it," said James A. Duke, Ph.D. "I based this on centuries of folklore about the African tree bark and a few small clinical trials that showed that the herb produced erections in about half of men with psychological impotence, and about 40 percent with physical erection problems. Unfortunately, the side effects were a little unnerving. . . . This is not an herb that you want to mess around with."[5]

In addition to the side effects mentioned, there seems to be only one case in the literature in which yohimbine caused sinusitis. This was reported in a 59-year-old male who was evaluated at the Whiteley Wood Clinic in Sheffield, England. Three days after beginning the treatment, he developed sinusitis pain above the eyes and tenderness to the touch. Symptoms ended 24 hours after he stopped the yohimbine therapy. He rechallenged himself a week later with the herb. The symptoms returned, but they again went away after he stopped using the herb.[6]

Of 26 over-the-counter samples of yohimbine, 9 contained none of the herb and

7 were found to have only trace amounts. The remaining 10 contained "negligible amounts." Consumers should read labels carefully to ensure that they are getting potent amounts of yohimbine.[7]

When opting to use yohimbine, it is best to consult with a professional who can suggest suitable products and dosages. It is also a good idea to review the potential side effects, especially for patients with heart, blood pressure, kidney, and other health problems.

References

1. Hendler, Sheldon Saul, *The Doctors' Vitamin and Mineral Encyclopedia* (New York: Simon & Schuster, 1990), 331–32.

2. Giller, Robert M., and Kathy Matthews, *Natural Prescriptions* (New York: Carol Southern Books, 1994), 210–12.

3. Rowland, David L., "Yohimbine, Erectile Capacity, and Sexual Response in Men," *Archives of Sexual Behavior* 26(1): 49–62, 1997.

4. Whitaker, Julian, *Dr. Whitaker's Guide to Natural Healing* (Rocklin, Calif.: Prima Publishing, 1995), 287–88.

5. Duke, James A., *The Green Pharmacy* (Emmaus, Pa.: Rodale Press, 1997), 188.

6. Wylie, K. R., "Yohimbine and Sinusitis," *British Journal of Psychiatry* 169: 384–85, 1996.

7. Betz, J., et al. "Chemical Analysis of 26 Commercial Yohimbe Products," *Journal of the American Chemical Society* 78: 1189–94, 1995.

100

Zinc

According to the U.S. Department of Agriculture, 50 percent of those who follow the Dietary Guidelines for Americans have zinc intakes that are less than 75 percent of the RDA. Meat, poultry, and fish provide about 50 percent of the zinc in an omnivore diet. Red meat contains twice as much zinc as white meat. Cereals and legumes provide about 30 percent of dietary zinc, but phytate and fiber in those foods may impede zinc absorption. Foods prepared from cow's milk contribute only about 20 percent of dietary zinc. The most likely cause of zinc deficiency, such as that found in diabetics, is a diet low in bioavailable zinc. The deficiency causes dermatitis, abnormal pregnancy, immature sex glands, poor eyesight, abnormal sense of taste and smell, macular degeneration, senile dementia, and other health problems.[1]

Ram Singh, M.D., and colleagues at the Center of Nutrition and Heart Research Laboratory in Moradabad, India, have found that a zinc deficiency may put some people at greater risk for heart disease and diabetes. Those who consumed less than 7 mg/day of zinc were more likely to suffer from diabetes, and city dwellers who ate less zinc had higher rates of heart disease. It was speculated that urban Indians are getting less zinc in their diets because they have replaced grains such as millet with refined cereals.[2]

At the University of California at Davis and the University of California Medical Center at Sacramento, high doses of zinc monomethionine complex (30 mg/day) were found to improve zinc status without adversely affecting copper levels in immune-deficient diabetics. Previously, it was believed that high doses of zinc might affect copper levels, thereby causing a copper deficiency. In the study, 14 diabetics were given zinc for 30 days. While this increased plasma zinc levels by 20 percent, it did not affect copper levels in the blood. There was also a beneficial change in white blood cell activity. The study, said Carl Keen, M.D., one of the researchers, has important implications for those with compromised immune systems, such as diabetics, who may need to add zinc to their diets.[3]

A study in Milan evaluated 18 patients who were receiving irradiation treatments for cancers of the head and neck region. The patients were given 45 mg of zinc sulfate tablets or a placebo three times daily and for one month afterward because of alterations in their sense of taste. One month after the study was concluded, those receiving zinc tablets had a quicker recovery of taste acuity than those given a placebo.[4]

At Waikato Hospital, Hamilton, New Zealand, researchers evaluated 48 patients with rheumatoid arthritis who had a mean age of 64.5 years. It was found that many of the patients were deficient in essential nutrients. For example, those getting recommended daily intakes were: calcium, 23 percent; folic acid, 46 percent; vitamin E, 29 percent; zinc, 10 percent; and selenium, 6 percent.[5]

In Haifa, Israel, Naveh Yekezkel and colleagues reported that in rheumatoid arthritis patients there is apparent zinc malabsorption and consequently zinc deficiency. The study involved 29 patients with rheumatoid arthritis and eight healthy controls, between the ages of 40 and 70, who were given 50 mg/day of zinc.[6]

Between 1995 and 1997, Japanese researchers studied 46 females and 28 males with tinnitus, or ringing in the ears. Twenty-two volunteers were in the control group. A significant reduction in blood levels of the mineral was found in the patients with tinnitus, compared to controls. Those with low levels of zinc were given 34 to 68 mg/day of zinc for over two weeks, and blood levels of the mineral went up following treatment. The researchers concluded that zinc is useful in treating some patients with tinnitus.[7]

Fifty out of 100 employees at the Cleveland Clinic in Ohio, who had cold symptoms, took a zinc lozenge containing 13.3 mg of zinc from zinc gluconate every two hours while they were awake. The remaining 50 were given lozenges containing calcium lactate pentahydrate. Time of recovery in the treated group was 4.4 days, compared to 7.6 days in the control group. Some in the treatment group experienced nausea and a bad taste in their mouths.[8]

At a public home for seniors in Rome, researchers found that zinc supplements (25 mg/day) boosted the immune systems of the volunteers. The controls were given a look-alike pill containing starch. Vitamin A, which was also tested, had a deleterious effect in this study.[9]

In a study of AIDS patients by Canadian researchers, 12 volunteers were given 200 mg/day of zinc for 30 days, while the controls were given the drug AZT. The zinc supplement brought a stabilization of body weight, an increase in helper cells, and an increase of plasma active zinc-bound thymulin concentrations. The number of infections was reduced in some of the patients as well. Zinc seems to be beneficial in treating infections caused by *Pneumocystis carinii* and *Candida,* which are serious problems for AIDS patients.[10]

Zinc supplements have proven beneficial for sterility and in reducing complications during pregnancy, according to researchers in France. In addition, zinc has very low risk when given in conjunction with other nutrients. The suggested dosage ranges from 10 to 60 mg/day.[11]

Zinc is the backbone of Robert M. Giller's treatment for men with prostate problems. Men with benign prostatic hypertrophy have low levels of zinc in their prostatic fluids. Zinc supplements can raise these levels and reduce the enlargement. In one study, 14 out of 19 men treated with zinc supplements had shrinkage of the prostate after two months of therapy. Other supplements for prostate problems include flaxseed oil, vitamin E, and saw palmetto. Giller's zinc recommendation is 60 mg/day.[12]

Researchers studied the effect of 10 mg/day of zinc or a placebo in a double-blind trial of 609 children between 6 and 35 months of age, concerning lower respiratory infections. Zinc supplements were given to 298 of the children, who had 0.19 episodes/child/year of acute lower respiratory infections, compared with 0.35 episodes/child/year in the controls. After adjusting for variables, a 45 percent reduction was found in the incidence of acute lower respiratory tract infections in the zinc-treated children.[13]

Although breast milk is the preferred milk for infants, it does not supply an abundant amount of zinc. Therefore, supplementation with zinc and other micronutrients may be beneficial in some situations, according to Lindsay H. Allen, a researcher at the University of California at Davis. Those situations include: a diet low in animal products and based on high-phytate cereals and legumes; severe growth stunting; low plasma zinc concentrations; and bouts of persistent diarrhea, which would remove zinc stores from the body.[14]

"Animal products are usually the best sources of dietary zinc, in terms of both content and bioavailability," said Allen. "Because diets in developing countries are predominantly based on plants and often high in phytates, which inhibit zinc absorption strongly, it can be difficult for children in these countries to obtain their recommended intake of zinc from their usual diets. Zinc requirements for children 6 to 24 months of age are 2.8 mg/day."

A study at the Laboratory of Metabolic and Hormonal Physiology in Paris indicates that strenuous exercise depletes body stores of zinc, in spite of adequate calorie and iron intake. Iron and zinc are found in many of the same foods, such as meat. The deficiencies might be related to increased turnover in protein, redistribution of zinc in the tissues, and/or increased zinc losses in perspiration.[15]

Abnormal zinc stores are responsible for some of the hematologic (blood) abnormalities found in female endurance runners. The zinc-deficient runners needed 100 mg/day of supplements for two months, followed by 40 mg/day of zinc sulfate as a maintenance dose to increase the amount of the mineral in their blood.[16]

In evaluating 104 children between the ages of four months and 18 years with sickle cell anemia, it was found that 44 percent of the patients had low blood levels of zinc. Those with low levels had lower standard deviation scores for height, weight, arm circumference, muscle area, fat-free mass, and delay in skeletal maturation. Children older than age nine with low zinc levels had decreased amounts of pubic hair and maturation of breasts and genitals.[17]

Vegetarian diets in the United States typically contain between 10 and 30 percent less zinc than nonvegetarian diets. Approximately 44 percent of the zinc in most American diets comes from meat, fish, and poultry. Lacto-ovo-vegetarians, while at a greater risk for zinc deficiency, can meet their requirements by eating plenty of whole grains and legumes.[18]

As indicated by the research, many Americans are deficient in zinc. You can find zinc supplements in a variety of formulations in health food and other stores. The RDA for the mineral is 15 mg/day for most men and 12 mg/day for most women.

References

1. Sandstead, Harold H., and Norman G. Egger, "Is Zinc Nutriture a Problem in Persons with Diabetes Mellitus?" *American Journal of Clinical Nutrition* 66: 681–82, 1997.

2. Heins, Catherine, "Decreased Zinc Intake Linked to Heart Disease," *Medical Tribune,* Jan. 7, 1999, 17.

3. Trainer, E. L., et al., "Effects of Zinc Methionine Supplemental on Trace Mineral Status and Neutrophil Function in Type 1 Diabetes," paper presented at Federation of American Societies for Experimental Biology Meeting, April 1, 1993, New Orleans, Louisiana.

4. Ripamonti, Carla, et al., "A Randomized, Controlled Clinical Trial to Evaluate the Effects of Zinc Sulfate on Cancer Patients with Taste Alterations Caused by Head and Neck Irradiation," *Cancer* 82(10): 1938–45, May 15, 1998.

5. Stone, Jonathan, et al., "Inadequate Calcium, Folic Acid, Vitamin E, Zinc, and Selenium Intake in Rheumatoid Arthritis Patients: Results of a Dietary Survey," *Seminars in Arthritis and Rheumatism* 27(3): 180–85, Dec. 1997.

6. Yekezkel, Naveh, et al., "Zinc Metabolism in Rheumatoid Arthritis: Plasma and Urinary Zinc and Relationship to Disease Activity," *Journal of Rheumatology* 24(4): 643–46, 1997.

7. Ochi, K., et al., "The Serum Zinc Level in Patients with Tinnitus and the Effect

of Zinc," *Nippon Jibinkoka Gakkai Kaiho* 100(9): 915–19, Sept. 1997.

8. Mossad, Sherif B., M.D. "Zinc Gluconate Lozenges for Treating the Common Cold: A Randomized, Double-Blind, Placebo-Controlled Study," *Annals of Internal Medicine* 125(2): 81–88, July 15, 1996.

9. Fortes, Cristina, et al., "The Effect of Zinc and Vitamin A Supplementation on Immune Response in an Older Population," *Journal of the American Geriatrics Society* 46: 19–26, 1998.

10. Mocchegiani, E., et al., "Benefit of Oral Zinc Supplementation as an Adjunct to Zidovudine (AZT) Therapy Against Opportunistic Infections in AIDS," *International Journal of Immunology* 17(9): 719–27, 1995.

11. Favier, Alain-Emile, "The Role of Zinc in Reproduction: Hormonal Mechanisms," *Biological Trace Element Research* 32: 363–82, 1992.

12. Giller, Robert M., and Kathy Matthews, *Natural Prescriptions* (New York: Carol Southern Books, 1994), 284–87.

13. Sazawal, S., et al., "Zinc Supplementation Reduces the Incidence of Acute Lower Respiratory Infections in Infants and Preschool Children: A Double-Blind, Controlled Trial," *Pediatrics* 102(1): 1–5, July 1998.

14. Allen, Lindsay H., "Zinc and Micronutrient Supplements for Children," *American Journal of Clinical Nutrition* 68: 495S–98S, Aug. 1998.

15. Couzy, F., et al., "Zinc Metabolism in the Athlete: Influence of Training, Nutrition, and Other Factors," *International Journal of Sports Medicine* 11: 263–66, 1990.

16. Nishiyama, Soroku, et al., "Zinc Status Relates to Hematological Deficits in Women Endurance Runners," *Journal of the American College of Nutrition* 15(4): 359–63, 1996.

17. Leonard, Mary B., et al., "Plasma Zinc Status, Growth, and Maturation in Children in Sickle Cell Disease," *Journal of Pediatrics* 132: 467–71, March 1998.

18. McBride, Judy, "Vegetarians, Watch Your Zinc!" *Agricultural Research,* March 1998, 13.

Index